TRENDING TOPICS IN MULTIPLE SCLEROSIS

Edited by **Alina González-Quevedo**

Trending Topics in Multiple Sclerosis
http://dx.doi.org/10.5772/61417
Edited by Alina González-Quevedo

Contributors

Manuel J Rodriguez, Nicole Mahy, Marco Pugliese, Juan Francisco Espinos-Parrilla, Genaro Gabriel Ortiz, Fermín Pacheco-Moisés, Mario Mireles-Ramírez, Alfredo León-Gil, Héctor González-Usigli, J Luis Flores-Alvarado, Erica Daniela González-Renovato, Angelica Sánchez-López, Erandis D Tórres-Sánchez, Tania E Gómez-Sorto, Margarita Cid-Hernández, Ema Kantorova, Egon Kurča, Daniel Cierny, Dušan Dobrota, Georgy Nevinsky, Valentina Ignatova, Lyudmila Todorova, Jivko Surchev, Masaaki Murakami, Daisuke Kamimura, Yasunobu Arima, Andrea Stofkova, Naoki Nishikawa, Kotaro Higuchi, Takuto Ohki, Ozgul Ekmekci, Anastasiya G. Trenova, Dafin F. Muresanu, Mickael Bonnan, Ján Lehotský, Jozef Michalik, Alena Javůrková, Jaroslava Raudenská, Denisa Zimová, Katarína Tomašovičová, Ehtishamul Haq, Insha Zahoor, Mushfiquddin Khan

Published by InTech

Janeza Trdine 9, 51000 Rijeka, Croatia

Publishing Process Manager Edi Lipovic

Technical Editor SPi Global

Cover InTech Design team

First published September, 2016

Printed in Croatia

Additional hard copies can be obtained from orders@intechopen.com

Trending Topics in Multiple Sclerosis, Edited by Alina González-Quevedo

p. cm.

Print ISBN 978-953-51-2656-0
Online ISBN 978-953-51-2657-7

For EU product safety concerns:
IN TECH d.o.o., Prolaz Marije Krucifikse Kozulić 3, 51000 Rijeka, Croatia,
info@intechopen.com or visit our website at intechopen.com.

Meet the editor

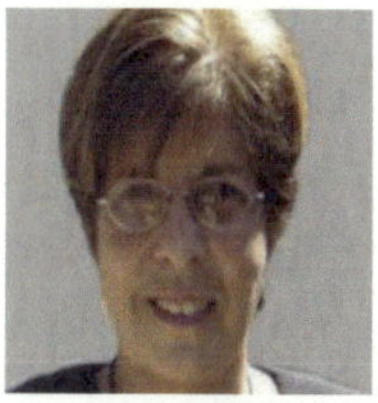

Alina González-Quevedo graduated from medical school at the University of Havana in 1972 with specialization in Clinical Biochemistry. Since 1977, she is a full-time professor of Biochemistry at the Medical University of Havana and senior researcher at the Institute of Neurology and Neurosurgery, where she occupied the positions of Head of the Department of Neurochemistry (1977–2009) and Assistant Director of Research (1995–2010). Her doctoral thesis engaged in the pathophysiological mechanisms of Cuban epidemic optic neuropathy in collaboration with the Venezuelan Institute for Scientific Research (1997–2002). She has also worked in other research areas such as brain barrier systems, demyelinating diseases, blood and CSF biomarkers for brain damage in essential hypertension and stroke and has published more than 100 scientific papers in peer-reviewed journals.

Contents

Preface

Multiple sclerosis (MS) is a chronic inflammatory disease characterized by progressive demyelination and neurodegeneration in the central nervous system (CNS), constituting the most common demyelinating disease of the CNS in humans. Oligodendrocytes and myelin appear to be the primary targets of the immune-mediated attack, but neurons are also damaged. Resident oligodendrocyte progenitor cells can remyelinate damaged axons during the first stages of the disease, where total or partial recovery is possible, but with time this mechanism fails. Axonal transection and degeneration occurring in the setting of acute inflammatory demyelination and as a consequence of chronic demyelination are considered to underlie permanent disability in MS patients.

Although intensive research over many decades has unveiled many pathophysiological mechanisms in the development of MS, the cause is still unknown. Nevertheless, it does seem clear that genetic susceptibility and environmental factors play crucial roles.

Trending Topics in Multiple Sclerosis is a book that provides an insight into some of the main problems currently debated in this area of research, focusing on topics that deal with genetic and environmental risk factors, pathophysiological mechanisms, neurocognitive findings, and neuroprotective strategies. The book is divided in two sections: the first section is dedicated mainly to **genetics and pathophysiology, while the second section deals largely with environmental risk factors and clinical and neurocognitive studies**.

Despite the fact that there is no evidence implicating classical Mendelian genetic inheritance with the risk for MS, numerous studies have offered results strongly supporting a genetic component of susceptibility to the disease. The first chapter deals with the possible role of genetic and biochemical markers in the modulation of the immune response in MS patients, which could thus be associated with MS risk and disability progression. The contribution of *HLA* and *non-HLA* genes and vitamin D in the pathogenesis of MS is reviewed, and the authors also present their personal experience in a Central European Slovak population.

The following chapters deal with gateway mechanisms for the entrance of immune cells to the CNS, oxidative stress, production of harmful catalytic antibodies, and intrathecal immunoglobulin synthesis.

In MS, demyelination often occurs at specific and discrete foci, suggesting that a certain signal might guide autoreactive T cells to particular site(s), regardless of the fact that brain autoantigens are widely distributed throughout the CNS. Chapter 2 engages in reviewing the gateway reflex, which can be triggered by various neural stimulations (gravity, electric stimulation, and pain), inducing gateways for immune cells to circumvent the blood-brain barrier (BBB), all of which involve sensory-sympathetic communication.

MS pathogenesis continues to be debated, but the most widely accepted theory recognizes that myelin destruction is mainly related to autoimmunity. While activated CD4+ myelin-reactive T cells are considered the major mediators in the pathogenesis of MS, the role of B cells and autoantibodies (auto-Abs) against myelin autoantigens has recently gained widespread recognition. Intrathecal synthesis (ITS) of immunoglobulins (Igs) is the strongest biological marker in MS. Nevertheless, since no specific target has been revealed, this synthesis has been persistently considered to be disease irrelevant. In Chapter 3, a very interesting review is presented, providing pertinent information on the possible role of B cells and subsequently ITS of Igs in the pathophysiology of MS. On the other hand, Chapter 4 deals with a novel concept considering that IgG, IgA, and/or IgM autoantibodies with catalytic activities directed to DNA, RNA, polysaccharides, and myelin basic protein (abzymes) could cooperatively promote important neuropathological mechanisms in MS.

Chapter 5 reviews the relationship of oxidative stress, glutathione redox and ATPase systems, and membrane fluidity with the development of MS. Based on the results of clinical studies suggesting that omega-3 long-chain polyunsaturated fatty acids (PUFAs) have anti-inflammatory, antioxidant, and neuroprotective effects in MS and animal models of MS. The authors also describe the effects of PUFA supplementation on the parameters indicated above in patients with relapsing-remitting MS.

The second section of this book starts by presenting in Chapter 6 Pediatric MS. Although MS is very infrequent in children and adolescents, pediatricians and neurologists should have this diagnosis in mind and need to know the differences, concerning clinical presentation, magnetic resonance imaging (MRI) findings, and neuroimmunologic features, between pediatric and adult MS patients.

The next two chapters deal with the influence of environmental factors, such as HIV infection and nutrition, in the development of MS. Chapter 7 deals with the association between HIV (or its treatment) and a reduced risk of developing MS, a fact that could contribute to the development of more promising treatment strategies for MS. On the other hand, Chapter 8 engages in the importance of understanding how nutritional epigenetic factors could influence the risk for developing MS and how this could help in establishing dietary interventions.

There is increasing recognition of cerebral cortical demyelination in MS and the role that this pathology may play in the neurological dysfunction—including cognitive deficits—experienced by most MS patients. Chapters 9 and 10 contend with the importance of neuropsychological assessment and social cognition in MS, respectively.

Chapter 11 is aimed to provide evidence on the immunomodulatory and neuroprotective effects of sex hormones on the pathological processes in MS and their importance for the development of new disease-modifying strategies.

Significant advances have been achieved in MS therapy with the use of disease-modifying drugs (DMDs), which are immunomodulatory or immunosuppressive, but these advances have been limited to the prevention of relapses, and long-term results are controversial. Neuroprotective strategies focusing simultaneously on several pathogenic mechanisms have been receiving increased attention. In this context, Chapter 12 approaches direct and indirect neuroprotective effects of DMDs and current knowledge of potential neuroprotective therapies and remyelination strategies. Chapter 13 mainly focuses on new drugs with proposed neuroprotective or neuroregenerative effects, highlighting the effect of diazoxide on neuroinflammation and the results of a clinical trial with this drug.

Alina González-Quevedo, MD, PhD
Department of Neurobiology
Institute of Neurology and Neurosurgery
University of Medical Sciences of Havana, Cuba

Section 1

Genetics and Pathophysiology

Genetic and Biochemical Factors Related to the Risk and Disability Progression in Multiple Sclerosis

Daniel Čierny, Jozef Michalik, Ema Kantorová,
Egon Kurča and Ján Lehotský

Additional information is available at the end of the chapter

http://dx.doi.org/10.5772/63468

Abstract

Sclerosis multiplex (multiple sclerosis, MS) is a chronic autoimmune inflammatory disease of the central nervous system. The immune regulatory defects lead to the process of inflammation and neurodegenerationthat results in the deterioration of neurological functions. It is still unclear as to why MS is so devastating and rapidly progressive in one patient and less so in another. It is known that the etiopathogenesis of MS is very complex, and many factors can be involved in the risk and character of the disease and its progression. In this chapter, we discuss the general molecular and cellular mechanisms of action of genetic and biochemical factors that are related to immune system regulation and thus can be connected to the individually varying risk and disability progression of MS. We found that gene variants of the gene polymorphism rs6897932 in interleukin 7 receptor α chain gene rs10735810 in vitamin D receptor gene and *HLA-DR* and *HLA-DQ* genes as well as the serum level of vitamin D are associated with MS risk or disability progression in Central European Slovak population.

Keywords: multiple sclerosis, risk, disability progression, gene polymorphism, biochemical marker

1. Introduction

In triggering an autoimmune response in multiple sclerosis (MS), environmental factors have a strong effect and interact with complex risk-conferring genetic variants [1–3]. In this process, the myelin reactive Tcells with altered functional characteristics are formed and activated [4]. The immune regulatory defects and increased migration of autoreactive lymphocytes within the brain, that are the typical traits in MS, lead to the process of inflammation, myelin sheath breakdown, demyelination, remyelination, neuronal and axonal degeneration, and subsequent deterioration of neurological functions [5]. Neurodegeneration, neuronal and axonal damage that correlate with the progression of the disease can be a process partly independent from inflammation and demyelination or even can be the cause of demyelination occurring from the disease onset. Axonal damage in MS is a result of many pathological processes [6, 7].

It is still unclear as to why MS is so devastating and rapidly progressive in one patient and less so in another. Because the etiopathogenesis of MS is very complex, disease development as well as the characteristics of disease progression is probably the consequence of multifactorial interaction. Our work is dedicated to genetic and biochemical markers that were chosen according to their possible role in the modulation of the immune response in MS patients and thus could be associated with MS risk and disability progression. In our work, we discuss the immune response-related genetic factors associated with MS that can be generally classified into *HLA* genes and *non-HLA* genes. Since vitamin D can have an important role in the pathogenesis of MS, great part of our work is dedicated to its metabolism, functions, mechanisms of action in MS and genetic factors that can modify these effects. In this work, we also present the results of our own analysis of genetic and biochemical markers that we found to be associated with MS risk or progression in the group consisting of MS patients with clinically diagnosed MS and healthy individuals from the region of Central Slovakia. To evaluate the disease progression rate, we used the widely accepted multiple sclerosis severity score (MSSS, score range 0.01–9.99) [8] that considers the neurological impairment of the functional systems (expanded disability status scale score) [9] together with disease duration. For the purpose of the association analysis of these markers with the rate of disease disability progression, we stratified MS patients by MSSS scores to three groups—slowly progressing MS (MSSS < 3), mid-rate progressing MS (MSSS 3–6) and rapidly progressing MS (MSSS > 6) [10].

2. Immune response-related genetic factors in the risk and progression of multiple sclerosis

MS is a typical gender-dependent disease; a higher risk of MS is observed in women than in men in all populations and races. A study conducted in Canada found female to male ratio in individuals affected by MS to be 3:1 [11]. The risk of MS development in siblings of an affected individual is estimated to be 5%, in children 2%, in monozygotic twins 25% [5]. However, it has been shown that genetic predisposition is not strong enough to induce disease development, and appropriate environmental triggers are necessary to start the disease process [1, 12]. In general, the MS-associated genes can be classified into genes of the HLA-complex and*non-HLA* genes [3].

3. Gene polymorphisms and haplotypes in the aetiology of multiple sclerosis

The single-nucleotide polymorphism (SNP) is a variation of a single nucleotide, which is present in the population in a frequency higher than 0.01. SNPs are the most common type of genetic variation and are usually caused by somatic or gametic mutations. Nucleotide change can cause the formation or loss of restriction sites for bacterial endonucleases that are able to cleave the specific DNA sequence. The identification of gene polymorphisms that are in correlation with other risk factors, including biochemical markers, can be useful in establishing the risk of MS development, prognosis, clinical course of the disease and response to therapy. Haplotype (haploid genotype) is a certain combination of alleles or SNPs in the sequence of the DNA, whichis localized on one chromosome and is inherited together. When two alleles are in linkage disequilibrium, they are inherited together in a higher frequency than expected randomly [13]. The combination of more alleles, known as tagging SNPs, enables us to identify the other associated alleles. For example, the allele A of gene polymorphism rs3135388 corresponds to the incidence of allele HLA-DRB1*1501, which is the most common genetic risk factor for MS development [14–16].

4. *HLA* genes and MS

Antigen expression that is inducible by cytokines is different on the various immune cells. Major histocompatibility complex II (MHCII) antigens are transmembrane proteins localized on the immune cells, thus having an important role in the process of exogenous antigen presentation to Tcells. MHCII molecules are coded by the gene of human leucocyte antigens D (*HLA-D* gene) that is localized on chromosome 6 and has three regions—HLA-DP, HLA-DQ and HLA-DR [17]. The susceptibility of the population to autoimmune diseases depends on the individual ability to express HLA-DQ and HLA-DR antigens. This expression can be induced by virus infection, most likely by EBV, influenza or paramyxovirus [18]. *MHCII* gene expression is regulated by vitamin D through its binding to the *vitamin D–responsive elements(VDREs)* that are localized in the promoter region of *HLA-DRB1* gene. This fact can explain the interaction between vitamin D, that is an important factor modifying MS development and disease course, and genetic predisposition to MS represented mainly by a highly conservative allele HLA-DRB1*1501. HLA-DRB1*1501 allele is in general considered to be the most important susceptibility allele of MS [19–24]. This allelewas found to be present in over 50% of MS cases [25, 26]. The increased frequencies of the DRB1*15 allele in MS patients have been described in Northern Europeans [23, 27], South and North Americans [20, 28], Mediterraneans [29, 30] and African Americans [21]. In Spanish cohorts, the DRB1*03 was the second most frequent allele associated with MS, but only after eliminating HLA-DRB1*15 [29]. The DRB1*03 allele has also been found to be significantly associated with the increased risk of MS in Scandinavians [27], Sardinians [31], and Australians [32]. Fernández et al. [33] found that the DRB1*13 allele is protective against MS development in Spaniards. A protective effect of the alleles DRB1*01, DRB1*07, DRB1*12 and DRB1*14 was confirmed in the recent meta-analysis in Caucasians [24]. The allele DRB1*07 was found to be protective against MS also in Scandinavians [34]. The DRB1*13.03 allele was found to be the primary risk allele in MS patients of European descent [23]. The protective effect against MS has also been shown for the HLA-DRB1*11 allele [24, 29].

The DQB1*06:02 allele was found to be linked to the increased risk of MS with a proved tight linkage disequilibrium between DRB1*15 and DQB1*06 in Caucasians [35]. As the risk factor of MS, DQB1*06:02 allele has also been identified in a cohort of Afro-Brazilians [36] and Spaniards [33]. Kaushansky et al. [37] suggested that the role of the DRB1*15:01 and DQB1*06:02 alleles in MS depends on the heterogeneous interaction of target antigen, genotype, and phenotype. On the contrary, Isobe et al. [38] found none of the HLA-DQB1 alleles to be associated with MS in African Americans. According to the combinations of HLA-alleles, the association of HLA-DRB1*15/*15 genotype with MS was identified by several studies [32, 34, 39]. In multi-case MS families, Barcellos et al. [39] identified a high risk DRB1*15/*08 genotype and protective DRB1*15/*14 genotype. The study of Sawcer et al. [23] indicates that in all populations of North-European ancestry, a predisposition to MS is linked with the DRB1*15:01-DQB1*06:02 haplotype. Furthermore, Link et al. [34] in a Scandinavian cohort showed that risk haplotypes for MS are almost all DRB1*15 bearing haplotypes, while protective effect against MS development are HLA class I A*02 allele-bearing haplotypes. In Sardinian MS patients, Cocco et al. [40] confirmed a positive association of the haplotype HLA DRB1*03:01-DQB1*02:01 with MS.

In the study from our laboratory, we analysed the association of the *HLA-DRB1/DQB1* genes, alleles and their combinations with susceptibility to MS in the population from central Slovakia. We found that the increased risk of MS is in individuals carrying alleles HLA-DRB1*15, DRB1*03 and DQB1*06, genotypes HLA-DRB1*15/*15 DQB1*06/*06 and haplotype DRB1*15-DQB1*06. In addition, we also found that HLA-DRB1/DQB1 class II alleles DRB1*07, DRB1*13, DQB1*03, genotypes DRB1*13/*11, DQB1*05/*03 and haplotypes DRB1*13-DQB1*06 and DRB1*11-DQB1*03 are associated with the protection against MS development. We cannot exclude that the proposed protective effects of the DRB1*11-DQB1*03 and DRB1*13-DQB1*06 haplotypes in our cohort could be, at least partially, due to the linkagedisequilibrium with alleles in the HLA class I region which is primarily associated with MS [41].

5. *Non-HLA* genes and MS

Gene products of *non-HLA* genes can contribute to the genetic risk of MS by modulation of different processes. These genes are involved in the regulation of functions of T- and Bcells, dendritic cells, NKcells, cytokine signalization, metabolism of interferons, vitamin D metabolism, neuronal regeneration and many others [3]. It has been found that these genes can contribute not only to the increased inherited risk of MS development but also to the risk of other autoimmune diseases [42, 43]. The examples of the SNPs involved in the etiopathogenesis of MS are summarised in **Table 1**.

Gene	*function*	*Localization*	*SNP*	*Alleles*
HLA-DRB1*1501*(human leucocyte antigen DRB1*1501)*	Antigen presentation	6p21	rs3135388	C/T
			rs3135005	C/T
IL-7Ra *(interleukin 7 receptor receptor alpha chain)*	Proliferation of memory Tcells, T- and B-cell development	5p13	rs6897932	C/T
IL-2Ra *(interleukin 2 receptor receptor alpha chain)*	Sensitization of Tcells to IL-2, proliferation of Tcells	10p15	rs2104286	A/G
			rs12722489	A/G
			rs11256369	C/G
			rs7076103	C/T
CD58 *(cluster of differentiation 58)*	Function of regulatory Tcells	1p13	rs2300747	A/G
			rs6677309	A/C
			rs12044852	A/C
CD6*(cluster of differentiation 6)*	Regulation, adhesion of T_{H17} and other Tcells	11q13	rs17824933	C/G
			rs12288280	G/T
CLEC16A *(C-type lectin domain family 16 member A)*	Cell receptor, induction of immune response	16p13	rs6498169	A/G
			rs12708716	A/G
VAV1 *(vav guanine nucleotide exchange factor 1)*	Lymphocyte survival, differentiation and proliferation	19p13	rs2546133	C/T
			rs2617822	A/G
PRKCA *(protein kinase C alpha)*	Regulation of IL-2 expression, receptor	17q22-q23	Allele variants in introns 3, 8	
EVI 5 *(ecotropic viral integration site 5 protein homolog)*	Nuclear protein, cell cycle regulation	1p22	rs6680578	A/T
			rs11808092	A/C
			rs11804321	C/T
IRF5 *(interferon regulatory factor 5)*	Regulation of cytokine activation	7q32	rs4728142	A/G
			rs3807306	A/C
IRF8 *(interferon regulatory factor8)*	Expression of interferon response genes, development of Bcells	16q24	rs17445836	A/G
TYK2 *(tyrosin kinase 2)*	Gene expression	19p13	rs34536443	C/G
			rs55762744	C/T
TNFRSF1A *(tumour necrosis factor receptor superfamily member 1A)*	Receptor for tumour necrosis factor	12p13	rs1800693	A/G
			rs4149584	A/C/G
			rs767455	C/T
			rs4149577	C/T
CD40 *(cluster of differentiation 40)*	Receptor for tumour necrosis factor	20q12-q13	rs1883832	C/T
CD226 *(cluster of differentiation 226)*	Activator of NKcells, lymphocyte adhesion, co-stimulator of Tcells	18q22	rs763361	C/T
KIF1B *(kinesin family member 1B) kinesin family member 1B)*	Neuronal regeneration	1p36	rs10492972	C/T
GPC 5 *(glypicane 5)*	Neuronal growth and reparation	13q32	rs9523762	A/G

Table 1. Gene polymorphisms involved in the etiopathogenesis of MS [3, 44–48].

6. Genetic variants in *interleukin 7 receptor α chain (IL-7Ra)* gene

IL7 is a type 1 short-chain cytokine of the haematopoietin family involved in the modulation of T- and B-cell development and T-cell homeostasis. To perform the immune system functions, IL7 binds to the transmembrane receptor that is formed by heterodimerisingthe common cytokine gamma chain and IL7 receptor alpha chain (IL7Ra or CD127). IL7Ra is a membrane glycoprotein folded to bind and mediate the action of IL7 and other alpha helical cytokines. IL7Ra consists of an extracellular domain, transmembrane region and cytoplasmic tail, which uses kinases for signal transduction [49]. The localization of the *IL7Ra* gene is chromosome 5p13.3. An increased expression of IL7Ra in peripheral blood mononuclear cells was found in MS patients when compared to controls [50, 51]. The IL7Ra and IL7 mRNA increased expression was found also in the cerebrospinal fluid of MS patients, possibly suggesting an altered balance between the isoforms of IL7Ra and a higher signal-inducing immune cell proliferation and survival [52]. According to the alternative splicing of exon 6 in *IL7Ra* gene, membrane-bound or soluble isoforms of IL-7Ra are produced [53]. A significantly increased ratio of the membrane-bound to soluble isoforms of IL7Ra in MS patients can facilitate the aberrant activation of potentially auto-reactive T cells [54].

Single-nucleotide polymorphisms in *IL7Ra* gene are involved in the dysregulation of immune homeostasis and thus can be associated with susceptibility to MS [55]. A genome-wide study in a large group of subjects from the UK and USA identified the strong association between SNP rs6897932 in *IL7Ra* gene and the risk of MS [2]. The non-conservative aminoacid change on position 244 (Ile→Thr) ofIL7Ra is a result of the SNP rs6897932 (ATC → ACC) in exon 6 of *IL7Ra* gene [56]. This aminoacid change has a functional effect on the product of expression of alternative spliced *IL7Ra* gene, which is manifested by changes in the proportion of the soluble versus membrane-bound isoforms of IL7Ra. The change of this ratio can be followed by a different regulation of the IL7 signal transduction pathway and directly associates the SNP rs6897932 with MS [57].

It has been found that allele C of SNP rs6897932 in *IL7Ra* gene contributes to the increased genetic risk of MS in groups of MS patients from the USA [57, 58], South Spain [59], Nordic countries—Denmark, Finland, Norway and Sweden [52], France [60], Netherlands [61] and Japan [62]. The homozygosity for C allele was identified as a risk genotype for MS susceptibility in Netherlands [61] and Spain [59]. A genotype association was also confirmed by the finding of increased counts of CC genotype of rs6897932 in MS patients compared to controls in the cohorts from the USA [58] and Japan [62]. Corresponding with the contribution of allele C to the risk of MS, the protective effect of allele T for MS risk in a Nordic case-control group has been reported by Lundmark et al. [52]. The protective effect of allele T has been reported also in Spain by Alcina et al. [59]. On the contrary, no association between SNP rs6897932 and MS was found in cohorts of MS patients from Northern Ireland [58], Germany [44] and Western Balkan countries—Serbia, Croatia and Slovenia [63].

Only a few studies addressed the question whether the rs6897932 in *IL7Ra* gene contributes only to the genetic risk of MS, or whether it can also affect the disease course and disability progression [44, 57, 61, 64]. Groups of patients with different forms of MS were compared in

http://dx.doi.org/10.5772/63468

several studies. In Northern European primary-progressive MS cases (PP MS), the underexpression of *IL7Ra* gene as well as different allele frequencies of IL7Ra promoter SNP was confirmed. Moreover, *IL7Ra* gene expression was found to be up-regulated in secondary-progressive MS (SP MS) patients [64]. In a study by Akkad et al. [44] in German MS patients, it was found that the soluble IL7Ra reduced the expression and allelic and genotypic association between rs6897932 and SP or PP MS but not with RR MS. In their study, a significantly higher frequency of allele C and genotype CC of rs6897932 in SP and PP MS patients was found, but not in RR MS patients compared to controls. The assessment of the severity of MS by MSSS did not show any association between rs6897932 genotype and disease severity in the USA [57]. Differences in allele frequencies in SP MS patients compared to healthy controls were reported in Dutch MS patients by Sombekke et al. [61]. In spite of that, no association between rs6897932 genotype and disease severity (MSSS, EDSS, other clinical tests) and disease activity (relapse rate and MRI markers) was found.

Results of our own work suggest the relevance of rs6897932 allele and gene variants in MS pathogenesis in Slovaks [10]. Our results have revealed that allele C is present in a higher frequency in MS patients (77.4%) as compared to the control group (72.3%), which indicates an increased risk of MS development (OR=1.314, 95% CI=1.004–1.720, p=0.047). Interestingly, allele T was manifested in MS patients in a significantly lower frequency representing only 22.6% as compared to 27.7% in controls. This suggeststhat allele T seems to be protective against MS development (OR = 0.761, 95% CI= 0.582–0.996, p = 0.047). The additive model fitted the best to assess association between genotypes and MS risk. Logistic regression analysis adjusted for sex and age revealed that there is a significant associationbetween IL7Ra rs6897932 genotype and MS risk (OR = 0.764, 95% CI = 0.586–0.995, $p_{\log}$ = 0.045). The genotype analysis showed that MS patients manifested a lower frequency of genotype CT when compared to controls (34.8% vs. 36.3) and genotype TT (5.2% vs. 9.9%) and a higher frequency of genotype CC (60.0% vs. 54.1%). When we used the additive genetic model, we found a significantly decreased risk of MS development in carriers of allele T with genotype CT (OR = 0.865, 95% CI = 0.609–1.228, p = 0.05) as well as with genotype TT (OR = 0.565, 95% CI = 0.282–1.132, p = 0.05).

After stratification of MS patients according to the disease disability progression rate, we found a significantly lower frequency of allele T in the subgroup of rapidly progressing MS patients (18.1%) as compared to 27.7% in controls. These results suggest that allele T is associated with protection against rapid disability progression of MS (OR = 0.576, 95% CI = 0.348–0.955, p = 0.031). An additive genetic model adjusted for sex and age fitted the best to assess the association between genotypes and the rate of disease disability progression. Linear logistic regression with disease disability rate as the dependent variable—MSSS (1, 2, 3 and 0 for controls) revealed that there is a significant association between IL7Ra rs6897932 genotype and disability progression of MS ($p_{\log}$ = 0.034). Genotype analysis showed that the frequency of genotype TT is higher in controls (9.6%) and lower in MS patients with rapid disability progression (3.5%). Frequency of genotype CC was higher in rapidly progressing MS patients (67.2%) and lower in controls (54.1%). The data suggest that individuals carrying genotype TT are protected against rapid disease disability progression of MS.

We have shown for the first time in a Central European Slovak population that allele C of rs6897932 is associated with the risk of MS, and allele T has a protective additive effect against MS susceptibility. Moreover,we revealed that minor allele T and genotype TT of rs6897932 in the *IL7Ra* gene are protective against rapid disease disability progression in MS [65].

7. Vitamin D and its role in risk and progression of multiple sclerosis

In the past decades, much attention has been given to vitamin D and its role in MS and other autoimmune diseases. The following sectionsare dedicated to the metabolism and structure of vitamin D, its immunological effects, serum level and mechanisms of action of vitamin D in the prevention and treatment of MS. We also describe the genetic factors that can modulate the biological effects of vitamin D.

7.1. The structure and metabolism of vitamin D

Vitamin D in the human body undergoes a complex metabolism. Cholecalciferol (vitamin D_3), as a precursor of a hormonally active form, is produced in the skin from 7-dehydrocholesterol after sunlight exposure and can also be absorbed from the diet. Subsequently, cholecalciferol is hydroxylated in the liver forming 25-hydroxycholecalciferol, calcidiol. The hormonally active form of vitamin D, 1,25- dihydroxycholecalciferol, calcitriol, is produced by further hydroxylation especially in the kidneys and also in other tissues. The enzyme catalysing this hydroxylation is 25-hydroxyvitamin D-1α-hydroxylase, coded by *CYP27B1* (cytochrome P450 family 27 subfamily B member 1) gene [66, 67]. In various cells, the bioactive form of vitamin D binds to the vitamin D receptor (VDR) providing its physiological functions by modulation of the target gene's transcription [68]. The circulating serum level of vitamin D depends not only on environmental factors such as exposition to sunlight and vitamin D intake but also on genetic and epigenetic factors.The genetic factors can influence the effects of vitamin D through the variability of the genes participating in its activation and degradation, transport and receptor signalling [69].

7.2. The effect of vitamin D on the functions of immune cells

There is growing evidence that vitamin D not only regulates bone metabolism but also has large-scale immunomodulatory and anti-inflammatory effects. A linkage has been found between vitamin D deficiency and increased risk of autoimmune diseases [70]. The immunocompetent cells—macrophages, dendritic cells, Tcells and Bcells are able to produce calcitriol and express the VDR at the high rate. Through this, vitamin D modulates the synthesis of various cytokines and immunoglobulins and is involved in the regulation of innate and adaptive immune response. Autocrine and paracrine effects of vitamin D depend also on its serum level, and individuals with hypovitaminosis D are in a state of immune system dysfunction and are predisposed to the development of autoimmune diseases [71].

In Tcells, calcitriol inhibits the production of IL-12 and IFN-γ and subsequent differentiation of T_{H1} lymphocytes that are the key cells involved in the MS development. Calcitriol improves the immunosuppressive functions of T_{REG}cells and ameliorates the T_{H2}-cell development by the activation of the promotor region of *IL-4* gene [19, 72]. Vitamin D increases the expression of IL-4, IL-5 and IL-10 that are able to activate T_{H2} cells, decreases the production of IFN-γ, blocks the formation of T_{H1}cells after antigen stimulation and has positive effects on the T_{H1}-mediated autoimmune diseases [73, 74]. Bcells, which also participate in the demyelinating process and produce intrathecalimmunoglobulins, express VDR and vitamin D hydroxylases. In Bcells, calcitriol reduces the intracellular signal pathways of nuclear transcription factor NF-kappa B (NF-kB) and CD40 signalling [75]. Calcitriol inhibits the maturation and proliferation of Bcells, induces apoptosis of Bcells, inhibits the differentiation of plasma and memory cells and decreases the production of immunoglobulinsIgG and IgM [76]. Immature Bcells are more prone to regulation by calcitriol when compared to plasma cells. Calcitriol also decreases the expression of MHCII molecules and co-stimulatory molecules in Bcells [19].

Calcitriol formed in macrophages inhibits the immune response by suppressing proliferation of T_{H1}- and T_{H17}cells and promoting the functions of T_{H2}- and T_{REG}cells [71]. Calcitriol inhibits the secretion of IL-12 by antigen-presenting cells and monocytes [77]. Vitamin D blocks the differentiation of immature dendritic cells and the expression of co-stimulatory molecules CD40, CD80, CD86 and MHC II, thus decreasing the capacity of dendritic cells to activate autoreactive Tcells. Vitamin D also ameliorates the spontaneous apoptosis of mature dendritic cells [73]. In macrophages, calcitriolsuppresses intracellular oxidative burst and listericidal activity. It also suppresses the expression of Fc and TLR receptors induced by IFN-γ that are important for antigen recognition [78]. Vitamin D suppresses the proliferation of antigen-specific Tcells and chemotaxisof dendritic cells by decreasing the expression of differentiation antigens CD80, CD86 and HLA-DR molecules [79].

7.3. The murine model of MS and vitamin D

In mice that lack the *VDR* gene or the gene of the enzyme catalysing vitamin D activation, an abnormal development and function of T_{H1}-lymphocytes and deficiency of peripheral T-lymphocytes have been observed [80, 81]. Calcitriol treatment can prevent the induction and progression of autoimmune diseases including experimental autoimmune encephalomyelitis (EAE), a murine model of MS [82, 83]. Calcitriol can also decrease the severity of EAE symptoms, and its deficiency causes an increased susceptibility of animals to EAE induction [77, 82]. In mice with chronic EAE, vitamin D administration suppresses the proliferation of specific T_{H1} cells, inhibits IL-12 dependent production of IFN-γ, prevents relapses and reduces perivascular infiltration, demyelination plaque formation and axonal degeneration in the brain and spinal cord [84].

7.4. Serum level of vitamin D and dose management

To reflect vitamin D status in the human body, calcidiol plasma level measurement is usually used. Calcidiol is the main circulating form of vitamin D in plasma, and its biological half-time is 19 days [85]. The recommended daily dose of vitamin D is approximately 10times higher than in the past. The optimal serum level of vitamin D is 75–250 nmol/l (30–100 ng/ml). In countries with less sunny climate, the necessary daily dose of vitamin D is 1000–4000 IU/day (1 μg = 40 IU) [86].

The risk of vitamin D overdosing is hypercalcaemia and subsequent organ and tissue damage. Whole body exposure to sunlight results in the production of around 10,000 IU of vitamin D, so it is not simple to cause vitamin D intoxication by its short-term peroral supplementation. The results of several studies suggest that even high-dose vitamin D_3 supplementation in MS patients is safe and clinically useful. Burton et al. [87] administered high peroral doses of vitamin D to healthy individuals and MS patients. The initial dose was 40,000 IU/dayduring 28 weeks, followed by 10,000 IU/day during 12 weeks; later it was gradually decreased to 0 IU/day, combined with 1.2 grams of calcium per day. During the period of 40,000 IU of vitamin D per day, the serum levels reached 413 nmol/l, which was higher than the conventional limit established for vitamin D toxicity (250 nmol/l). Calcidiol serum levels remained around this limit for 18 weeks without any observed negative effects. The serum level of calcium was in the physiological reference range during the whole study duration. Moreover, no cardiac rhythm abnormalities or impairment of hepatic or renal functions was observed. Kimball et al. [88] administered 4000–40,000 IU/day to patients in the active phase of MS together with 1.2 grams of calcium. Medium serum level of calcidiol was 78 ± 35 nmol/l and rose to 386 ± 157 nmol/l. Serum calcium level and urinary calcium to creatinine ratio did not exceed the physiological reference values. Vitamin D supplementation in this study did not cause any change in the serum level of hepatic enzymes, creatinine, electrolytes, proteins and parathormone. Although the serum level of calcidiol doubled the physiological upper range value, hypercalcaemia or hypercalciuria was not observed.

Although the significant toxicity of vitamin D_3 was not observed even in doses of 40,000 IU/day, its daily dose in healthy individuals should not exceed 2000 IU. The optimal daily dose of vitamin D_3 that should be routinely recommended to women during pregnancy and lactation is 1000 IU. Children born in families with MS history should be administered daily 200–400 IU of vitamin D_3 [66].

7.5. Vitamin D and the course, prevention and treatment of MS

The role of vitamin D in the prevention of MS development has been confirmed by many experimental, epidemiological, genetic and immunological studies. Vitamin D insufficiency during the whitematter development can alter the pathways of axonal differentiation and adhesion and increase the apoptosis of oligodendrocytes that express VDR. This results in local microenvironmental changes and altered regeneratory and remyelinating capacity [66]. In individuals with an increased genetic risk of MS, it is possible to prevent the demyelination process by preventive vitamin D administration. This preventive strategy would be better than reparation of already developed myelin and axonal damage [12, 66].

High-dose peroral vitamin D intake has been found to be inversely associated with the risk of MS in a cohort of more than 90,000 women. Peroral vitamin D supplementation in a dose higher than 400 IU/day leads to the reduction of MS risk when compared to the individuals with no vitamin D intake (RR = 0.59, 95% CI = 0.38–0.91,p = 0.006) [89]. Also,calcidiol plasma levels are inversely correlated with MS risk. This association is particularly obvious in whites, while among blacks and Hispanics with lower 25-hydroxyvitamin D levels than whites, there was no significant association between vitamin D and MS risk [90]. Vitamin D also has reparative effects for the nervous tissue, especially in patients in the early phases of the disease. In countries with low sun exposure, food supplementation of vitamin D could be a simple and cheap method of MS prevention [86]. The incidence of MS could be reduced by the administration of vitamin D to pregnant women, and all children living in mild climates should be more exposed to sunlight and should be on a vitamin D–rich diet [66].

Vitamin D is not only a factor modifying MS risk, but it can also have a role in the modulation of disease course. It has been observed that in relapsing remitting MS, calcidiol plasma levels are lower during relapses compared to the periods of remission [91]. In addition, there is evidence that lower calcidiol levels are associated with higher relapse rates and higher risk of exacerbation, as well as higher expanded disability status scale (EDSS) scores and progressive forms of MS [92–94]. Vitamin D can improve memory and cognitive impairments in patients with MS, Alzheimer disease and in patients after chemotherapeutical treatment [95]. High-dose peroral vitamin D supplementation has immunomodulatory effects and leads to reduction in the number of relapses and suppression of the inflammatory activity and proliferation of Tcells [87], as well as the decrease in the number of gadolinium-enhancing lesions in brain [88].

In our study, we examined the serum levels of calcidiol in a group of MS patients from the Central-Northern part of Slovakia. We found that hypovitaminosis D is more frequent in MS patients, when compared to healthy individuals. Serum levels of calcidiol were significantly lower in MS patients when compared to controls (15.0 ± 6.1 ng/ml vs. 18.2 ± 8.3 ng/ml, $p_{(K-W)}$= 0.001). Moreover, we found that there is an association of the serum level of vitamin D with the rate of MS disability progression ($p(K-W)$ = 0.000). We detected similar serum levels of calcidiol in slow progressing and mid-rate progressing MS patients (15.7 ± 5.0 ng/ml vs. 15.8 ± 6.6 ng/ml), but interestingly we noticed a marked decrease of calcidiol serum levels in rapidly progressing MS patients (12.8 ± 5.9 ng/ml). In addition, calcidiol levelwas significantly lower in all subgroups of MS patients when compared to controls (18.2 ± 8.3 ng/ml). Thus we can conclude that decreased serum level of calcidiol in MS patients can be one of the factors related to increased risk of MS development, as well as increased risk of rapid disease disability progression.

7.6. Genetic factors related to vitamin D effects in MS

Nucleotide exchange in DNA sequence can cause the production of protein products with different activities. Polymorphisms of the genes involved in the activation, transport, signalling and degradation of vitamin D can, together with other factors, modify the individual immune response and thus can be related to MS. Because of the beneficial effects of vitamin D, in individuals with genes predisposing to its higher serum levels, the risk of MS should be reduced [96]. The serum level of vitamin D can be modified by *VDR* gene polymorphisms [97–99]. The fact that serum levels of vitamin D are similar in twins, and especially when they are monozygotic twins, speaks in favour of a genetic regulation. Gene polymorphisms FokI in

VDR gene, rs4646536 and rs703842 in the *CYP27B1* gene and rs10741657 in the *CYP2R1* gene are the significant predictors of caldiciol serum level [99]. Hypovitaminosis D is common in higher latitudes because of the lack of sun exposure [100]. The fact that not all vitamin D–deficient individuals develop MS is probably the result of the complexity of the etiopathogeneis of MS and the interaction of many factors. The positive effects of vitamin D in MS can be dampened for example by the allele HLA-DRB1*15 [96]. In MS patients, it is necessary to find out the link between the genotype and the vitamin D serum level and also the genetic interactions among the genes *CYP27B1, VDR* and *HLA* [19]. The gene polymorphisms associated with vitamin D metabolism are summarized in **Table 2**.

Gene	*function*	*Localization*	*SNP*	*Allele*
CYP27B1 *(cytochrome P450 family 27 subfamily B member 1, 25-hydroxyvitamin D_3 1-alpha-hydroxylase)*	Hydroxylation	12q13	rs703842	C/T
			rs10877012	G/C
			rs4646536	C/T
			rs10877015	A/G
			rs118204009	A/G
			rs118204012	A/G
			rs118204011	C/T
CYP2R1 *(cytochrome P450 family 2 subfamily R member 1, vitamin $D_3$25-hydroxylase)*	Hydroxylation	11p15	rs10741657	A/G
			rs10500804	G/T
			rs12794714	A/G
DBP *(vitamin D binding protein)*	Transport in plasma	4q12	rs7041	G/T
			rs4588	A/C
VDR *(vitamin D receptor)*	Receptor	12q13	rs1544410 (BsmI)	A/G (B/b)
			rs7975232 (ApaI)	T/C (A/a)
			rs731236 (TaqI)	T/C (T/t)
			rs10735810 (FokI)	C/T (F/f)
			rs11568820 (Cdx2)	G/A
			rs2254210	A/G
			rs98784	C/T
CYP24A1 *(cytochrome P450 family 24 subfamily A polypeptide, vitamin D 24-hydroxylase)*	Deactivation	20q13	rs2296241	A/G

Table 2. The gene polymorphisms associated with vitamin D metabolism [19, 98, 99, 101].

7.6.1. Genetic variants in vitamin D receptor gene in MS

According to the effects of vitamin D in MS, the molecular mechanisms of vitamin D function should be considered. As mentioned earlier, vitamin D executes its physiological effect via binding and activation of VDR. Interestingly, the activation of VDR by calcitriol can suppress the induction of EAE, while animals that lack VDR are not protected against EAE [102]. The gene for VDR is located on the 12q13 chromosomal region and consists of 11 exons. Non-coding exons 1A, 1B and 1C are located in the 5′ end of the VDR gene, and exons 2–9 encode the structural portion of the VDR protein [103]. VDR sequence is similar to that of the receptors for steroid hormones and hormones of the thyroid gland. VDR is a regulatory transcription factor and consists of highly conservative DNA-binding and ligand-binding domains. The signal pathways associated with the VDR regulate the transcription of genes involved in the regulation of bone metabolism, immune response and cancer [83]. The polymorphisms in the initiation codon of the *VDR* gene can cause the formation of transcription variants coding different proteins [104]. In the *VDR* gene, SNPs ApaI (rs7975232), BsmI (rs1544410), FokI (rs10735810) and TaqI (rs731236) have functional biological effects and are mostly studied in MS as well as in other diseases. These gene polymorphisms can alter mRNA level, its stability and alternative splicingand also the stability of the final gene product, amount of protein isoforms and their interactions [105]. FokI gene polymorphism is located in exon 2 of the *VDR* gene, and its variants result in a change of protein structure. There are two possible allele variants, f (presence of a restriction site for FokI endonuclease) and F (absence of a restriction site for FokI endonuclease). It has been confirmed that the f (T) allele leads to the expression of a VDR protein, which is three amino acids longer (427 amino acids) than the F (C) allele (424 amino acids). The shorter isoform of the receptor is more transcriptionally potent through a more efficient interaction with transcription factor TFIIB [105, 106]. Near the 3′ end of the *VDR* gene, we can find the ApaI and BsmI polymorphism in the intron between exon 8 and 9 and TaqI gene polymorphism in exon 9 [107]. The allele variants of these gene polymorphisms and their combinations regulate the functions of VDR through the modulation of mRNA stability. In Caucasians, TaqI, ApaI and BsmI polymorphisms are in strong linkage disequilibrium and are present in five haplotype blocks. Haplotype2 (t-A-B) probably results in a lower number of 'A' in polyA variable number of tandem repeats (VNTR), while haplotype 1 (T-A-b) is connected to a large number of 'A', thus modulating mRNA stability [106]. Morrison et al. [108] found that allele b (G) of the BsmI polymorphism causes a decreased expression of VDR mRNA.

Interestingly, several studies have found an association between *VDR* gene polymorphisms and the risk of MS. Differences in allele frequency of the BsmI polymorphism in the *VDR* gene were found in Japan by Fukazawa et al. [109], who for the first time pointed out the involvement of *VDR* gene polymorphisms in the pathogenesis of MS. The association of *VDR* gene polymorphisms with MS has been confirmed in cohorts of MS patients from Japan [110], theUK [111, 112], Australia [107] and the USA [98]. On the contrary, no association of VDR gene polymorphisms with the risk of MS was found by studies in MS patients from Canada [113], Netherlands [114], Greece [115], Spain [116, 117], Tasmania [118] and Iran [119]. The presence of specific haplotypes of the *VDR* gene can increase the risk of MS development, especially its progressive forms. Tajouri et al. [107] in Australia found haplotype A-t (T-C) of ApaI and TaqI polymorphism to increase the risk of MS development, especially its progressive forms. The carriership of allele t (C) in their study increased MS risk twice. Fukazawa et al. [109] found allele b (G) and genotype bb (GG) of BsmI polymorphism to increase MS risk, but without any association with the form and severity of MS (EDSS, magnetic resonance imaging (MRI)). Allele b (G) of BsmI polymorphism of VDR has been found to be associated with MS risk in combination with allele A (T) of ApaI polymorphism by Niino et al. [110]. However, in their study, they did not find any association of ApaI gene polymorphism with clinical form and severity of MS evaluated by the EDSS score, disease duration and MRI findings. Agliardi et al. [120] in Italy found that allele T (T) and genotype TT (TT) are protective against MS development, supported by the finding that the expression of VDR mRNA is increased four times by genotype Tt (TC) and eight times by genotype TT (TT) when compared to genotype tt (CC). The observed effect is present especially when the protective allele Tis present in the combination with HLA-DRB1*15 allele.

The role of VDR gene polymorphisms is still not completely understood, and it seems to vary among different populations. For proper cell signalling to decrease the risk of MS, it is probably necessary to reach a certain level of the transcriptional activity of VDR that is also modified genetically. For proper immunoregulation, the individuals that have the genotype causing the decreased VDR protein activity can need a higher peroral vitamin D intake or higher level of sun exposure. Contrarily, in individuals with higher transcriptional activity of VDR, a lower sun exposure or vitamin D intake can be sufficient for proper immune system regulation.

The findings of our previous study in MS patients from the Central-Northern region of Slovakia have confirmed the association of FokI heterozygous genotype Ff with an increased risk of MS in women [10]. Although we found no statistically significant differences in the proportions of FokI genotypes or allele frequencies between total MS patient and the control group, we have observed significant differences in the FokI genotype distribution between women with MS and the female control group ($p = 0.042$). Our results have shown a significantly higher frequency of heterozygous Ff genotypes in FokI polymorphism in the female MS group (53.4%) as compared to 43.7% in the female control group (OR = 1.48, 95% CI = 1.01–2.16). In spite of this fact, when we compared the subgroup of rapidly progressing MS patients with the subgroup of slow progressing MS patients, allele and genotype counts were not significantly different between them (allele f: 34.5 vs. 43.3%, allele F: 65.5 vs. 56.7%, genotype ff: 10.3 vs. 13.4%, genotype Ff: 48.3 vs. 59.8%). Since we have not shown any significant association between FokI VDR gene polymorphism and the rate of disease disability progression in our cohort of Slovak MS patients, we observed a trend of higher frequency of homozygotes FF to be 41.4% in MS patients with rapid progression of disease as compared to 26.8% in slow progressing MS patients (OR = 1.93, 95% CI=0.94–3.94) with a marginal level of significance ($p = 0.071$). From the results of our study, it seems that contributions from genetic and allelic variants of FokI VDR gene polymorphism have only a small impact in a disease as complex as MS, andits role in the etiopathogenesis of MS still remains controversial.

8. Conclusions

In summary, we can conclude that many genetic and biochemical factors can be involved in the etiopathogenesis of MS. These markers could be used to evaluate the risk of MS development and the risk of rapid disease disability progression.

http://dx.doi.org/10.5772/63468

The proposed markers that have been found to be associated with MS risk or disability progression in Central European Slovak population are summarized in **Table 3**. In our studies, we identified decreased serum level of vitamin D, allele C and genotype CC of polymorphism rs6897932 in the *IL7Ra* gene, genotype Ff of rs10735810 in the *VDR* gene (only in women); HLA-alleles DRB1*15, DRB1*03, DQB1*06; HLA-genotypes DRB1*15/*15, DQB1*06/*06 and HLA-haplotype DRB1*15-DQB1*06 as the main risk factors for MS development. On the contrary, allele T of rs6897932 in the *IL7Ra* gene (in individuals with genotype CT and TT); HLA-alleles DRB1*07, DRB1*13, DQB1*03; HLA-genotypes DRB1*13/*11, DQB1*05/*03 and HLA-haplotypes DRB1*13-DQB1*06 and DRB1*11-DQB1*03 displayed a protective effect against MS development. Genotype CC of rs6897932 in the *IL7Ra* gene and decreased serum level of vitamin D were identified as negative prognostic factors for rapid disability progression in MS, while minor allele T of rs6897932 in the *IL7Ra* gene (especially in individuals with TT genotype) was identified as a protective factor disability progression.

	MS development	*Rapid disease disability progression*
Risk factors	Decreased serum vitamin D	Decreased serum vitamin D
	rs6897932 in *IL7Ra* gene—allele C, genotype CC	rs6897932 in *IL7Ra* gene—genotype CC
	HLA-alleles DRB1*15, DRB1*03, DQB1*06; HLA-genotypes DRB1*15/*15, DQB1*06/*06; HLA-haplotype DRB1*15-DQB1*06	
	rs10735810 in *VDR* gene —genotype Ff (only women)	
Protective factors	rs6897932 in *IL7Ra* gene—allele T, genotype CT and TT	rs6897932 in *IL7Ra* gene—allele T, genotype TT
	HLA-alleles DRB1*07, DRB1*13, DQB1*03; HLA-genotypes DRB1*13/*11, DQB1*05/*03; HLA-haplotypes DRB1*13-DQB1*06, DRB1*11- DQB1*03	

Table 3. The proposed markers associated with the MS risk or disability progression in Slovaks [10, 41, 65].

From the results of our study, we conclude that rs6897932 of the *IL7Ra*gene, rs10735810 in the *VDR* gene, HLA-DR and DQ genotypes, as well as serum level of vitamin D may be the important markers that could be used as part of a panel of markers to evaluate the risk of MS development and disability progression. The relevance of these markers identified in our study should be verified in larger groups of individuals not only in Slovakia but also in other different populations. The relevant positive or negative prognostic genetic or biochemical markers can improve the diagnostic and therapeutic procedure and can help to minimize neurological damage in predisposed individuals.

Acknowledgements

The work was supported by the projects '"Centre for Translational Medicine' code: 6220220021, 'Identification of Novel Markers in Diagnostic Panel of Neurological Diseases' code: 26220220114, 'Martin Biomedical Center (BioMed Martin)' ITMS code: 26220220187 co-financed from EU sources and European Regional Development Fund and the grant of Ministry of Health, 2012/30-UKMA-7 and APVV No. 15/0107.

Author details

Daniel Čierny[1], Jozef Michalik[2], Ema Kantorová[2], Egon Kurča[2] and Ján Lehotský[3*]

*Address all correspondence to: lehotsky@jfmed.uniba.sk

1 Department of Clinical Biochemistry, Jessenius Faculty of Medicine and University Hospital Martin, Comenius University in Bratislava, Martin, Slovak Republic

2 Department of Neurology, Jessenius Faculty of Medicine and University Hospital Martin, Comenius University in Bratislava, Martin, Slovak Republic

3 Department of Medical Biochemistry and BioMed, Jessenius Faculty of Medicine in Martin, Comenius University in Bratislava, Martin, Slovak Republic

References

[1] Kakalacheva K, Lünemann JD. Environmental triggers of multiple sclerosis. FEBS Lett. 2011; 585(23):3724–9. doi: 10.1016/j.febslet.2011.04.006

[2] International Multiple Sclerosis Genetics Consortium, Hafler DA, Compston A, Sawcer S, Lander ES, Daly MJ, De Jager PL, de Bakker PI, Gabriel SB, Mirel DB, Ivinson AJ, Pericak-Vance MA, Gregory SG, Rioux JD, McCauley JL, Haines JL, Barcellos LF, Cree B, Oksenberg JR, Hauser SL. Risk alleles for multiple sclerosis identified by a genome-wide study. N Engl J Med. 2007;357(9):851-62. PMID: 17660530

[3] Nischwitz S, Müller-Myhsok B, Weber F. Risk conferring genes in multiple sclerosis.FEBS Lett. 2011; 585(23):3789–97. doi: 10.1016/j.febslet.2011.03.037

[4] Stinissen P, Hellings N.Activation of myelin reactive T cells in multiple sclerosis: a possible role for T cell degeneracy? Eur J Immunol. 2008; 38(5):1190–3. doi: 10.1002/eji.200838371

[5] Compston A, Coles A. Multiple sclerosis.The Lancet. 2008; 372(9648):1502–17. doi: 10.1016/S0140-6736(08)61620-7

[6] Levin MC, Douglas JN, Meyers L, Sangmin L, Yoojin S, Gardner LA.Neurodegeneration in multiple sclerosis involves multiple pathogenic mechanisms. DegenerNeurolNeuromuscul Dis. 2014; 2014(4):49–63. doi: http://dx.doi.org/10.2147/DNND.S54391

[7] Kostic MS, Rajkovic JS, PoticFloranovic MS, Dimov ID, Pavlovic DD. Multiple sclerosis and oxidative stress—a clinical perspective.Neurochem J. 2013; 7(1):76–86. doi: 10.1134/S1819712412040083

[8] Roxburgh RH, Seaman SR, Masterman T, Hensiek AE, Sawcer SJ, Vukusic S, Achiti I, Confavreux C, Coustans M, le Page E, Edan G, McDonnell GV, Hawkins S, Trojano M, Liguori M, Cocco E, Marrosu MG, Tesser F, Leone MA, Weber A, Zipp F, Miterski B, Epplen JT, Oturai A, Sørensen PS, Celius EG, Lara NT, Montalban X, Villoslada P, Silva AM, Marta M, Leite I, Dubois B, Rubio J, Butzkueven H, Kilpatrick T, Mycko MP, Selmaj KW, Rio ME, Sá M, Salemi G, Savettieri G, Hillert J, Compston DA. Multiple sclerosis severity score: using disability and disease duration to rate disease severity. Neurology. 2005; 64(7):1144–51. PMID: 15824338

[9] Kurtzke JF. Rating neurologic impairment in multiple sclerosis: an expanded disability status scale (EDSS). Neurology. 1983; 33(11):1444–52. PMID: 6685237

[10] Čierny D, Michalik J, Kurča E, Dobrota D, Lehotský J.FokI vitamin D receptor gene polymorphism in association with multiple sclerosis risk and disability progression in Slovaks. Neurol Res. 2015; 37(4):301–8. doi: 10.1179/1743132814Y.0000000459

[11] Orton SM, Herrera BM, Yee IM, Valdar W, Ramagopalan SV, Sadovnick AD, Ebers GC; Canadian Collaborative Study Group. Sex ratio of multiple sclerosis in Canada: a longitudinal study. Lancet Neurol. 2006; 5(11):932–6. PMID: 17052660

[12] Hayes CE. Vitamin D: a natural inhibitor of multiple sclerosis. ProcNutr Soc. 2000; 59(4):531–5. PMID: 11115787

[13] Wall JD, Pritchard JK. Assessing the performance of the haplotype block model of linkage disequilibrium.Am J Hum Genet. 2003; 73(3):502–15. PMID: 12916017

[14] De Bakker PI, McVean G, Sabeti PC, Miretti MM, Green T, Marchini J, Ke X, Monsuur AJ, Whittaker P, Delgado M, Morrison J, Richardson A, Walsh EC, Gao X, Galver L, Hart J, Hafler DA, Pericak-Vance M, Todd JA, Daly MJ, Trowsdale J, Wijmenga C, Vyse TJ, Beck S, Murray SS, Carrington M, Gregory S, Deloukas P, Rioux JD. A high-resolution HLA and SNP haplotype map for disease association studies in the extended human MHC. Nat Genet. 2006; 38(10):1166–72. PMID: 16998491

[15] Sombekke MH, Lukas C, Crusius JB, Tejedor D, Killestein J, Arteta D, Martínez A, Uitdehaag BM, Knol DL, Peña AS, Geurts JJ, De Jager PL, Barkhof F, Vrenken H, Polman

CH. HLA-DRB1*1501 and spinal cord magnetic resonance imaging lesions in multiple sclerosis. Arch Neurol. 2009; 66(12):1531–6. doi: 10.1001/archneurol.2009.278

[16] Benešová Y, Vašků A, Stourač P, Hladíková M, Fiala A, Bednařík J. Association of HLA-DRB1*1501 tagging rs3135388 gene polymorphism with multiple sclerosis. J Neuroimmunol. 2013; 255(1–2):92–6. doi: 10.1016/j.jneuroim.2012.10.014

[17] Mehra NK, Kaur G. 2003.Gene map of the human leukocyte antigen (HLA) region.In Expert RevMol Med.2003; 5:1. Available from: http://journals.cambridge.org/fulltext_content/ERM/ERM5_07/S1462399403005957sup001.pdf

[18] Jedlička P. Onemocneníbíléhmotymozkomíšní. In: Jedlička P, Keller O. editors. Speciálníneurologie. 1st ed. Praha: Galén; 2005. p. 203–212. ISBN 80-7262-312-5.

[19] Sundqvist E, Bäärnhielm M, Alfredsson L, Hillert J, Olsson T, Kockum I. Confirmation of association between multiple sclerosis and CYP27B1. Eur J Hum Genet. 2010; 18(12): 1349–52. doi: 10.1038/ejhg.2010.113

[20] Dyment DA, Herrera BM, Cader MZ, Willer CJ, Lincoln MR, Sadovnick AD, Risch N, Ebers GC. Complex interactions among MHC haplotypes in multiple sclerosis: susceptibility and resistance. Hum Mol Genet. 2005; 14(14):2019–26. PMID: 15930013

[21] Oksenberg JR, Barcellos LF, Cree BA, Baranzini SE, Bugawan TL, Khan O, et al. Mapping multiple sclerosis susceptibility to the HLA-DR locus in African Americans. Am J Hum Genet. 2004; 74(1):160–7.

[22] Lincoln MR, Montpetit A, Cader MZ, Saarela J, Dyment DA, Tiislar M, Ferretti V, Tienari PJ, Sadovnick AD, Peltonen L, Ebers GC, Hudson TJ. A predominant role for the HLA class II region in the association of the MHC region with multiple sclerosis. Nat Genet. 2005; 37(10):1108–12.

[23] Sawcer S, Hellenthal G, Pirinen M, Spencer CCA, Patsopoulos NA, Moutsianas L, et al. The International Multiple Sclerosis Genetics Consortium (IMSGC), Wellcome Trust Case Control Consortium 2 (WTCCC2).Genetic risk and a primary role for cell-mediated immune mechanisms in multiple sclerosis.Nature. 2011; 476(7359):214–9. doi: 10.1038/nature10251

[24] Zhang Q, Lin CY, Dong Q, Wang J, Wang W. Relationship between HLA-DRB1 polymorphism and susceptibility or resistance to multiple sclerosis in Caucasians: a meta-analysis of non-family-based studies. Autoimmun Rev. 2011; 10(8):474–81. doi: 10.1016/j.autrev.2011.03.003

[25] Schmidt H, Williamson D, Ashley-Koch A. HLA-DR15 haplotype and multiple sclerosis: a HuGE review. Am J Epidemiol. 2007; 165(10):1097–109. PMID: 17329717

[26] Ramagopalan SV, Morris AP, Dyment DA, Herrera BM, DeLuca GC, Lincoln MR, Orton SM, Chao JM, Sadovnick AD, Ebers GC.The inheritance of resistance alleles in multiple sclerosis.PLoS Genet. 2007; 3(9):e150. doi: 10.1371/journal.pgen.0030150

[27] Masterman T, Ligers A, Olsson T, Andersson M, Olerup O, Hillert J. HLA-DR15 is associated with lower age at onset in multiple sclerosis. Ann Neurol. 2000; 48(2):211–9. PMID: 10939572

[28] Kaimen-Maciel DR, Reiche EM, Borelli SD, Morimoto HK, Melo FC, Lopes J, Dorigon RF, Cavalet C, Yamaguchi EM, Silveira TL, Da Silva WV, Comini-Frota ER, Brum Souza DG, Donadi EA. HLA-DRB1* allele-associated genetic susceptibility and protection against multiple sclerosis in Brazilian patients. Mol Med Rep. 2009; 2(6):993–8. doi: 10.3892/mmr_00000204.

[29] Romero-Pinel L, Pujal JM, Martínez-Yélamos S, Gubieras L, Matas E, Bau L, Torrabadella M, Azqueta C, Arbizu T. HLA-DRB1: genetic susceptibility and disability progression in a Spanish multiple sclerosis population. Eur J Neurol. 2011; 18(2):337–42. doi: 10.1111/j.1468-1331.2010.03148.x

[30] Kouri I, Papakonstantinou S, Bempes V, Vasiliadis HS, Kyritsis AP, Pelidou HS.HLA associations with multiple sclerosis in Greece. J Neurol Sci. 2011; 308(1–2):28–31. doi: 10.1016/j.jns.2011.06.037

[31] Marrosu MG, Murru R, Murru MR, Costa G, Zavattari P, Whalen M, Cocco E, Mancosu C, Schirru L, Solla E, Fadda E, Melis C, Porru I, Rolesu M, Cucca F. Dissection of the HLA association with multiple sclerosis in the founder isolated population of Sardinia. Hum Mol Genet. 2001; 10(25):2907–16. PMID: 11741834

[32] Stankovich J, Butzkueven H, Marriott M, Chapman C, Tubridy N, Tait BD, Varney MD, Taylor BV, Foote SJ; ANZgene Consortium, Kilpatrick TJ, Rubio JP. HLA-DRB1 associations with disease susceptibility and clinical course in Australians with multiple sclerosis. Tissue Antigens. 2009; 74(1):17–21. doi: 10.1111/j.1399-0039.2009.01262.x

[33] Fernández O, Fernández V, Alonso A, Caballero A, Luque G, Bravo M, León A, Mayorga C, Leyva L, de Ramón E. DQB1*0602 allele shows a strong association with multiple sclerosis in patients in Malaga, Spain. J Neurol. 2004; 251(4):440–4. PMID: 15083289

[34] Link J, Kockum I, Lorentzen AR, Lie BA, Celius EG, Westerlind H, Schaffer M, Alfredsson L, Olsson T, Brynedal B, Harbo HF, Hillert J. Importance of human leukocyte antigen (HLA) class I and II alleles on the risk of multiple sclerosis. PLoS One. 2012; 7(5):e36779. doi: 10.1371/journal.pone.0036779

[35] Kaushansky N, Ben-Nun A. DQB1*06:02-associated pathogenic anti-myelin autoimmunity in multiple sclerosis-like disease: potential function of DQB1*06:02 as a disease-predisposing allele. Front Oncol. 2014; 4:280.doi: 10.3389/fonc.2014.00280

[36] Caballero A, Alves-Leon S, Papais-Alvarenga R, Fernandez O, Navarro G. Alonso, A. DQB1*0602 confers genetic susceptibility to multiple sclerosis in Afro-Brazilians. Tissue Antigens. 1999; 54(5):524–26. PMID: 10599893

[37] Kaushansky N, Altmann DM, David CS, Lassmann H, Ben-Nun A. DQB1*0602 rather than DRB1*1501 confers susceptibility to multiple sclerosis-like disease induced by proteolipid protein (PLP). J Neuroinflammation.2012; 9:29.doi: 10.1186/1742-2094-9-29

[38] Isobe N, Gourraud PA, Harbo HF, Caillier SJ, Santaniello A, Khankhanian P, Maiers M, Spellman S, Cereb N, Yang S, Pando MJ, Piccio L, Cross AH, De Jager PL, Cree BA, Hauser SL, Oksenberg JR. Genetic risk variants in African Americans with multiple sclerosis. Neurology. 2013; 81(3):219–27. doi: 10.1212/WNL.0b013e31829bfe2f

[39] Barcellos LF, Sawcer S, Ramsay PP, Baranzini SE, Thomson G, Briggs F, et al. Heterogeneity at the HLA-DRB1 locus and risk for multiple sclerosis. Hum Mol Genet. 2006; 15(18):2813–24. PMID: 16905561

[40] Cocco E, Murru R, Costa G, Kumar A, Pieroni E, Melis C, Barberini L, Sardu C, Lorefice L, Fenu G, Frau J, Coghe G, Carboni N, Marrosu MG. Interaction between HLA-DRB1-DQB1 Haplotypes in Sardinian multiple sclerosis population. PloS One. 2013; 8(4):e59790. doi: 10.1371/journal.pone.0059790

[41] Michalik J, Čierny D, Kantorová E, Kantárová D, Juraj J, Párnická Z, Kurča E, Dobrota D, Lehotský J. The association of HLA-DRB1 and HLA-DQB1 alleles with genetic susceptibility to multiple sclerosis in the Slovak population. Neurol Res. 2015; 37:1060–67 doi: 10.1080/01616412.2015.1115212.

[42] D'Netto MJ, Ward H, Morrison KM, Ramagopalan SV, Dyment DA, DeLuca GC, Handunnetthi L, Sadovnick AD, Ebers GC. Risk alleles for multiple sclerosis in multiplex families.Neurology. 2009; 72(23):1984–8. doi: 10.1212/WNL.0b013e3181a92c25

[43] Hoffjan S, Akkad DA. The genetics of multiple sclerosis: an update 2010. Mol Cell Probes. 2010; 24(5):237–43. doi: 10.1016/j.mcp.2010.04.006

[44] Akkad DA, Hoffjan S, Petrasch-Parwez E, Beygo J, Gold R, Epplen JT. Variation in the IL7RA and IL2RA genes in German multiple sclerosis patients. J Autoimmun. 2009; 32(2):110–5. doi: 10.1016/j.jaut.2009.01.002

[45] Brynedal B, Bomfim IL, Olsson T, DuvefeltK,Hillert J. Differential expression, and genetic association, of CD58 in Swedish multiple sclerosis patients. ProcNatlAcadSci U S A. 2009; 106(23):E58. doi: 10.1073/pnas.0904338106

[46] De Jager PL, Jia X, Wang J, de Bakker PI, Ottoboni L, Aggarwal NT, Piccio L, Raychaudhuri S, Tran D, Aubin C, Briskin R, Romano S; International MS Genetics Consortium, Baranzini SE, McCauley JL, Pericak-Vance MA, Haines JL, Gibson RA, Naeglin Y, Uitdehaag B, Matthews PM, Kappos L, Polman C, McArdleWL, Strachan DP, Evans D, Cross AH, Daly MJ, Compston A, Sawcer SJ, Weiner HL, Hauser SL, Hafler DA, Oksenberg JR. Meta-analysis of genome scans and replication identify CD6, IRF8 and TNFRSF1A as new multiple sclerosis susceptibility loci. Nat Genet. 2009; 41(7):776–82. doi: 10.1038/ng.401

[47] Dyment DA, Cader MZ, Chao MJ, Lincoln MR, Morrison KM, Disanto G, Morahan JM, De Luca GC, Sadovnick AD, Lepage P, Montpetit A, Ebers GC, Ramagopalan SV. Exome sequencing identifies a novel multiple sclerosis susceptibility variant in the TYK2 gene. Neurology. 2012; 79(5):406–11. doi: 10.1212/WNL.0b013e3182616fc4

[48] Park TJ, Kim HJ, Kim JH, Bae JS, Cheong HS, Park BL, Shin HD. Associations of CD6, TNFRSF1A and IRF8 polymorphisms with risk of inflammatory demyelinating diseases.NeuropatholApplNeurobiol. 2013; 39(5):519–30. doi: 10.1111/j.1365-2990.2012.01304.x

[49] Fry TJ, Mackall CL. 2002. Interleukin-7: from bench to clinic. Blood. 2002; 99(11):3892–904

[50] Bomprezzi R, Ringnér M, Kim S, Bittner ML, Khan J, Chen Y, Elkahloun A, Yu A, Bielekova B, Meltzer PS, Martin R, McFarland HF, Trent JM. Gene expression profile in multiple sclerosis patients and healthy controls: identifying pathways relevant to disease. Hum Mol Genet. 2003; 12(17):2191–9. PMID: 12915464

[51] Ramanathan M, Weinstock-Guttman B, Nguyen LT, Badgett D, Miller C, Patrick K, Brownscheidle C, Jacobs L. In vivo gene expression revealed by cDNA arrays: the pattern in relapsing–remitting multiple sclerosis patients compared with normal subjects. J Neuroimmunol. 2001; 116(2):213–9.116: 213–219. PMID: 11438176

[52] Lundmark F, Duvefelt K, Iacobaeus E, Kockum I, Wallström E, Khademi M, Oturai A, Ryder LP, Saarela J, Harbo HF, Celius EG, Salter H, Olsson T, Hillert J. Variation in interleukin 7 receptor alpha chain (IL7R) influences risk of multiple sclerosis. Nat Genet. 2007; 39(9):1108-13. PMID: 17660816

[53] Goodwin RG, Friend D, Ziegler SF, Jerzy R, Falk BA, Gimpel S, Cosman D, Dower SK, March CJ, Namen AE, et al. Cloning of the human and murine interleukin-7 receptors: demonstration of a soluble form and homology to a new receptor superfamily. Cell. 1990; 60(6):941–51. PMID: 2317865

[54] Kreft KL, Verbraak E, Wierenga-Wolf AF, van Meurs M, Oostra BA, Laman JD, Hintzen RQ. Decreased systemic IL-7 and soluble IL-7Rα in multiple sclerosis patients. Genes Immun. 2012; 13(7):587–92. doi: 10.1038/gene.2012.34

[55] Zhang Z, Duvefelt K, Svensson F, Masterman T, Jonasdottir G, Salter H, Emahazion T, Hellgren D, Falk G, Olsson T, Hillert J, Anvret M. Two genes encoding immune-regulatory molecules (LAG3 and IL7R) confer susceptibility to multiple sclerosis. Genes Immun. 2005; 6(2):145–52. PMID: 15674389

[56] Teutsch SM, Booth DR, Bennetts BH, Heard RN, Stewart GJ. Identification of 11 novel and common single nucleotide polymorphisms in the interleukin-7 receptor-alpha gene and their associations with multiple sclerosis.Eur J Hum Genet. 2003; 11(7):509–15. PMID: 12825072

[57] Gregory SG, Schmidt S, Seth P, Oksenberg JR, Hart J, Prokop A, Caillier SJ, Ban M, Goris A, Barcellos LF, Lincoln R, McCauley JL, Sawcer SJ, Compston DA, Dubois B, Hauser

SL, Garcia-Blanco MA, Pericak-Vance MA, Haines JL; Multiple Sclerosis Genetics Group. Interleukin 7 receptor alpha chain (IL7R) shows allelic and functional association with multiple sclerosis. Nat Genet. 2007; 39(9):1083–91. PMID: 17660817

[58] O'Doherty C, Kantarci O, Vandenbroeck K. IL7RA polymorphisms and susceptibility to multiple sclerosis. N Engl J Med. 2008; 358(7):753–4. doi: 10.1056/NEJMc0707553

[59] Alcina A, Fedetz M, Ndagire D, Fernández O, Leyva L, Guerrero M, Arnal C, Delgado C, Matesanz F. The T244I variant of the interleukin-7 receptor-alpha gene and multiple sclerosis.Tissue Antigens. 2008; 72(2):158–61. doi: 10.1111/j.1399-0039.2008.01075.x

[60] Weber F, Fontaine B, Cournu-Rebeix I, Kroner A, Knop M, Lutz S, Müller-Sarnowski F, Uhr M, Bettecken T, Kohli M, Ripke S, Ising M, Rieckmann P, Brassat D, Semana G, Babron MC, Mrejen S, Gout C, Lyon-Caen O, Yaouanq J, Edan G, Clanet M, Holsboer F, Clerget-Darpoux F, Müller-Myhsok B. IL2RA and IL7RA genes confer susceptibility for multiple sclerosis in two independent European populations. Genes Immun. 2008; 9(3):259–63. doi: 10.1038/gene.2008.14

[61] Sombekke MH, van der Voort LF, Kragt JJ, Nielsen JM, Guzel H, Visser A, Oudejans CB, Crusius JB, Peña AS, Vrenken H, Polman CH, Killestein J. Relevance of IL7R genotype and mRNA expression in Dutch patients with multiple sclerosis. MultScler. 2011; 17(8):922–30. doi: 10.1177/1352458511402411

[62] Fang L, Isobe N, Yoshimura S, Yonekawa T, Matsushita T, Masaki K, Doi H, Ochi K, Miyamoto K, Kawano Y, Kira J; South Japan Multiple Sclerosis Genetics Consortium. Interleukin-7 receptor alpha gene polymorphism influences multiple sclerosis risk in Asians. Neurology. 2011; 76(24):2125–7. doi: 10.1212/WNL.0b013e31821f466c

[63] Stanković A, Dincić E, Ristić S, Lovrecić L, StarcevićCizmarević N, Djurić T, Sepcić J, KapovićM, RaicevićR, PeterlinB, AlavantićD, ZivkovićM. Interleukin 7 receptor alpha polymorphism rs6897932 and susceptibility to multiple sclerosis in the Western Balkans. MultScler. 2010; 16(5):533–6. doi: 10.1177/1352458509360548

[64] Booth DR, Arthur AT, Teutsch SM, Bye C, Rubio J, Armati PJ, Pollard JD, Heard RN, Stewart GJ; Southern MS Genetics Consortium. Gene expression and genotyping studies implicate the interleukin 7 receptor in the pathogenesis of primary progressive multiple sclerosis. J Mol Med. 2005; 83(10):822–30. PMID: 16075257

[65] Čierny D, Hányšová S, Michalik J, Kantorová E, Kurča E, Škereňová M, Lehotský J. Genetic variants in interleukin 7 receptor α chain (IL-7Ra) are associated with multiple sclerosis risk and disability progression in Central European Slovak population. J Neuroimmunol.2015; 282:80–4.doi: 10.1016/j.jneuroim.2015.03.010

[66] Chaudhuri A. Why we should offer routine vitamin D supplementation in pregnancy and childhood to prevent multiple sclerosis. Med Hypotheses. 2005; 64(3):608–18. PMID: 15617877

[67] Saccone D, Asani F, Bornman L. Regulation of the vitamin D receptor gene by environment, genetics and epigenetics. Gene. 2015; 561(2):171–80. doi: 10.1016/j.gene.2015.02.024

[68] Norman AW.Minireview: vitamin D receptor: new assignments for an already busy receptor. Endocrinology. 2006; 147(12):5542–8. PMID: 16946007

[69] Ascherio A, Munger KL, Simon KC. Vitamin D and multiple sclerosis. Lancet Neurol. 2010; 9(6):599–612. doi: 10.1016/S1474-4422(10)70086-7

[70] Adorini L, Penna G. Control of autoimmune diseases by the vitamin D endocrine system. Nat ClinPractRheumatol. 2008; 4(8):404–12.doi: 10.1038/ncprheum0855

[71] Bikle DD. Vitamin D regulation of immune function.VitamHorm. 2011; 86:1–21.doi: 10.1016/B978-0-12-386960-9.00001-0

[72] Smolders J, Thewissen M, Peelen E, Menheere P, Tervaert JW, Damoiseaux J, Hupperts R. Vitamin D status is positively correlated with regulatory T cell function in patients with multiple sclerosis. PLoS One. 2009; 4(8):e6635. doi: 10.1371/journal.pone.0006635.

[73] Penna G, Adorini L. 1 Alpha,25-dihydroxyvitamin D3 inhibits differentiation, maturation, activation, and survival of dendritic cells leading to impaired alloreactive T cell activation. J Immunol. 2000; 164(5):2405–11. PMID: 10679076

[74] Boonstra A, Barrat FJ, Crain C, Heath VL, Savelkoul HF, O'Garra A. 2001. 1α,25-Dihydroxyvitamin D3 has a direct effect on naive CD4+ T cells to enhance the development of Th2 cells. JImmunol. 2001; 167(9):4974–80. PMID: 11673504

[75] Geldmeyer-Hilt K, Heine G, Hartmann B, Baumgrass R, Radbruch A, Worm M. 1,25-dihydroxyvitamin D3 impairs NF-kB activation in human naïve B cells. BiochemBiophys Res Commun. 2011; 407(4):699–702. doi: 10.1016/j.bbrc.2011.03.078

[76] Chen S, Sims GP, Chen XX, Gu YY, Chen S, Lipsky PE. Modulatory effects of 1,25-dihydroxyvitamin D3 on human B cell differentiation. J Immunol. 2007; 179(3):1634–47. PMID: 17641030

[77] Lemire JM, Archer DC, Beck L, Spiegelberg HL. Immunosuppressive actions of 1,25-dihydroxyvitamin D3: preferential inhibition of Th1 functions. J Nutr. 1995; 125(6 Suppl):1704S–8S. PMID: 7782931

[78] Helming L, Böse J, Ehrchen J, Schiebe S, Frahm T, Geffers R, Probst-Kepper M, Balling R, Lengeling A. 1alpha,25-Dihydroxyvitamin D3 is a potent suppressor of interferon gamma-mediated macrophage activation. Blood. 2005; 106(13):4351–8. PMID: 16118315

[79] Bartels LE, Hvas CL, Agnholt J, Dahlerup JF, Agger R. Human dendritic cell antigen presentation and chemotaxis are inhibited by intrinsic 25-hydroxy vitamin D activation. IntImmunopharmacol. 2010;10(8):922–8. doi: 10.1016/j.intimp.2010.05.003

[80] O'Kelly J, Hisatake J, Hisatake Y, Bishop J, Norman A, Koeffler HP. Normal myelopoiesis but abnormal T lymphocyte responses in vitamin D receptor knockout mice. J Clin Invest. 2002; 109(8):1091–9. PMID: 11956247

[81] Panda DK, Miao D, Tremblay ML, Sirois J, Farookhi R, Hendy GN, Goltzman D. Targeted ablation of the 25-hydroxyvitamin D 1alpha -hydroxylase enzyme: evidence for skeletal, reproductive, and immune dysfunction. ProcNatlAcadSci U S A. 2001; 98(13):7498–503. PMID: 11416220

[82] Cantorna MT, Hayes CE, DeLuca HF. 1,25-Dihydroxyvitamin D3 reversibly blocks the progression of relapsing encephalomyelitis, a model of multiple sclerosis. ProcNatlAcadSci U S A. 1996; 93(15):7861–4. PMCID: PMC38839

[83] Kamen DL, Tangpricha V. Vitamin D and molecular actions on the immune system: modulation of innate and autoimmunity. J Mol Med (Berl). 2010; 88(5):441–450. doi: 10.1007/s00109-010-0590-9

[84] Mattner F, Smiroldo S, Galbiati F, Muller M, Di Lucia P, Poliani PL, Martino G, Panina-Bordignon P, Adorini L. Inhibition of Th1 development and treatment of chronic-relapsing experimental allergic encephalomyelitis by a non-hypercalcemic analogue of 1,25-dihydroxyvitamin D(3). Eur J Immunol. 2000; 30(2):498–508. PMID: 10671205

[85] Haynes RC Jr. Vitamin D. In Gilman AG, Rall TW, Nies AR, Taylor P. editors. Goodman and Gilman's the pharmacological basis of therapeutics. 8th ed. New York: McGraw-Hill; 1992. p. 1515

[86] Pierrot-Deseilligny C, Souberbielle JC. Widespread vitamin D insufficiency: a new challenge for primary prevention, with particular reference to multiple sclerosis. Presse Med. 2011; 40(4 Pt 1):349–56. doi: 10.1016/j.lpm.2011.01.003

[87] Burton JM, Kimball S, Vieth R, Bar-Or A, Dosch HM, Cheung R, Gagne D, D'Souza C, Ursell M, O'Connor P. A phase I/II dose-escalation trial of vitamin D3 and calcium in multiple sclerosis. Neurology. 2010; 74(23):1852–9. doi:10.1212/WNL.0b013e3181e1cec2

[88] Kimball SM, Ursell MR, O'Connor P, Vieth R. Safety of vitamin D3 in adults with multiple sclerosis. Am J ClinNutr. 2007; 86(3):645–51. PMID: 17823429

[89] Munger KL, Zhang SM, O'Reilly E, Hernán MA, Olek MJ, Willett WC, Ascherio A.Vitamin D intake and incidence of multiple sclerosis. Neurology. 2004; 62(1):60–5. PMID: 14718698

[90] Munger KL, Levin LI, Hollis BW, Howard NS, Ascherio A. Serum 25-hydroxyvitamin D levels and risk of multiple sclerosis. JAMA. 2006; 296(23):32–8. PMID: 17179460

[91] Soilu-Hänninen M, Airas L, Mononen I, Heikkilä A, Viljanen M, Hänninen A. 25-Hydroxyvitamin D levels in serum at the onset of multiple sclerosis. MultScler. 2005; 11(3):266–71.

[92] Ozgocmen S, Bulut S, Ilhan N, Gulkesen A, Ardicoglu O, Ozkan Y. Vitamin D deficiency and reduced bone mineral density in multiple sclerosis: effect of ambulatory status and functional capacity. J Bone MinerMetabol. 2005; 23(4):309–13. PMID: 15981027

[93] Smolders J, Menheere P, Kessels A, Damoiseaux J, Hupperts R. Association of vitamin D metabolite levels with relapse rate and disability in multiple sclerosis.MultScler. 2008; 14(9):1220–4. doi: 10.1177/1352458508094399

[94] Runia TF, Hop WC, de Rijke YB, Buljevac D, Hintzen RQ. Lower serum vitamin D levels are associated with a higher relapse risk in multiple sclerosis. Neurology. 2012; 79(3): 261–6. doi: 10.1212/WNL.0b013e31825fdec7

[95] Cadden MH, Koven NS, Ross MK. Neuroprotective effects of vitamin D in multiple sclerosis.NeurosciMed. 2011; 2(3):198–207. doi: 10.4236/nm.2011.23027

[96] Simon KC, Munger KL, Kraft P, Hunter DJ, De Jager PL, Ascherio A. Genetic predictors of 25-hydroxyvitamin D levels and risk of multiple sclerosis. J Neurol. 2011; 258(9): 1676–82. doi: 10.1007/s00415-011-6001-5

[97] Smolders J, Damoiseaux J, Menheere P, Tervaert JW, Hupperts R. Fok-I vitamin D receptor gene polymorphism (rs10735810) and vitamin D metabolism in multiple sclerosis. J Neuroimmunol. 2009; 207(1–2):117–21. doi: 10.1016/j.jneuroim.2008.12.011

[98] Simon KC, Munger KL, Xing Yang, Ascherio A. Polymorphisms in vitamin D metabolism related genes and risk of multiple sclerosis. MultScler. 2010; 16(2):133–8. doi: 10.1177/1352458509355069

[99] Orton SM, Morris AP, Herrera BM, Ramagopalan SV, Lincoln MR, Chao MJ, Vieth R, Sadovnick AD, Ebers GC. Evidence for genetic regulation of vitamin D status in twins with multiple sclerosis.Am J ClinNutr. 2008; 88(2):441–7. PMID: 18689381

[100] Holick MF, Chen TC. Vitamin D deficiency: a worldwide problem with health consequences. Am J ClinNutr. 2008; 87(4):1080S–6S. PMID: 18400738

[101] Ramagopalan SV, Dyment DA, Cader MZ, Morrison KM, Disanto G, Morahan JM, Berlanga-Taylor AJ, Handel A, De Luca GC, Sadovnick AD, Lepage P, Montpetit A, Ebers GC. Rare variants in the CYP27B1 gene are associated with multiple sclerosis. Ann Neurol. 2011; 70(6):881–6. doi: 10.1002/ana.22678

[102] Meehan TF, DeLuca HF. The vitamin D receptor is necessary for 1alpha,25-dihydroxyvitamin D(3) to suppress experimental autoimmune encephalomyelitis in mice. Arch BiochemBiophys. 2002; 408(2):200–4. PMID: 12464272

[103] Miyamoto K, Kesterson RA, Yamamoto H, Taketani Y, Nishiwaki E, Tatsumi S, Inoue Y, Morita K, Takeda E, Pike JW. Structural organization of the human vitamin D receptor chromosomal gene and its promoter.MolEndocrinol. 1997; 11(8):1165–79. PMID: 9212063

[104] Wang TT, Tavera-Mendoza LE, Laperriere D, Libby E, MacLeod NB, Nagai Y, Bourdeau V, Konstorum A, Lallemant B, Zhang R, Mader S, White JH. Large-scale in silico

and microarray-based identification of direct 1,25-dihydroxyvitamin D3 target genes. MolEndocrinol. 2005; 19(11):2685–95. PMID: 16002434

[105] Uitterlinden AG, Fang Y, Van Meurs JB, Pols HA, Van Leeuwen JP. Genetics and biology of vitamin D receptor polymorphisms. Gene. 2004; 338(2):143–56. PMID: 15315818

[106] Jurutka PW, Remus LS, Whitfield GK, Thompson PD, Hsieh JC, Zitzer H, Tavakkoli P, Galligan MA, Dang HT, Haussler CA, Haussler MR. The polymorphic N terminus in human vitamin D receptor isoforms influences transcriptional activity by modulating interaction with transcription factor IIB. MolEndocrinol. 2000; 14(3):401–20. PMID: 10707958

[107] Tajouri L, Ovcaric M, Curtain R, Johnson MP, Griffiths LR, Csurhes P, Pender MP, Lea RA. Variation in the vitamin D receptor gene is associated with multiple sclerosis in an Australian population. J Neurogenet. 2005; 19(1):25–38. PMID: 16076630

[108] Morrison NA, Qi JC, Tokita A, Kelly PJ, Crofts L, Nguyen TV, Sambrook PN, Eisman JA. Prediction of bone density from vitamin D receptor alleles.Nature. 1994; 367(6460): 284–7. PMID: 8161378

[109] Fukazawa T, Yabe I, Kikuchi S, Sasaki H, Hamada T, Miyasaka K, Tashiro K. Association of vitamin D receptor gene polymorphism with multiple sclerosis in Japanese. J Neurol Sci. 1999; 166(1):47–52. PMID: 10465499

[110] Niino M, Fukazawa T, Yabe I, Kikuchi S, Sasaki H, Tashiro K. Vitamin D receptor gene polymorphism in multiple sclerosis and the association with HLA class II alleles. J Neurol Sci. 2000; 177(1):65–71. PMID: 10967184

[111] Partridge JM, Weatherby SJ, Woolmore JA, Highland DJ, Fryer AA, Mann CL, Boggild MD, Ollier WE, Strange RC, Hawkins CP. Susceptibility and outcome in MS: associations with polymorphisms in pigmentation-related genes. Neurology. 2004; 62(12): 2323–5. PMID: 15210908

[112] Cox MB, Ban M, Bowden NA, Baker A, Scott RJ, Lechner-Scott J. Potential association of vitamin D receptor polymorphism Taq1 with multiple sclerosis. MultScler. 2012; 18(1):16–22. doi: 10.1177/1352458511415562

[113] Steckley JL, Dyment DA, Sadovnick AD, Risch N, Hayes C, Ebers GC. Genetic analysis of vitamin D related genes in Canadian multiple sclerosis patients. Canadian Collaborative Study Group.Neurology. 2000; 54(3):729–32. PMID: 10680811

[114] Smolders J, Damoiseaux J, Menheere P, Tervaert JW, Hupperts R. Association study on two vitamin D receptor gene polymorphisms and vitamin D metabolites in multiple sclerosis. Ann N Y Acad Sci. 2009; 1173:515–20. doi: 10.1111/j.1749-6632.2009.04656.x

[115] Sioka C, Papakonstantinou S, Markoula S, Gkartziou F, Georgiou A, Georgiou I, Pelidou SH, Kyritsis AP, Fotopoulos A.Vitamin D receptor gene polymorphisms in

multiple sclerosis patients in northwest Greece. J Negat Results Biomed.2011; 10:3.doi: 10.1186/1477-5751-10-3

[116] Irizar H, Muñoz-Culla M, Zuriarrain O, Goyenechea E, Castillo-Triviño T, Prada A, Saenz-Cuesta M, De Juan D, Lopez de Munain A, Olascoaga J, Otaegui D. HLA-DRB1*15:01 and multiple sclerosis: a female association? MultScler. 2012; 18(5):569–77. doi: 10.1177/1352458511426813

[117] García-Martín E, Agúndez J. A. G., Martínez C, Benito-León J, Millán-Pascual J, Calleja P, Díaz-Sánchez M, Pisa D, Turpín-Fenoll L, Alonso-Navarro H, Ayuso-Peralta L, Torrecillas D, Plaza-Nieto JF, Jiménez-Jiménez FJ. Vitamin D3 Receptor (VDR) Gene rs2228570 (Fok1) and rs731236 (Taq1) variants are not associated with the risk for multiple sclerosis: results of a new study and a meta-analysis. PLoS One. 2013; 8(6): e65487. doi: 10.1371/journal.pone.0065487

[118] Dickinson JL, Perera DI, van der Mei AF, Ponsonby AL, Polanowski AM, Thomson RJ, Taylor BV, McKay JD, Stankovich J, Dwyer T. Past environmental sun exposure and risk of multiple sclerosis: a role for the Cdx-2 vitamin D receptor variant in this interaction. MultScler. 2009; 5(5):563–70. doi: 10.1177/1352458509102459

[119] Niksresht AR, Dadkhah B, KamaliSarverstani E. The association of vitamin D receptor gene BsmIpolymorphism with multiple sclerosis in Iranian patients.J Kerman Univ MedSci Health Serv. 2009; 16(2):116–23. doi: http://jkmu.kmu.ac.ir/en/index.php/kmus/article/view/245

[120] Agliardi C, Guerini FR, Saresella M, Caputo D, Leone MA, Zanzottera M, Bolognesi E, Marventano I, Barizzone N, Fasano ME, Al-Daghri N, Clerici M. Vitamin D receptor (VDR) gene SNPs influence VDR expression and modulate protection from multiple sclerosis in HLA-DRB1*15-positive individuals. Brain Behav Immun. 2011; 25(7):1460–7. doi: 10.1016/j.bbi.2011.05.015

Chapter 2

The Gateway Reflex, a Novel Neuro-immune Interaction, is Critical for the Development of Mouse Multiple Sclerosis (MS) Models

Daisuke Kamimura, Yasunobu Arima,
Andrea Stofkova, Naoki Nishikawa, Kotaro Higuchi,
Takuto Ohki and Masaaki Murakami

Additional information is available at the end of the chapter

http://dx.doi.org/10.5772/62938

Abstract

The central nervous system (CNS) is an immune-privileged tissue protected by the brain–blood barrier (BBB), which limits the absorption of substances and cells from blood flow. In the case of inflammatory diseases in the CNS, such as multiple sclerosis (MS), however, autoreactive T cells that attack brain autoantigens, including myelin proteins, circumvent the BBB. Despite the wide distribution of brain autoantigens, demyelination often occurs as discrete foci. This fact suggests that there might be a certain cue that guides autoreactive T cells to particular site(s) in the CNS. In other words, there exists a mechanism that facilitates a site-specific accumulation of autoreactive T cells in the CNS. Using a murine model of MS, experimental autoimmune encephalomyelitis (EAE), we identified dorsal vessels of the fifth lumbar (L5) spinal cord as the initial entry site of immune cells. The formation of a gateway for immune cells is defined by local neural stimulations. For example, neural stimulation by gravity creates this gateway by increasing the expression of chemokines that attract autoreactive T cells. Regional neural activation by the other stimuli, such as electric pulses or pain sensation, also induces gateway formation, but at different blood vessels via chemokine expression. These neuro-immune interactions are examples of the gateway reflex and are extensively reviewed in this chapter.

Keywords: gateway reflex, inflammation amplifier, NF-κB, STAT, multiple sclerosis

1. Introduction

Multiple sclerosis (MS) is a common neurological disease that is estimated to inflict more than 2.5 million patients worldwide [1–4]. MS is associated with chronic inflammation of the central nervous system (CNS) with myelin antigens as the immune target during the inflammation processes. The clinical manifestations of MS are variable and often include both symptoms of upper motor neurons, such as hyperreflexia, ataxia, spasticity, and visual defects, and lower motor neuron symptoms, such as sensory neuron defects and paralysis [5]. Given the uniform presence of myelin antigens in the CNS, however, variable local, rather than systemic clinical symptoms raise the possibility that there exists specific sites in the CNS that are vulnerable to immune cells thus triggering auto-reactivity. As discussed below, we observed using a murine model of MS, experimental autoimmune encephalomyelitis (EAE), that regional neural stimulations permit entry of immune cells into the CNS, which may explain the variable MS symptoms among patients.

Genetic susceptibility of MS is well studied, and major histocompatibility complex (MHC) genes and genes associated with CD4+ helper T-cell activation and homeostasis are identified as susceptible genes. The strongest genetic linkage was found at certain alleles of MHC class II, which suggests a relationship between autoreactive CD4+ T cells and MS development in humans [6]. Consistently, autoreactive CD4+ T cells have important roles in the development and relapse of animal models of MS [4, 7–13]. In addition to MHC genes, several genome-wide association studies (GWAS) of MS patients have identified additional genetic loci including interleukin (IL)-17, IL-2 receptor (CD25), and IL-7 receptor (CD127), which are important for CD4+ T-cell effector function, activation, and survival [14–16]. These lines of genetic evidence suggest that blocking CD4+ T-cell entry into the CNS, thereby blocking subsequent inflammation in the CNS, would be an effective way for the treatment of MS. Indeed, drugs that target T-cell migration such as fingolimod (FTY720) and natalizumab (anti-VLA4 antibody) have shown clinical success in the treatment of MS. Fingolimod is an orally available sphingosine-1-phosphate receptor modulator, which reduces CD4+ T-cell invasion to the CNS due to the inhibition of lymphocyte egress from lymph nodes [17]. Natalizumab, on the other hand, targets alpha4 integrin (a subunit of VLA4), which is required for the migration of CD4+ T cells to inflamed CNS [4, 18]. The prominent clinical effects of these drugs provide a proof of concept for therapeutic strategies to suppress the invasion of autoreactive CD4+ T cells into the CNS. Because side effects such as progressive multifocal leukoencephalopathy warrant caution for the use of fingolimod and natalizumab [19, 20], a novel strategy including a blockade of the entry site, or gateway, of immune cells to the CNS is desired.

It is widely known that the CNS is an immune-privileged site, protected by the blood–brain barrier (BBB), which restricts the exchange of substances and cell migration into and out of the organ. However, CNS invasion by immune cells occurs in not only neuropathologic conditions including MS, but also normal healthy conditions. We have been studying where and how immune cells can enter the CNS using EAE models. In this chapter, our

http://dx.doi.org/10.5772/62938

recent findings about these gateways, a mechanism to operate them, and perspectives are discussed.

2. Blood–brain barrier and inflammation

The BBB is a specialized blood vessel formed by several cell types including vascular endothelial cells, pericytes, and astrocyte endfeet. In addition, tight junctions are critical for barrier development and are established through interactions of tight junction molecules, such as ZO-1, claudins, and occludins, between the vascular endothelial cells to cause a size exclusion of about 500 daltons [21, 22]. Despite this rigid barrier system, autoreactive T cells can enter to the CNS and cause autoimmune diseases such as MS. The breakdown of the BBB is also observed in neurodegenerative disorders such as Alzheimer's disease and Parkinson's disease [23]. Because neuroinflammation is associated with almost all diseases in the CNS [24], the relationship between a dysfunctional BBB and inflammatory cytokines has been well studied. For example, TNFαincreases BBB permeability during sepsis, and IL-1β regulates the BBB via reactivation of the HIF-VEGF axis in MS [25, 26]. IFNγ and TNFα decrease the expression of TWIK-related potassium channel-1 in human brain microvascular endothelial cells, which leads to increase the transmigration of various immune cells across the endothelial cells in vitro [27]. IL-17A, which is a signature cytokine of Th17 cells, also contributes to BBB leakage in vitro and in vivo. EAE was significantly suppressed in IL-17A-deficient mice [28], and IL-17A-deficient CD4+ T cells hardly invade the CNS through the fifth lumbar (L5) spinal cord unlike normal ones [12]. IL-17A-mediated BBB dysfunction involves the formation of reactive oxygen species by cellular oxidases, which down-regulate tight junction molecules and the activation of the endothelial contractile machinery in vitro [29, 30]. Seeing that GWAS and animal model data have revealed that autoreactive CD4+ T cells producing many cytokines play a central role in MS, understanding the in vivo behavior of disease-causing CD4+ T cells offers crucial insights about the pathophysiology of MS. Intravital two-photon imaging using a rat transfer EAE model showed that there are at least three stages for CNS invasion by autoreactive CD4+ T cells: intraluminal scanning, perivascular scanning, and CNS-surface scanning [31]. This study also suggested that the reactivation of CNS-invading CD4+ T cells by perivascular/meningeal antigen-presenting cells is followed by parenchymal infiltration of pathogenic CD4+ T cells [31]. Chemokine guidance and cellular adhesion events of pathogenic CD4+ T cells are also critical for the CNS invasion [12, 31]. Myelin autoantigen candidates associated with MS including Myelin Basic Protein (MBP), myelin-oligodendrocyte protein (MOG) and proteolipid proteins (PLP) [32–35] are present throughout CNS white matter, while MS lesions are often observed by MRI as focal plaques [36]. These facts suggest that there exists an additional signal that directs pathogenic CD4+ T cells to initiate inflammatory reactions at particular region(s) of the CNS. We recently demonstrated that this signal is provided by several types of neural activations. We also defined a molecular mechanism of the resulting neuro-immune interactions for the development and relapse of murine models of MS, as discussed in the following sections.

3. Gravity-mediated gateway reflex

We first considered the initial site where the autoreactive CD4+ T cells invade the CNS. In EAE models, mice or rats are generally immunized with various CNS antigens such as myelin-oligodendrocyte protein (MOG) emulsified with complete Freund's adjuvant (CFA) in the presence of pertussis toxin administration, which are critical for the generation of autoreactive CD4+ T cells and the induction of MS-like symptoms, including a progressive paralysis that usually begins at the tip of the tail. EAE can also be induced in wild-type animals by the transfer of autoreactive CD4+ T cells isolated from other EAE mice. This transfer EAE model is induced without antigens, CFA, or pertussis toxin treatment, making this model suitable for investigating the behavior of the disease-causing CD4+ T cells in detail. Whole-mount sagittal sections of adult mice at a preclinical stage of the transfer EAE model (day 4 or 5 after MOG-reactive CD4+ T-cell transfer) revealed that MOG-reactive pathogenic CD4+ T cells preferentially accumulated at the L5 spinal cord, but not in the brain at this early stage. This observation suitably explains the first clinical symptom of typical EAE, a weakness of the tail tip. A closer analysis of the L5 spinal cord revealed that the accumulation of MOG-reactive CD4+ T cells occurred around the dorsal vessels. Various chemokines including Th17-attracting CCL20 were up-regulated at the L5 dorsal vessels during EAE compared with dorsal vessels from other spinal cords. Indeed, anti-CCL20 antibody treatment or transfer of MOG-reactive CD4+ T cells lacking its receptor, CCR6, compromised the L5 accumulation of these CD4+ T cells and subsequent development of EAE, which is consistent with a published study [37]. Interestingly, the selective up-regulation of chemokines at the L5 dorsal vessels was observed even at steady state, albeit to a lesser degree than in the EAE condition. These results suggested that the L5 dorsal vessels are the first gateway for pathogenic CD4+ T cells in this transfer EAE system (**Figure 1**), and some physiological effects under steady state that modulate chemokine levels at the L5 dorsal vessels are enhanced during EAE.

Further investigation revealed that the selective up-regulation of chemokines at the L5 dorsal vessels at steady state were the result of neuro-immune interactions. It is known that neurons in the dorsal root ganglion (DRG) beside the L5 spinal cord are connected to the soleus muscles, the main anti-gravity muscles [38]. Consistent with a constant stimulation of the soleus muscles by Earth's gravity, the L5 DRG is the largest among all DRGs in mice and humans [39]. We hypothesized that constant stimulation by gravity might mediate the uniqueness of the L5 spinal cord in establishing the gateway of immune cells including autoreactive CD4+ T cells. Consistent with this hypothesis, we found two peaks of CCL20 expression at the dorsal vessels of the cervical and lumbar cords, although CCL20 expression was higher at the latter. To examine the effect of gravity, mice were suspended by their tails so that their hind legs were released from gravity. This treatment resulted in a reduced accumulation of MOG-specific CD4+ T cells at the L5 cord. Instead, these CD4+ T cells invaded the cervical cords as if a new gateway was created by the additional gravitational burden on the forefeet muscles due to the tail suspension [12]. Consistently, the tail suspension downregulated CCL20 levels in the L5 dorsal blood vessels, but up-regulated CCL20 in the cervical cords. Moreover, electric stimulations to the soleus muscles in tail-suspended mice restored CCL20 levels and CD4+ T-cell

http://dx.doi.org/10.5772/62938

accumulation at the L5 spinal cord [12]. These results suggest that a certain neural activation triggered by gravity contributes to the gateway at the L5 dorsal blood vessels for autoreactive CD4+ T cells to infiltrate the CNS (**Figure 1**).

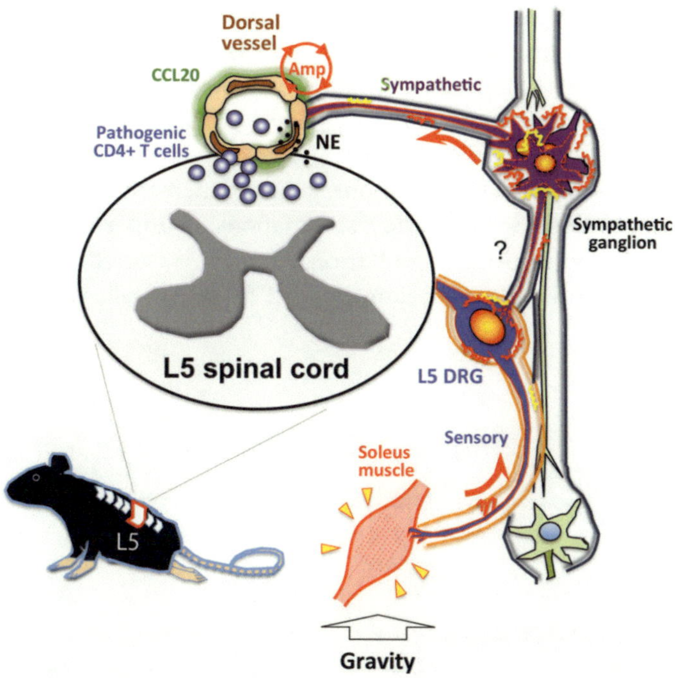

Figure 1. Gravity-mediated gateway reflex. Constant gravity-mediated stimulation of the soleus muscles induces the activation of sensory nerves, whose cell bodies are located at the dorsal root ganglion (DRG) of the fifth lumbar (L5) spinal cord. Signals via L5 DRG neurons travel to sympathetic neurons located nearby, resulting in norepinephrine (NE) secretion at the dorsal vessels there. NE enhances the inflammation amplifier (Amp) in the L5 dorsal vessel endothelium, causing an up-regulation of CCL20 and subsequent accumulation of pathogenic CD4+ T cells.

Sympathetic nerve activation was involved in the gravity-mediated chemokine expressions at the L5 dorsal vessels. c-Fos expression, which is a marker of neural activation, was higher in L5 sympathetic ganglions than in L1 sympathetic ganglions. Blood flow speeds at the L5 dorsal vessels, but not at other blood vessels including L1 dorsal vessels, femoral artery, and portal vein, became slower when mice were tail suspended, while electronic stimulation of the soleus muscles increased the flow speed, suggesting an involvement of autonomic nerves including sympathetic ones in this response [12]. Furthermore, pharmacological blockade of adrenergic receptors significantly inhibited CCL20 levels, NF-κB activation and MOG-reactive pathogenic CD4+ T-cell accumulation at the L5 dorsal vessels, and also suppressed clinical signs of EAE [12]. Thus, sensory nerve activation due to anti-gravity responses leads to a sympathetic nerve stimulation that creates a gateway for immune cells to pass through the CNS via the L5 dorsal vessels [12]. This neuro-immune response, which leads to change in the status of the vascular endothelium, is named the "gateway reflex" [40–42]. Other examples of the gateway reflex are described below.

4. Electric stimulation-mediated gateway reflex

Neural activations can be artificially induced by various methods including electric stimulations and treatment with reagents. We wondered if electric stimulation of different muscles could create gateways in blood vessels at distinct positions via regional neural activations. As discussed earlier, weak electric stimulation to the soleus muscles restored chemokine expression at the L5 dorsal vessels of tail-suspended mice, because the cell body of sensory neurons in the soleus muscles is mainly located in the L5 DRG. We applied this methodology to other muscles. As expected, electric stimulations to thigh muscles including the quadriceps, which are known to be regulated by L3 DRG neurons, led to an increased expression of chemokines in L3 dorsal vessels in mice, while electric stimulations of upper regions, such as forefoot muscles including the epitrochlearis and triceps brachii, resulted in an up-regulation of chemokines in the fifth cervical to fifth thoracic cord dorsal vessels, which is where the DRG

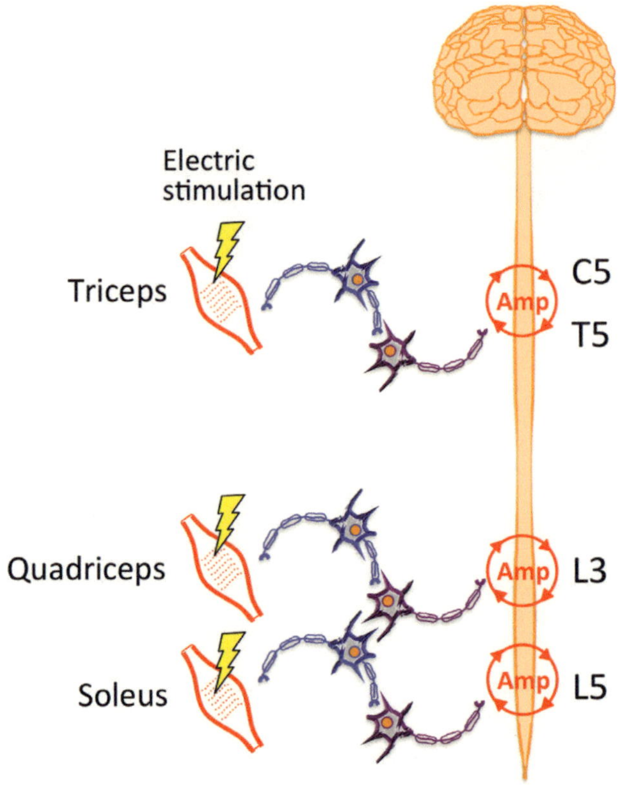

Figure 2. Electric stimulation-mediated gateway reflex. Artificially induced neural activation by weak electric stimulation followed by sensory-sympathetic cross talk can trigger the gateway reflex. Electric pulses to the triceps induce chemokine up-regulation at the dorsal vessels of the fifth cervical (C5) to fifth thoracic (T5) spinal cord through activation of the inflammation amplifier (Amp). Similarly, stimulation of the quadriceps induces a gateway at the dorsal vessels of the third lumbar (L3) cord, whereas the gateway dorsal vessels of the L5 cord are created by electric pulses to the soleus muscles.

neurons of the C5-T5 spinal cords project to/from these muscles. These results established the electric stimulation-mediated gateway as another example of the gateway reflex (**Figure 2**). In addition, they offer an important implication that the gateway reflex can be controlled by artificially stimulating specific neurons, providing a promising opportunity for a novel therapeutic strategy against inflammatory diseases in the CNS.

5. Pain-mediated gateway reflex

It is reported that many MS patients experience pain, and some patients take pain relief medication to improve their quality of life [43]. Pain is a common symptom in many diseases and disorders, but it is often considered a symptomatic effect that arises from tissue damage caused by the disease. However, it is known that pain triggers neural inputs via sensory neurons expressing nociceptors such as TRPV1 [44, 45]. Therefore, we assumed that a pain-mediated gateway reflex might exist, which would affect the disease status of MS and EAE. In EAE, modulations of nociception (pain sensation) are reported during the disease development [46]. Adoptive transfer of MOG reactive, pathogenic CD4+ T cells induces a transient EAE within a week after transfer, followed by a remission phase. Mice that experienced the first episode of EAE and are in the remission phase, which we termed EAE-recovered mice, never develop EAE symptoms again under normal conditions. We experimentally induced pain sensation in these EAE-recovered mice by ligating the middle branch of the trigeminal nerves, which has been reported as being composed of only sensory neurons [47]. Pain induction at the time of pathogenic T-cell transfer resulted in a persistence of EAE symptoms and caused considerable delay of the remission phase. On the contrary, suppressing pain by medication inhibited EAE development in several mouse models including an active immunization model in SJL mice. Because a majority of MS progresses with relapse and it is reported that pain is more intense in MS patients with higher disease scores [48], we examined whether pain induction triggers EAE relapse in mice. EAE-recovered mice were subjected to trigeminal nerve ligation to induce pain sensation. In separate experiments, pain-processing nerves were also chemically activated by the injection of capsaicin and substance P at the cheek or forefeet of EAE-recovered mice. All these treatments induced relapse of EAE, indicating that pain is not a simple by-product of the disease, but significantly contributes to the development and EAE relapse [13]. Similar to the gravity-mediated gateway reflex, a sensory-sympathetic pathway is involved in the pain-mediated EAE relapse, because pharmacological or genetic inhibition of pain-processing molecules such as TRPV1 and Nav1.8, and chemical ablation of sympathetic neurons by 6-hydroxydopamine (6-OHDA) suppressed EAE relapse induced by trigeminal nerve ligation. Interestingly, stress-mediated events, including immobilization stress and forced swimming stress (about 20 minutes/day), did not trigger EAE relapse although serum corticosterone, norepinephrine, and epinephrine were induced at a similar level to pain induction, suggesting that specific sensory-sympathetic nerve pathways, rather than systemic hormonal stress responses, mediate the relapse of EAE (**Figure 3**).

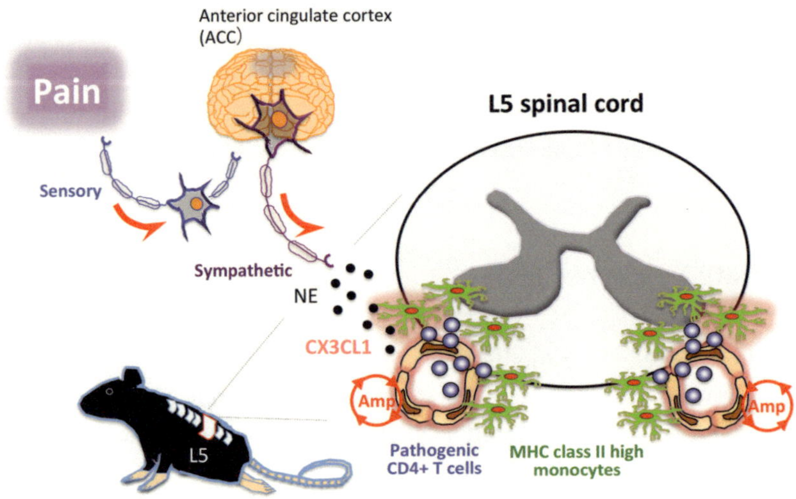

Figure 3. Pain-mediated gateway reflex. Pain-induced sensory neuron activation results in the activation of specific sympathetic neurons that control norepinephrine (NE) expression around the ventral vessels of every level of the spinal cords. This system is regulated by the anterior cinculate cortex (ACC) in the brain. Because the fifth lumbar (L5) spinal cord abundantly contains MHC class II high activated monocytes, this region is affected significantly during pain sensation. NE from pain-specific sympathetic neurons at the ventral vessels induces the production of CX3CL1 from the activated monocytes, further recruiting these cells in an auto/paracrine manner. The MHC class II high activated monocytes are able to present MOG antigens to pathogenic CD4+ T cells, which in turn activate the inflammation amplifier (Amp) in regional endothelial cells and subsequently cause a relapse in the disease.

During the first episode of EAE, MOG-reactive CD4+ T cells enter the CNS from the dorsal vessels of the L5 spinal cord [12]. The transferred CD4+ T cells are then found at the upper levels of the spinal cord and brain, which matches typical clinical manifestations of EAE including the initial tail tip weakness and subsequent ascending paralysis. Intriguingly, after pain induction in apparently normal EAE-recovered mice, the relapse also starts from the loss of tonicity of the tail tip, suggesting that the L5 cord could again be a gateway for relapse. However, an immunohistochemical examination of the L5 spinal cord from EAE-recovered mice showed differences with naïve mice, with many MHC class II high monocytes around the meningeal region. After pain induction, these cells accumulated at the L5 ventral vessels, but not dorsal vessels within a day. This accumulation is dependent on a chemokine CX3CL1, which is secreted from the MHC class II high monocytes themselves and astrocytes after norepinephrine stimulation. Therefore, the pain-mediated gateway reflex induces norepinephrine secretion from sympathetic neurons around the L5 ventral vessels and subsequent auto/paracrine induction of CX3CL1 followed by MHC class II high monocyte accumulations. Because these monocytes are able to present MOG peptides, circulating MOG-reactive pathogenic CD4+ T cells can recognize the L5 ventral vessels as an entry site to the CNS. Indeed, a depletion of CD4+ T cells including pathogenic ones from EAE-recovered mice abrogated the clinical symptoms of EAE relapse (i.e. paralysis), but the accumulation of MHC class II high monocytes around the L5 ventral vessels remained intact. These results suggested that the activated monocyte accumulation is an upstream event relative to pathogenic CD4+ T-cell invasion and required for EAE relapse induced by pain sensation [13].

The sympathetic nerve activation caused by pain appeared to be relatively systemic compared with that via the sensory pathway, since the expression levels of neural activation marker c-Fos increased in certain nerve cells in sympathetic ganglions at all spinal levels investigated, which is in contrast to the gravity-mediated gateway reflex in which the L5 sympathetic ganglion alone showed the highest expression of c-Fos. However, the pain-mediated gateway reflex affects blood vessels at the ventral sides of the L5 spinal cord. Why does the pain-mediated gateway reflex influence the L5 level alone, similar to the gravity-mediated gateway reflex? We assume that this property is related to the fact that the L5 cord is the first lesion in the transfer EAE model. Even at the remission phase of transfer EAE, MHC class II high monocytes that have infiltrated in the CNS during the initial episode remained mostly in the L5 spinal cord despite the disappearance of clinical symptoms [13]. Otherwise, gravity-mediated neural inputs might make the L5 environment different from other CNS regions. Whichever the explanation, we found that pain induction similarly triggers sympathetic neural activation to some neuron cells of every spinal level, but the L5 spinal cord responded strongest, most likely due to an abundance of activated monocytes.

It is known that pain-sensing neurons activate sympathetic neurons at least partially via the anterior cingulate cortex (ACC) in the somatosensory area of the brain [49, 50]. Blockade of this sensory-sympathetic connection by the injection of an N-methyl-D-aspartate (NMDA) receptor antagonist at the ACC suppressed the accumulation of MHC class II high monocytes at the L5 ventral vessels even after pain induction, and conversely, injection of an NMDA agonist at the ACC induced the accumulation of these cells without pain stimulation in EAE-recovered mice. These results clearly suggest that the sensory-sympathetic connection at the ACC is involved in pain-mediated EAE relapse. Thus, we showed a third pain-mediated gateway reflex where neural signals travel from a TRPV1 and Nav1.8-dependent sensory circuit to sympathetic neurons via the ACC, reaching the dorsal vessels of the spinal cords [13] (**Figure 3**).

The study of the pain-mediated gateway reflex also highlights the importance of MHC class II high monocytes for EAE relapse. Parabiosis experiments, in which two different congenically marked mice are joined together surgically to share blood circulation, revealed that MHC class II high monocytes that accumulated at the L5 ventral vessels were derived from the peripheral blood stream during the first EAE development and stayed in the CNS, but not from resident microglia in the CNS [13]. These infiltrated MHC class II high monocytes survive in the CNS during the remission phase and play a pathogenic role upon relapse when the mice have a pain sensation. Therefore, in addition to controlling neural pathways and/or molecular machinery of the gateway reflexes, MHC class II high monocytes could also be a potential cellular target for treatment of relapse-remitting MS and progressive-relapsing MS.

6. Other gateway reflexes

In addition to the sensory perceptions described above, including gravity-, electric stimulation-, and pain-mediated stimuli, neural excitations occur in response to emotional alterations and physical/mental stresses. These physiological events too are often associated with MS symptoms [51]. Worsening of the clinical symptoms of neurological diseases including MS when the body is exposed to high ambient temperatures, called Uhthoff's phenomenon, is another well-known example [52]. It is also known that stress burdens are associated with activation of the sympathetic nervous system, such as increased noradrenaline levels in the peripheral blood. Despite these correlations, a mechanical link between stress and disease development remains elusive. Neuronal activations, noradrenaline surge, and disease development are fundamental of the gateway reflex. Stress-induced neural signals traveling to the CNS might modulate specific blood vessels depending on stress type, opening or closing a gateway for immune cells in the CNS. To examine this possibility, we have been testing the effects of various stresses on the pathogenesis of EAE. Although restraint stress and forced swim stress did not provoke EAE relapse [13], some stresses were found to worsen the clinical symptoms, whereas another stress prevented EAE development. These phenomena represent the fourth and fifth examples of the gateway reflex. The effects of good stress, or eustress, have also been reported in cancer models, in which tumor growth is delayed when mice are reared under an enriched environment with running wheels, tunnels, etc. in a larger cage [53, 54]. We suggest it may be possible to prevent diseases if stimulating the appropriate neurons can trigger a good gateway reflex.

Kevin Tracey and his colleagues have reported that activation of the vagus nerves, which mainly consist of parasympathetic nerves, leads to the suppression of systemic inflammation during septic shock in mice. This neural reflex is specifically called the "inflammatory reflex." In this context, lipopolysaccharide treatment in mice leads to norepinephrine release in the spleen via vagus and splenic nerves. A subset of T cells that receive norepinephrine signaling produces acetylcholine, which acts on macrophages to suppress the lipopolysaccharide-induced expression of inflammatory mediators such as TNFα [55], thus acting as a negative feedback system for excessive inflammatory reactions such as septic shock. It is also reported that electro-acupuncture in mice at the ST36 Zusanli acupoint, which is located close to the common peroneal and tibial branches of the sciatic nerve, or directly to the sciatic nerve prevents a sepsis model through vagal activation and dopamine production [56]. A similar strategy may generate the gateway reflex in humans.

7. Inflammation amplifier

As described above, regional sensory neural activations transmit neural signals to sympathetic neurons, which then secrete norepinephrine at the target blood vessels to establish a gateway and recruit immune cells. Because chemokines have a critical role in immune cell recruitment, we hypothesized that machinery responsible for the production of chemokines could act as an interface between neural signals and immune reactions. Indeed, we discovered the inflammation amplifier, which is a local chemokine inducer. In this section, we describe the inflammation amplifier as a molecular mechanism for neuro-immune interactions in blood vessels.

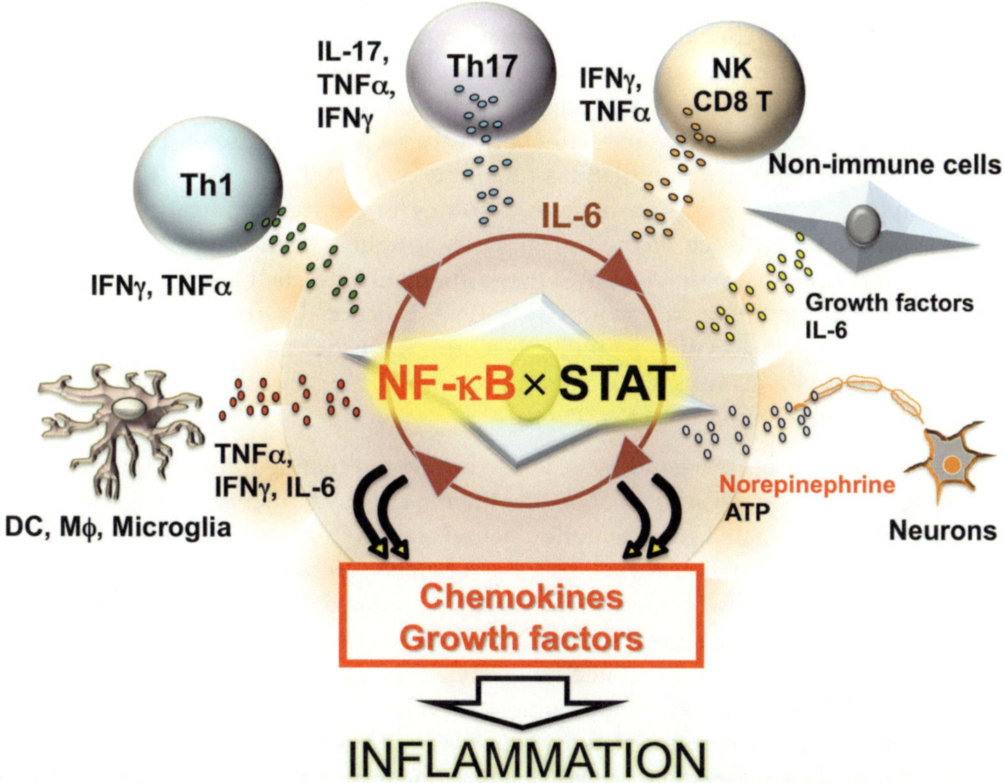

Figure 4. Inflammation amplifier. Simultaneous activation of the transcription factors NF-κB and STATs creates a synergistic effect on the production of inflammation mediators, such as chemokines, growth factors, and IL-6, in nonimmune cells, such as vascular endothelial cells and fibroblasts. Factors activating NF-κB and STATs are various and include IL-6, TNFα, and IL-17. IL-6 is expected to act on nonimmune cells to form a positive feedback loop that amplifies this synergistic effect. Massive chemokine and growth factor production by this mechanism, called the inflammation amplifier, plays a central role in the pathogenesis of many inflammatory diseases and disorders.

To establish an IL-6-dependent autoimmune mouse model, we previously generated a knock-in mouse strain called F759 mice, which lacks the SOCS3 binding site of the IL-6 signal transducer, gp130, thereby inhibiting SOCS3-dependent negative signaling and excessive STAT3 activation [57]. Accordingly, F759 mice developed spontaneous rheumatoid arthritis-like joint disease and autoantibody production [58], which is consistent with the high levels of IL-6 and clinical success of its signaling blockade in rheumatoid arthritis patients [59, 60]. Using these autoimmune-prone F759 mice, we performed mechanistic analyses for the pathogenesis of their autoimmunity and found that IL-6 signaling in nonimmune cells, such as vascular endothelial cells and fibroblasts, rather than immune cells, is important for the exaggerated inflammation [61, 62]. Mechanistically, coactivation of the transcription factors NF-κB and STATs in nonimmune cells led to a synergistic production of inflammatory agents, including chemokines and growth factors, compared with NF-κB or STAT activation alone (**Figure 4**). Factors that activate NF-κB and STATs and therefore trigger the inflammation amplifier include IL-17A, TNFα, IL-22, IL-6, and IFNγ. Furthermore, neurotransmitters, including norepinephrine and several growth factors, augment the amplifier by enhancing NF-κB activation [12, 63]. Since chemokines can recruit immune cells and promote inflammation, we named this synergistic mechanism in nonimmune cells the "inflammation amplifier" [64, 65]. Mice lacking gp130 or STAT3 in type 1 collagen+ cells including various nonimmune cells were highly resistant to animal models of rheumatoid arthritis, MS, and chronic graft rejection via suppression of the regional accumulation of immune cells [12, 13, 62, 63, 66, 67]. The inflammation amplifier is also seen in astrocytes, resulting in the development of EAE [68]. In addition, we found evidence of the inflammation amplifier activation in human clinical specimens, and human disease-associated genes are highly enriched in inflammation amplifier-related genes according to genome-wide RNA functional screening [67]. These data suggested that the inflammation amplifier is a critical mechanism for the development of various inflammatory diseases via excessive expression of inflammatory chemokines and growth factors from nonimmune cells (**Figure 4**).

Subsequent studies about the gateway reflex demonstrated that neural signals translate into inflammatory signals by the inflammation amplifier in target vascular endothelial cells. In the case of the gravity-mediated gateway reflex, neural signals from the soleus muscles reached the L5 dorsal vessel endothelium via sensory-sympathetic cross talk, where norepinephrine from the activated sympathetic neurons excessively stimulated the inflammation amplifier by increasing NF-κB activity to secrete various NF-κB-targets including chemokines. Moreover, the L5 but not L1 dorsal vessel endothelium showed activation of STAT3. Pharmacological inhibition of beta-adrenergic receptors suppressed NF-κB activation, chemokine production, and pathogenic CD4+ T-cell accumulation in the L5 dorsal vessels and EAE development [12]. Similarly, during the pain-mediated gateway reflex, treatment with a beta-adrenergic receptor antagonist resulted in no accumulation of activated monocytes or pathogenic CD4+ T cells around the target dorsal vessels of the L5 spinal cord. Neutralization of cytokines that activate the inflammation amplifier such as IL-6 and IL-17A also suppressed the pain-induced EAE relapse and pathogenic CD4+ T-cell accumulation [13]. These results indicate that the inflammation amplifier is a foundation of the immunological response induced by the gateway reflex.

8. Future directions

The CNS is an immune-privileged site protected by the BBB, but the gateway reflex, which can be triggered by various neural stimulations, can induce gateways for immune cells to circumvent the BBB. So far, three kinds of gateway reflex have been identified: gravity, electric stimulation, and pain-induced, all of which involve sensory-sympathetic communication. Further study of the mechanisms driving the gateway reflex should consider the neural network involved and whether it is present in other organs and tissues. Newly developed imaging techniques and tools including a tissue decolorization reagent, CUBIC [69, 70], will help elucidate the former. For the latter, it is recently reported there exists barrier architecture with similar components to the BBB in the gut endothelium, the so-called gut-vascular barrier [22]. A similar system may explain how immune cells breach this barrier. Because neuronal circuits run throughout the body, the gateway reflex could have a tremendous

http://dx.doi.org/10.5772/62938

clinical benefit, as closing a specific gateway would dampen autoimmune inflammation in a target organ without massive systemic immune suppression, while opening it in tumors could enhance cancer immunotherapy.

Acknowledgements

We thank the excellent assistance by Ms. Chiemi Nakayama, Ms. Mitsue Ezawa and Ms. Satomi Fukumoto (Hokkaido University, Sapporo, Japan), and Dr. Peter Karagiannis for reading the manuscript. This work was supported by KAKENHI (D. K., Y. A., T. A., and M. M.), Takeda Science Foundation (M. M. and D. K.), Institute for Fermentation Osaka (M. M.), Mitsubishi Foundation (M. M.), Uehara Memorial Foundation (M. M.), Mochida Memorial Foundation for Medical and Pharmaceutical Research (D. K.), Suzuken Memorial Foundation (D. K. and Y. A.), Japan Prize Foundation (Y. A.), Ono Medical Research Foundation (Y. A.), Kanzawa Medical Research Foundation (Y. A.), Kishimoto Foundation (Y. A.), Nagao Takeshi Research Foundation (Y. A.), Tokyo Medical Research Foundation (M. M. and Y. A.), JSPS Postdoctoral Fellowship for Foreign Researchers (A.S.), JST-CREST program (M. M.), and the Osaka Foundation for the Promotion of Clinical Immunology (M. M.). The authors declare they have no conflicting financial interests.

Author details

Daisuke Kamimura*, Yasunobu Arima, Andrea Stofkova, Naoki Nishikawa, Kotaro Higuchi, Takuto Ohki and Masaaki Murakami

*Address all correspondence to: murakami@igm.hokudai.ac.jp

Molecular Neuroimmunology, Graduate School of Medicine, Institute for Genetic Medicine, Hokkaido University, Sapporo, Hokkaido ,Japan

References

[1] Noseworthy JH, Lucchinetti C, Rodriguez M, Weinshenker BG. Multiple sclerosis. N Engl J Med 2000;343(13):938–952. DOI: 10.1056/NEJM200009283431307

[2] Hafler DA, Slavik JM, Anderson DE, O'Connor KC, De Jager P, Baecher-Allan C. Multiple sclerosis. Immunol Rev 2005;204:208–231. DOI: 10.1111/j.0105-2896.2005.00240.x

[3] McFarland HF, Martin R. Multiple sclerosis: a complicated picture of autoimmunity. Nat Immunol 2007;8(9):913–919. DOI: 10.1038/ni1507

[4] Steinman L. Immunology of relapse and remission in multiple sclerosis. Annu Rev Immunol 2014;32:257–281. DOI: 10.1146/annurev-immunol-032713-120227

[5] Keegan BM, Noseworthy JH. Multiple sclerosis. Ann Rev Med 2002;53:285–302. DOI: 10.1146/annurev.med.53.082901.103909

[6] International Multiple Sclerosis Genetics C, Wellcome Trust Case Control C, Sawcer S, Hellenthal G, Pirinen M, Spencer CC, et al.: Genetic risk and a primary role for cell-mediated immune mechanisms in multiple sclerosis. Nature 2011;476(7359):214–219. DOI: 10.1038/nature10251

[7] Kuchroo VK, Anderson AC, Waldner H, Munder M, Bettelli E, Nicholson LB. T cell response in experimental autoimmune encephalomyelitis (EAE): role of self and cross-reactive antigens in shaping, tuning, and regulating the autopathogenic T cell repertoire. Annu Rev Immunol 2002;20:101–123. DOI: 10.1146/annurev.immunol.20.081701.141316

[8] Sospedra M, Martin R. Immunology of multiple sclerosis. Annu Rev Immunol 2005;23:683–747. DOI: 10.1146/annurev.immunol.23.021704.115707

[9] Steinman L, Zamvil SS. Virtues and pitfalls of EAE for the development of therapies for multiple sclerosis. Trends Immunol 2005;26(11):565–571. DOI: 10.1016/j.it.2005.08.014

[10] Goverman J. Autoimmune T cell responses in the central nervous system. Nat Rev Immunol 2009;9(6):393–407. DOI: 10.1038/nri2550

[11] Rangachari M, Kuchroo VK. Using EAE to better understand principles of immune function and autoimmune pathology. J Autoimmun 2013;45:31–39. DOI: 10.1016/j.jaut.2013.06.008

[12] Arima Y, Harada M, Kamimura D, Park JH, Kawano F, Yull FE, et al.: Regional neural activation defines a gateway for autoreactive T cells to cross the blood–brain barrier. Cell 2012;148(3):447–457. DOI: 10.1016/j.cell.2012.01.022

[13] Arima Y, Kamimura D, Atsumi T, Harada M, Kawamoto T, Nishikawa N, et al.: A pain-mediated neural signal induces relapse in murine autoimmune encephalomyelitis, a multiple sclerosis model. eLife 2015;4. DOI: 10.7554/eLife.08733

[14] Gregory SG, Schmidt S, Seth P, Oksenberg JR, Hart J, Prokop A, et al.: Interleukin 7 receptor alpha chain (IL7R) shows allelic and functional association with multiple sclerosis. Nat Genet 2007;39(9):1083–1091. DOI: 10.1038/ng2103

[15] Lundmark F, Duvefelt K, Iacobaeus E, Kockum I, Wallstrom E, Khademi M, et al.: Variation in interleukin 7 receptor alpha chain (IL7R) influences risk of multiple sclerosis. Nat Genet 2007;39(9):1108–1113. DOI: 10.1038/ng2106

[16] Australia, New Zealand Multiple Sclerosis Genetics C. Genome-wide association study identifies new multiple sclerosis susceptibility loci on chromosomes 12 and 20. Nat Genet 2009;41(7):824–828. 10.1038/ng.396

[17] Cohen JA, Barkhof F, Comi G, Hartung HP, Khatri BO, Montalban X, et al.: Oral fingolimod or intramuscular interferon for relapsing multiple sclerosis. N Engl J Med 2010;362(5):402–415. DOI: 10.1056/NEJMoa0907839

[18] Steinman L. Blocking adhesion molecules as therapy for multiple sclerosis: natalizumab. Nat Reviews Drug Discov 2005;4(6):510–518. DOI: 10.1038/nrd1752

[19] Bloomgren G, Richman S, Hotermans C, Subramanyam M, Goelz S, Natarajan A, et al.: Risk of natalizumab-associated progressive multifocal leukoencephalopathy. N Engl J Med 2012;366(20):1870–1880. DOI: 10.1056/NEJMoa1107829

[20] Van Schependom J, Gielen J, Laton J, Nagels G. Assessing PML risk under immunotherapy: if all you have is a hammer, everything looks like a nail. Mult Scler 2015. DOI: 10.1177/1352458515596458

[21] Steed E, Balda MS, Matter K. Dynamics and functions of tight junctions. Trends Cell Biol 2010;20(3):142–149. DOI: 10.1016/j.tcb.2009.12.002.

[22] Spadoni I, Zagato E, Bertocchi A, Paolinelli R, Hot E, Di Sabatino A, et al.: A gut-vascular barrier controls the systemic dissemination of bacteria. Science 2015;350(6262):830–834. DOI: 10.1126/science.aad0135

[23] Zlokovic BV. The blood–brain barrier in health and chronic neurodegenerative disorders. Neuron 2008;57(2):178–201. DOI: 10.1016/j.neuron.2008.01.003.

[24] Wyss-Coray T, Mucke L. Inflammation in neurodegenerative disease--a double-edged sword. Neuron 2002;35(3):419–432.

[25] Tsao N, Hsu HP, Wu CM, Liu CC, Lei HY. Tumour necrosis factor-alpha causes an increase in blood–brain barrier permeability during sepsis. J Med Microbiol 2001;50(9): 812–821.

[26] Argaw AT, Zhang Y, Snyder BJ, Zhao ML, Kopp N, Lee SC, et al.: IL-1beta regulates blood–brain barrier permeability via reactivation of the hypoxia-angiogenesis program. J Immunol 2006;177(8):5574–5584.

[27] Bittner S, Ruck T, Schuhmann MK, Herrmann AM, Moha ou Maati H, Bobak N, et al.: Endothelial TWIK-related potassium channel-1 (TREK1) regulates immune-cell trafficking into the CNS. Nat Med 2013;19(9):1161–1165. DOI: 10.1038/nm.3303

[28] Komiyama Y, Nakae S, Matsuki T, Nambu A, Ishigame H, Kakuta S, et al.: IL-17 plays an important role in the development of experimental autoimmune encephalomyelitis. J Immunol 2006;177(1):566–573.

[29] Huppert J, Closhen D, Croxford A, White R, Kulig P, Pietrowski E, et al.: Cellular mechanisms of IL-17-induced blood–brain barrier disruption. FASEB J 2010;24(4):1023–1034. DOI: 10.1096/fj.09-141978

[30] Kebir H, Kreymborg K, Ifergan I, Dodelet-Devillers A, Cayrol R, Bernard M, et al.: Human TH17 lymphocytes promote blood–brain barrier disruption and central nervous system inflammation. Nat Med 2007;13(10):1173–1175. nm1651 [pii] 10.1038/nm1651

[31] Bartholomaus I, Kawakami N, Odoardi F, Schlager C, Miljkovic D, Ellwart JW, et al.: Effector T cell interactions with meningeal vascular structures in nascent autoimmune CNS lesions. Nature 2009;462(7269):94–98. DOI: 10.1038/nature08478

[32] Ota K, Matsui M, Milford EL, Mackin GA, Weiner HL, Hafler DA. T-cell recognition of an immunodominant myelin basic protein epitope in multiple sclerosis. Nature 1990;346(6280):183–187. DOI: 10.1038/346183a0

[33] Allegretta M, Nicklas JA, Sriram S, Albertini RJ. T cells responsive to myelin basic protein in patients with multiple sclerosis. Science 1990;247(4943):718–721.

[34] Zhang J, Markovic-Plese S, Lacet B, Raus J, Weiner HL, Hafler DA. Increased frequency of interleukin 2-responsive T cells specific for myelin basic protein and proteolipid protein in peripheral blood and cerebrospinal fluid of patients with multiple sclerosis. J Exp Med 1994;179(3):973–984.

[35] Reindl M, Di Pauli F, Rostasy K, Berger T. The spectrum of MOG autoantibody-associated demyelinating diseases. Nat Reviews Neurol 2013;9(8):455–461. DOI: 10.1038/nrneurol.2013.118

[36] Polman CH, Reingold SC, Banwell B, Clanet M, Cohen JA, Filippi M, et al.: Diagnostic criteria for multiple sclerosis: 2010 revisions to the McDonald criteria. Ann Neurol 2011;69(2):292–302. DOI: 10.1002/ana.22366

[37] Reboldi A, Coisne C, Baumjohann D, Benvenuto F, Bottinelli D, Lira S, et al.: C-C chemokine receptor 6-regulated entry of TH-17 cells into the CNS through the choroid plexus is required for the initiation of EAE. Nat Immunol 2009;10(5):514–523. DOI: 10.1038/ni.1716

[38] Ohira Y, Kawano F, Stevens JL, Wang XD, Ishihara A. Load-dependent regulation of neuromuscular system. J Gravit Physiol 2004;11(2):P127-128.

[39] Shen J, Wang HY, Chen JY, Liang BL. Morphologic analysis of normal human lumbar dorsal root ganglion by 3D MR imaging. AJNR Am J neuroradiol 2006;27(10):2098–2103.

[40] Tracey KJ. Immune cells exploit a neural circuit to enter the CNS. Cell 2012;148(3):392–394. DOI: 10.1016/j.cell.2012.01.025

[41] Andersson U, Tracey KJ. Neural reflexes in inflammation and immunity. J Exp Med 2012;209(6):1057–1068. DOI: 10.1084/jem.20120571

[42] Sabharwal L, Kamimura D, Meng J, Bando H, Ogura H, Nakayama C, et al.: The Gateway Reflex, which is mediated by the inflammation amplifier, directs pathogenic immune cells into the CNS. J Biochem 2014;156(6):299–304. DOI: 10.1093/jb/mvu057

[43] Feinstein A, Magalhaes S, Richard JF, Audet B, Moore C. The link between multiple sclerosis and depression. Nat Rev Neurol 2014;10(9):507–517. DOI: 10.1038/nrneurol.2014.139

[44] Morales-Lazaro SL, Simon SA, Rosenbaum T. The role of endogenous molecules in modulating pain through transient receptor potential vanilloid 1 (TRPV1). J Physiol 2013;591(Pt 13):3109–3121. DOI: 10.1113/jphysiol.2013.251751

[45] Bennett DL, Woods CG. Painful and painless channelopathies. Lancet Neurol 2014;13(6):587–599. DOI: 10.1016/S1474-4422(14)70024-9

[46] Khan N, Smith MT. Multiple sclerosis-induced neuropathic pain: pharmacological management and pathophysiological insights from rodent EAE models. Inflammopharmacology 2014;22(1):1–22. DOI: 10.1007/s10787-013-0195-3

[47] Thygesen TH, Baad-Hansen L, Svensson P. Sensory action potentials of the maxillary nerve: a methodologic study with clinical implications. J Oral Maxillofac Surg : official journal of the American Association of Oral and Maxillofacial Surgeons 2009;67(3):537–542. DOI: 10.1016/j.joms.2008.02.015

[48] Ehde DM, Gibbons LE, Chwastiak L, Bombardier CH, Sullivan MD, Kraft GH. Chronic pain in a large community sample of persons with multiple sclerosis. Mult Scler 2003;9(6):605–611.

[49] Ikemoto K, Kitahama K, Nishimura A, Jouvet A, Nishi K, Arai R, et al.: Tyrosine hydroxylase and aromatic L-amino acid decarboxylase do not coexist in neurons in the human anterior cingulate cortex. Neurosci Letters 1999;269(1):37–40.

[50] Critchley HD. Neural mechanisms of autonomic, affective, and cognitive integration. J Comp Neurol 2005;493(1):154–166. 10.1002/cne.20749

[51] Karagkouni A, Alevizos M, Theoharides TC. Effect of stress on brain inflammation and multiple sclerosis. Autoimmun Rev 2013;12(10):947–953. DOI: 10.1016/j.autrev.2013.02.006

[52] Frohman TC, Davis SL, Beh S, Greenberg BM, Remington G, Frohman EM. Uhthoff's phenomena in MS--clinical features and pathophysiology. Nat Rev Neurol 2013;9(9):535–540. DOI: 10.1038/nrneurol.2013.98

[53] Cao L, Liu X, Lin EJ, Wang C, Choi EY, Riban V, et al.: Environmental and genetic activation of a brain-adipocyte BDNF/leptin axis causes cancer remission and inhibition. Cell 2010;142(1):52–64. DOI: 10.1016/j.cell.2010.05.029.

[54] Li G, Gan Y, Fan Y, Wu Y, Lin H, Song Y, et al.: Enriched environment inhibits mouse pancreatic cancer growth and down-regulates the expression of mitochondria-related genes in cancer cells. Sci Rep 2015;5:7856. DOI: 10.1038/srep07856

[55] Andersson U, Tracey KJ. Reflex principles of immunological homeostasis. Annu Rev Immunol 2012;30:313–335. DOI: 10.1146/annurev-immunol-020711-075015

[56] Torres-Rosas R, Yehia G, Pena G, Mishra P, del Rocio Thompson-Bonilla M, Moreno-Eutimio MA, et al.: Dopamine mediates vagal modulation of the immune system by electroacupuncture. Nat Med 2014;20(3):291–295. DOI: 10.1038/nm.3479

[57] Ohtani T, Ishihara K, Atsumi T, Nishida K, Kaneko Y, Miyata T, et al.: Dissection of signaling cascades through gp130 in vivo: reciprocal roles for STAT3- and SHP2-mediated signals in immune responses. Immunity 2000;12(1):95–105.

[58] Atsumi T, Ishihara K, Kamimura D, Ikushima H, Ohtani T, Hirota S, et al.: A point mutation of Tyr-759 in interleukin 6 family cytokine receptor subunit gp130 causes autoimmune arthritis. J Exp Med 2002;196(7):979–990.

[59] Nishimoto N, Kishimoto T, Yoshizaki K. Anti-interleukin 6 receptor antibody treatment in rheumatic disease. Ann Rheum Dis 2000;59 Suppl 1:i21-27.

[60] Nishimoto N, Kishimoto T. Inhibition of IL-6 for the treatment of inflammatory diseases. Curr Opin Pharmacol 2004;4(4):386–391. DOI: 10.1016/j.coph.2004.03.005

[61] Sawa S, Kamimura D, Jin GH, Morikawa H, Kamon H, Nishihara M, et al.: Autoimmune arthritis associated with mutated interleukin (IL)-6 receptor gp130 is driven by STAT3/IL-7-dependent homeostatic proliferation of CD4+ T cells. J Exp Med 2006;203(6):1459–1470. DOI: 10.1084/jem.20052187

[62] Ogura H, Murakami M, Okuyama Y, Tsuruoka M, Kitabayashi C, Kanamoto M, et al.: Interleukin-17 promotes autoimmunity by triggering a positive-feedback loop via interleukin-6 induction. Immunity 2008;29(4):628–636. DOI: 10.1016/j.immuni.2008.07.018

[63] Harada M, Kamimura D, Arima Y, Kohsaka H, Nakatsuji Y, Nishida M, et al.: Temporal expression of growth factors triggered by epiregulin regulates inflammation development. J Immunol 2015;194(3):1039–1046. DOI: 10.4049/jimmunol.1400562

[64] Murakami M, Hirano T. The pathological and physiological roles of IL-6 amplifier activation. Int J Biol Sci 2012;8(9):1267–1280. DOI: 10.7150/ijbs.4828

[65] Atsumi T, Singh R, Sabharwal L, Bando H, Meng J, Arima Y, et al.: Inflammation amplifier, a new paradigm in cancer biology. Cancer Res 2014;74(1):8–14. DOI: 10.1158/0008-5472.CAN-13-2322

[66] Lee J, Nakagiri T, Oto T, Harada M, Morii E, Shintani Y, et al.: IL-6 amplifier, NF-kappaB-triggered positive feedback for IL-6 signaling, in grafts is involved in allogeneic rejection responses. J Immunol 2012;189(4):1928–1936. DOI: 10.4049/jimmunol.1103613

[67] Murakami M, Harada M, Kamimura D, Ogura H, Okuyama Y, Kumai N, et al.: Disease-association analysis of an inflammation-related feedback loop. Cell Rep 2013;3(3):946–959. DOI: 10.1016/j.celrep.2013.01.028

[68] Ma X, Reynolds SL, Baker BJ, Li X, Benveniste EN, Qin H. IL-17 enhancement of the IL-6 signaling cascade in astrocytes. J Immunol 2010;184(9):4898–4906. DOI: 10.4049/jimmunol.1000142

[69] Susaki EA, Tainaka K, Perrin D, Kishino F, Tawara T, Watanabe TM, et al.: Whole-brain imaging with single-cell resolution using chemical cocktails and computational analysis. Cell 2014;157(3):726–739. DOI: 10.1016/j.cell.2014.03.042

[70] Tainaka K, Kubota SI, Suyama TQ, Susaki EA, Perrin D, Ukai-Tadenuma M, et al.: Whole-body imaging with single-cell resolution by tissue decolorization. Cell 2014;159(4):911–924. DOI: 10.1016/j.cell.2014.10.034

Chapter 3

Intrathecal Immunoglobulin Synthesis in MS—A Complete Reappraisal

Mickael Bonnan

Additional information is available at the end of the chapter

http://dx.doi.org/10.5772/63201

Abstract

Multiple sclerosis (MS) is characterized by the intrathecal synthesis (ITS) of immunoglobulins (Igs), which, although nonspecific, is the strongest biological marker. Since no specific target has been elucidated, this synthesis is considered to be disease-irrelevant. We demonstrate that this synthesis provides pertinent information about the pathophysiological processes involved. Quantification of ITS is based on an approximation intrinsically underestimating its level and it remains constant in MS, albeit sometimes at a low level. B-cell maturation seems to be initiated within the cervical lymph nodes and B-cells traffic on both sides of the blood-brain barrier by rounds of bidirectional traffic. During this process, they undergo somatic hypermutation, which is the hallmark of antigen-driven antibody maturation, suggesting that most of the ITS is probably directed against as yet unknown targets. Alternatively, examining"non-disease-relevant" ITS in the light of meningeal tertiary lymphoid organs provides new insights into the pathophysiology of MS. Although no specific target has yet been identified in MS, recent developments in the search for targeted antigens point to non-conventional antigens (posttranslationally modified proteins or oxidized products) of which a few are promising for future research.

Keywords: multiple sclerosis, meningeal inflammation, intrathecal synthesis, immunoglobulins, autoantibody, epitopes, antigens

1. Introduction

The normal central nervous system (CNS) is completely devoid of resident plasma cells, so finding infiltrating B-cells in the CNS is rather exceptional. Infiltrating activated CD20+CD23+ B-cells in brain parenchyma number to less than 0.1–1.5 cell/cm^2 [1–3]. Therefore, no intrathecal immunoglobulin (Ig) synthesis (ITS) occurs in the basal state, and locally produced Igs testify to former or active CNS infection or inflammatory processes. Therefore, while it is easy to demonstrate high levels of ITS, quantifying low levels poses technical problems.

Although ITS is one of the most sensitive biological clues for MS, it was long considered to be nonspecific or a bystander of CNS inflammation since the latter mainly involves T-cells and no specific antibody target has yet emerged. The recent success of anti-CD20 therapy in relapsing and progressive MS sheds light on a more central role of non-CNS B-cells in the pathophysiology of MS. However, progressive MS pathophysiology is still poorly understood and CNS resident B-cells may play an even greater role. Since locally synthesized Igs are the main B-cell by-products, ITS offers a good opportunity for studying resident B-cells. The role of cerebrospinal fluid (CSF) B-cells has not yet been elucidated and is probably diverse as follows: (1) cytotoxic effect of antibodies; (2) local antigen presentation to T-cells; and (3) secretion of cytokines playing a complex regulating role, including a possible Ig-unrelated CNS cytotoxicity. Therefore, CNS-trapped B-cells not only synthesize oligoclonal bands (OCBs) but might also play a pivotal role in the slow-burning CNS inflammation.

2. Quantitative measures of CSF IgG

2.1. Pitfalls in assessing ITS level

Synthesis of Igs does not occur in the normal CNS and the tiny Ig concentration measured in normal CSF reflects a low-rate passive diffusion through the blood-brain barrier (BBB) to CSF. It was long thought that although virtually all the molecules may diffuse from serum to CSF, BBB permeability positively correlated with the molecular weight [4]. For example, the ratio decreases from 1:205 with albumin (65 kDa) to 1:440 with IgG (150 kDa) and 1:900 with IgM (970 kDa) [5]. Moreover, the permeability of the BBB commonly increases during CNS pathologies, leading to an increase in CSF concentrations of blood-borne proteins and Igs. As

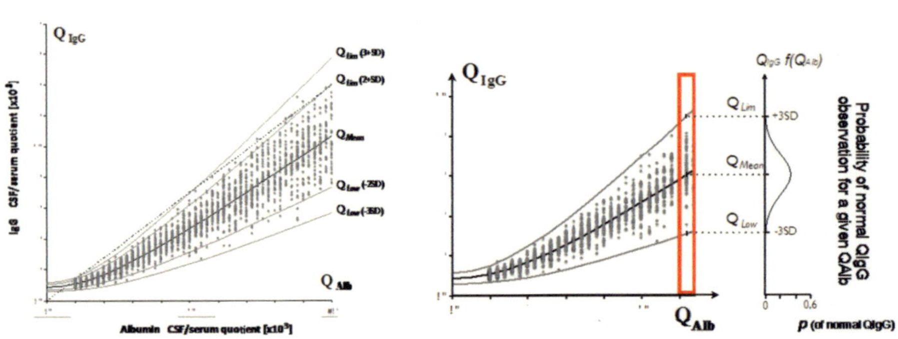

Figure 1. CSF IgG passively diffused from blood to CSF in normal population. Left panel (A). Plot of CSF/serum quotients with hyperbolic function of quotient ratios ("'Reibergram"). Reference range defined by Q_{Lim} : Q_{mean}±2SD or ±3SD involving, respectively, 96 and 99% of the normal population. Dotted line is the upper normal limit (>0.7) of IgG index, intersecting the Q_{Lim} curve at two points. **Right panel (B). Probability curve of basal Q_{IgG} for a given Q_{Alb}.** The maximum probability is obtained for Q_{mean}. Points are obtained from a simulated healthy population.

a consequence, the level of intrathecally synthesized Igs related to CNS inflammation is obscured by the passively diffused CSF Igs concentration and requires a mathematical approach that takes into account the permeability and blood concentration of the targeted molecules. The albumin quotient (or ratio), Q_{Alb} = $[Alb_{CSF}]/[Alb_{serum}]$, is indicative of BBB dysfunction and increases with its permeability. It is also influenced by the patient's age and underlying CNS pathologies. In the basal state, which is devoid of intrathecal IgG synthesis, the ratio $[IgG_{CSF}]/[IgG_{serum}]$ is proportional to Q_{Alb}.

The daily IgG synthesis rate can be assessed by Tourtellotte's formula (median value 29 mg/day), but inconsistent values are obtained at the individual level owing to assumptions [6]. The linear approach where the IgG index = Q_{IgG}/Q_{Alb} (normal values <0.7) does not take into account either normal Q_{IgG} variance nor nonlinear correlations with Q_{Alb}, leading to an approximation around the limit (**Figure 1**, left panel). Moreover, since Q_{Alb} increases with age, the IgG index is thought to decrease mechanically without any change in ITS [7]. Data are best fitted by an empiric hyperbolic function (the "Reibergram") [8] whose constant parameters were fitted with a large dataset of 4154 control patients [9]. From a theoretical point of view, the hyperbolic function is the application of Fick's laws of diffusion applied to albumin and Igs [9]. For a given Q_{Alb} in a population of normal patients, the distribution of Q_{IgG} follows a normal law around the mean curve as $Q_{mean}=f(Q_{Alb})$ (**Figure 1**, right panel) [9]. With intrathecal synthesis (ITS), the IgG concentration in the CSF is the sum of IgG passively diffused from the blood and synthesized intrathecally

$$Q_{IgG}=\left(\left[IgG_{CSF\_passive}\right]+\left[IgG_{CSF\_Loc}\right]\right)/\left[IgG_{serum}\right]=Q_{IgG\_basal}+Q_{IgG\_Loc},$$

where Q_{IgG_basal} is the Q_{IgG} of the same patient before the onset of ITS. In clinical practice, only Q_{IgG} is directly available but not Q_{IgG_basal}, so the exact IgG_{CSF_Loc} concentration can only be approximated by using Reiber's discrimination curve. The upper limit of the reference range, Q_{Lim}, is usually set arbitrarily as Q_{mean}+3SD and involves >99% of the normal population. By applying this definition, intrathecal IgG synthesis is considered to be present when $Q_{IgG}> Q_{Lim}$. The major drawback of this reference range is the loss of sensitivity for cases displaying a low level of ITS ($Q_{Lim}> Q_{IgG}> Q_{IgG\_basal}$). In common practice, demonstrating ITS in such cases requires a CSF-restricted OCBs positivity. As expected, restricting the reference range to Q_{Lim}+2SD instead of +3SD increases the percentage of abnormal Q_{IgG} in MS cohorts by 6–10% for IgG and up to 20% for IgM, which increases the risk of false positivity to 4% [7].

The true amount of intrathecally (or locally) synthesized IgG should be calculated as follows:

$$IgG_{Loc}\left(mg/L\right)=\left(Q_{IgG}-Q_{IgG\_basal}\right)x\left[IgG_{serum}\right].$$

However, since Q_{IgG_basal} is unavailable, it can be replaced by either Q_{Lim} or Q_{mean}. As previously demonstrated, replacing Q_{IgG_basal} by Q_{Lim} confers maximal specificity in single patient studies but with the drawback of an unavoidable underestimation of ITS. The range of IgG_{Loc}

underestimation may vary widely from 1 to 50 mg/L according to Q_{Alb} (unpublished results). In cohort studies, Q_{IgG_basal} is advantageously replaced by Q_{mean}, which provides a closer estimation of the exact IgG_{Loc} [7].

Lastly, inter-assay variability may directly impact Q_{IgG} or the IgG index. For example, a 10% decrease in serum IgG directly means a 10% increase in IgG index, and 10% variations of the IgG index from day to day are commonly reported [7, 10]. As a consequence, minor fluctuations in IgG levels may be translated into normal or abnormal Q_{IgG} results, although the intrathecal IgG synthesis rate is not really impacted. A final pitfall of ITS assessment relates to the properties of CNS-targeting antibodies themselves, which are capable of brain adsorption that can potentially abolish low levels of specific antibodies that are synthesized locally or spill over to the CSF [11].

2.2. Predicted changes in ITS measures in response to treatments

Using formulas and normal values obtained from the literature, we simulated results of a cohort with tunable ITS level (unpublished results). This model provides the advantage of being able to compare the calculated (approximated) IgG_{Loc} with the fixed IgG_{Loc}.

IgG_{Loc} estimation based on Q_{mean} fitted well with the exact IgG_{Loc}, even in small cohorts and for small ITS (<1 mg/L). On the other hand, individual or cohort estimations of IgG_{Loc} based on Q_{Lim} were strongly biased in a range dependent on Q_{Alb}.

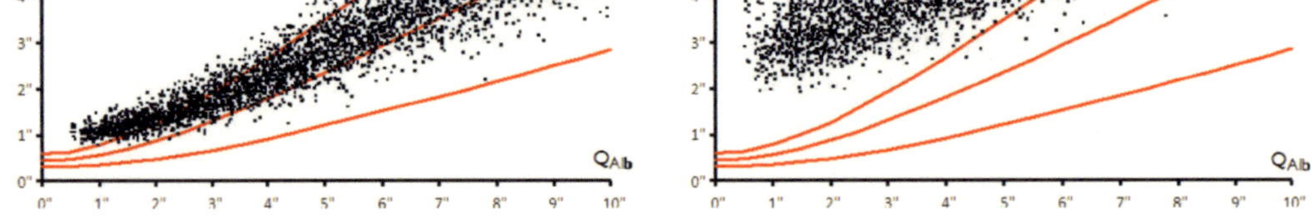

Figure 2. Effect of plasma exchange on Q_{IgG}. Simulated population with ITS +5 mg/L. Q_{IgG} values increase to abnormal range whereas ITS level remains unchanged.

Plasma exchange depletes both serum IgG and IgG passively transferred through the BBB. Therefore, assuming that ITS remains constant during the procedure, the contrast in locally synthesized and passively diffused IgG in CSF is dramatically tuned by plasma exchange (**Figure 2**). For example, after a 90% decrease in $[IgG_{serum}]$, IgG in CSF originates almost entirely from local synthesis. The IgG index increases whereas the precision of the IgG_{Loc} calculation (based on Q_{mean}) remains unchanged.

For a given level of ITS, a decrease in BBB permeability decreases Q_{IgG_basal} in a nonlinear response whereas Q_{Loc} remains constant. Therefore, Q_{IgG} and the IgG index may shift to abnormal values and $IgG_{Loc}(Q_{Lim})$ increases incorrectly, whereas $IgG_{Loc}(Q_{mean})$ remains constant.

As a consequence, monitoring of the ITS level should be based on the unbiased $IgG_{Loc}(Q_{mean})$.

3. Qualitative measures of CSF IgG—method and limitations of oligoclonal band analysis

3.1. Oligoclonal bands

CSF OCB analysis is based on an isoelectric focalization (IEF) technique fractionating Ig into multiple bands according to their respective pI. Structurally diverse antibodies sharing the same pI may cofocus in a single band [12]. Studying IgM OCBs is harder owing to the dissociation of pentamers before the F fragment and the arbitrary reassociation of the separated monomers [13].

Moreover, owing to differential posttranslational modifications (PTMs) (glycosylation or amino acid modifications), each particular IgG clone may display several pKs and may run in multiple bands in IEF conditions [14, 15]. Monoclonal antibodies occurring naturally (monoclonal gammopathy) or commercially available ones are resolved in multiple bands on IEF gel runs (ladder pattern) [15–17]. In a series of 20 myelomas, IEF identified 5–10 OCB in serum [18]. Commercial monoclonal antibodies produced by hybridomas (monoclonal mouse antibody) or monoclonal IgG produced in vivo by plasma cell tumors (multiple myeloma) are highly heterogeneous and present a clone-specific profile of glycosylation [17, 19]. Lastly, each OCB is a visual optical interpretation of a local contrast of color density differentiating OCB from the surrounding polyclonal background. Apart from the relative subjectivity of the technique, faint and ambiguous OCB may be obscured by a dense polyclonal background. Capillary IEF seems to increase sensitivity and demonstrated OCB in negative patients with classical IEF [20]. Therefore, immunoblotting against known antigens, for example, in association with viral encephalitis, unmasks specific OCB in cases failing to demonstrate any OCB with conventional IEF [21]. In MS patients explored for specific antibody anti-viral synthesis, OCB against multiple viruses may occur in the same migrating zone on IEF [22] and CSF OCB against myelin basic protein (MBP) or measles obtained with immunoblot detection does not comigrate with OCB obtained by IEF [23].

There may be several consequences of this as follows: (1) each OCB may be composed of multiple distinct IgG, which may share by chance the same isoelectric point [15]; (2) multiple OCB in MS may derive from one or a small number of cell clones [17]; (3) OCB count cannot predict the number or variety of B-cell clones; and (4) clonally expanded B-cell clones may precede OCB detection, thus reflecting the difficulty to detect very low levels of ITS.

ITS in MS is characterized by numerous unambiguous OCBs (≥10 OCB) that are highly specific of MS [24]. Monoclonal bands are exceptional and should be considered carefully. Repeated LP in these atypical cases demonstrates a broadening of ITS or a different diagnosis [25]. Owing to their lack of specificity [25], ≥2 OCB are required in most studies to define an oligoclonal pattern with optimal specificity.

Absence of OCB (type 1 pattern) is observed in less than 10% in recent studies, whereas most MS patients display the type 2 pattern and only some have type 3 (**Figure 3**). Among OCB+ patients, patterns 2 and 3 are observed in about 90 and 10% in relapsing-remitting (RR) and secondary progressive (SP) patients, respectively, whereas the distribution is 40 and 60% in primary progressive (PP) patients [27], suggesting that pattern responses may be linked to pathophysiology.

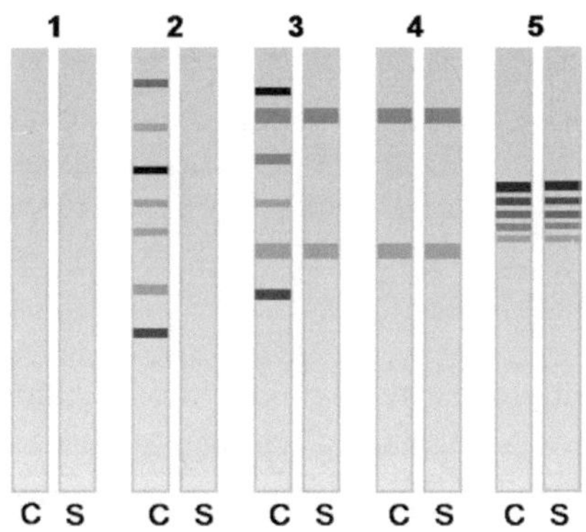

Figure 3. Types of isoelectric focusing patterns on agarose gels [26]: Type 1, no OCB in CSF or serum (normal pattern). Type 2, OCB restricted to CSF, absent in serum. Indicates low-level ITS. Typical pattern in MS. Type 3, Identical OCB in both serum and CSF with extra bands in CSF. Pattern seen during systemic synthesis associated with intrathecal synthesis. Seen in MS. Type 4, OCBs in CSF mirror those in serum. Indicates a systemic IgG synthesis and passive transfer of OCB from blood to CSF, without any local synthesis. From a purely theoretical point of view, a low local synthesis with similar B-cell clones cannot be completely deciphered from this situation. Type 5, Ladder-type identical OCB in both serum and CSF typically associated with monoclonal IgG proteins. Peripheral IgG synthesis without local synthesis.

3.2. Absence of OCB in MS patients is a technical limitation

OCB are almost always present when $Q_{IgG}> Q_{Lim}$, but are also commonly present when Q_{IgG} Q_{Lim} [26, 28, 29]. Nonetheless, about 5–10% of MS patients fail to demonstrate any OCB or an elevated IgG index. Nevertheless, the question remains whether ITS is really absent from such patients' CSF. Our short review argues for a probable faint ITS in the rare 'CSF-negative' patients, making ITS the most valuable marker of MS to date.

A high CSF IgA synthesis has been demonstrated in a few patients lacking the classical IgG synthesis [30, 31]. Free light chain (FLC) sensitivity seems to be near 100% but the (expected) specificity lower than OCB makes FLC less useful for routine clinical purposes [32, 33]. Oligoclonal κ-FLCs are detected in about 50% of MS patients without OCB [34, 35]. Isoelectric focusing with affinity blotting against known antigens overcomes the limitation induced by the background and unmasks specific ITS. OCBs against the neurotropic MRZ viruses, measles, rubella, and varicella zoster virus (VZV), which are commonly observed in MS for reasons that remain unclear, were present in the CSF of 72% of MS patients who otherwise failed to demonstrate OCB with IEF [36].

The specific antibody index (AI) is calculated by using the ratio of specific antibodies Q_{Spec}=[$Spec_{CSF}$]/[$Spec_{serum}$] in the formula, AI = Q_{Spec}/Q_{IgG}, where AI values >1.3–1.5 indicate the presence of ITS. An MRZ pattern, which is defined as an elevated AI against ≥2 neurotropic viruses, is observed in up to 90% of MS patients [37, 38]. However, the AI is not usually assessed in patients with Q_{IgG} Q_{Lim} and negative OCB, because they are thought to be MRZ-negative since AI correlates with Q_{IgG} [29]. When multiple AIs (VZV, herpes simplex virus (HSV), cytomegalovirus (CMV), measles, rubella, and Borrelia) were systematically assessed in MS patients without apparent ITS (Q_{IgG} Q_{Lim} and negative OCB), all of them showed ≥1 MRZ reactivity and up to 47% of patients had OCB against ≥1 MRZ [29, 36, 39–41]. Interestingly, AI results are not completely congruent with those obtained by IEF with affinity blotting, thus increasing the prevalence of ITS detected by ≥1 technique to 64% in the "CSF-negative" subgroup of MS patients [36]. Since the MRZ reaction is common but not exclusive and because reactions against many other viruses have been confirmed in MS (see below), a larger antigenic test panel might improve the frequency of ITS detection [29], for example, by the systematic use of antigen array [42] and the systematic assessment of IgM.

Studies combining all currently available techniques should be undertaken in MS patients, especially in those with "negative CSF", in order to establish the true prevalence of ITS in MS, especially in patients of non-Caucasian descent who are thought to harbor a lower CSF positivity [43, 44]. Future studies could combine quantitative techniques (IgG_{Loc}, FLC, AI against MRZ) and highly sensitive qualitative techniques (OCB) until the discovery of putative antigenic targets such as anti-CCP (cyclic citrullinated peptide) in rheumatoid arthritis. Criteria for standardizing intrathecal Ig synthesis should be based on the simultaneous normalization of all the tests. In view of the fluctuations of ITS in individual patients (up to 30% of IgG_{Loc} [45]), the action of a drug upon ITS should be statistically demonstrated in groups. To be able to demonstrate a successful intrathecal reset, a null Ig synthesis should be confirmed by using several techniques together.

4. Intrathecal Ig synthesis is a robust and predictive marker in MS

4.1. Factors influencing ITS level

About 95% of patients display OCB but a quantifiable IgG synthesis only occurs in about 70% of them. Several studies have shown that the level of ITS is highly variable from one patient to another, which suggests a genetic determinism. Females are more prone to OCB positivity (92% vs 84%) and to a higher IgG index (1.32 ± 0.92 vs 1.03 ± 0.54) [46, 47]. An ethnic influence on IgG index level and OCB status has also been confirmed by several studies. Black-ascending patients are more prone to a higher IgG index, a higher rate of IgG synthesis, and OCB positivity [48, 49]. The IgG index level is still higher in Afro-Americans after adjustment for OCB status [49]. The association of female sex to higher IgG index was also confirmed in this group [49].

Prevalence of abnormal OCB status and IgG_{Loc} is lower in Asian patients than in Caucasian patients [50–52]. In Asian patients having the strongest genetic risk factors (DRB1*1501), the prevalence of OCB positivity remains lower than in Caucasians (<72% vs 97%) [53, 54]. Moreover, irrespective of genetic background, extreme latitudes may exert a positive influence on OCB status whereas tropical latitudes exert a negative influence [53, 55].

Several studies have confirmed a strong association between OCB status and human leukocyte antigen (HLA). The DRB1*15 allele confers a higher risk of OCB positivity whereas the genotypes DRB1*04:04/*04:05 or DRB1*03:01/*04:01 are associated with OCB negativity [56, 57]. Interestingly, DRB1*1501 also increases the prevalence of abnormal IgG and IgA indexes but not of the IgM index [54]. In Asian patients, even though these determinants are conserved, OCB status is also driven by a strong interaction with latitude [53].

Genetic markers of γ chains (GMs) display 18 serologic specificities and all of the variants but two are expressed in the Fc region of γ chains. Some of these variations have been shown to strongly influence antibody-dependent cell-mediated cytotoxicity (ADCC) and complement-dependent cytotoxicity (CDC) [58]. In an animal model of rheumatoid arthritis, the recognition of collagen-II epitopes by VH chains strongly depended on GM haplotypes [59]. Interestingly, GM haplotypes are in almost total linkage disequilibrium among world populations and are therefore typical of geographic origin unless there is a genetic admixture [60]. Gm21* haplotypes were associated with high ITS in a Caucasian population although Gm5*;3 haplotypes are associated with a low level of ITS[96, 97]. Studies are required concerning non-Caucasian (African and Asian descent) haplotypes. Gm haplotypes are neither correlated with serum IgG level nor with the risk of MS [61, 62]. The causes of interaction between GM allotypes and ITS level remain elusive and the relationship between allotypes and CNS FcRn function (which enhances IgG clearance from CSF via Fc interaction) is unknown. Other non-HLA unknown genes also influence OCB status [56, 63].

Healthy siblings of MS patients display a hyperimmune condition termed "MS immunopathic trait" that is characterized by (1) one or more CSF OCB, (2) an exaggerated response to a variety of viral antigens, and (3) an increased BBB permeability [64, 65]. CSF OCB were found in up to 19% of MS siblings in contrast to 4% of an unrelated control population [66, 67], some of them also displaying an elevated IgG index [66] and up to half of these siblings having both OCB- and measles-specific IgG local synthesis [64, 67]. It is not clear whether ITS observed in these cases reflects a presymptomatic MS in high-risk patients, elite non-progressors, or an unrelated predisposition to ITS.

4.2. ITS is robust over time

ITS occurs as a very early disease event. In pediatric cohorts with very early onset MS (before 6 years), only 8% showed IgG OCB, a figure increasing to 90% with 69% of intrathecal production in two early onset cohorts (<15 y) and even more after a further relapse [68, 69]. In adults, the proportion of OCB positivity tends to appear at re-examination [70] or increases as the disease progresses (RR = 325/360, SP: 25/25, and PP: 39/39) [27]. In a longitudinal study of CSF from 19 patients taken at multiple time points up to 12 years (mean 8 years), OCB never abated with time and demonstrated a robust pattern [71]. Most of the changes concerned band intensity and the acquisition of a new band [25, 72], although band loss was sometimes described in earlier reports [25, 71]. The same stability of OCB over time was observed with IgG, IgM, and IgA [13, 71, 73].

When focusing on the clonal repertoire of CSF Ig, the highest number of clones was found in patients with the longest disease duration, suggesting a continuous clonal expansion over time [74]. However, the low number of patients included cannot totally rule out disease heterogeneity [74]. In a longitudinal study of CSF B-cells in two MS patients, clonal rearrangements on VH (VH3 and VH4), D segment, JH, and HCDR3 sequences were conserved at two time points 1 and 4 years apart [75]. The antibody index of phagotopes from the entire panel of clones extracted from a single patient was stable at 2 years [76]. The peptidic targets of the OCB IgG are constant over time [72] and the activity index (AI) against infectious agents also remained stable over several years [77, 78]. These findings are in line with a slightly delayed oligoclonal immune response immediately after the onset of MS. However, once initiated, CSF IgG secretion persists over time indefinitely and is little altered qualitatively at the clonal level [71]. Other CSF parameters such as albumin index, IgG, and IgM index remained essentially the same in the clinically isolated syndrome (CIS), RR-MS, and progressive MS groups [27, 79].

A few exceptions should be mentioned as follows: (1) IgM OCBs behave differently, if absent at onset, no further IgM OCBs appear [73]; when present, they tend to disappear after a few years (RR: 109/360, SP: 15/25, PP: 0/39) [27]. When oligoclonal IgMs are present, the disease lasts for less than 5 years in 90% of patients, but when IgMs are absent, it lasts for more than 5 years in 60% of patients. (2) Anti-MBPs in CSF are high during relapses in about 90% of patients but vanish during the 6 weeks following onset, relapse treatment appearing to precipitate this event [80, 81].

Each patient has a private and unique CSF OCB pattern, the so-called OCB fingerprint [82, 83]. The pattern persists even though the total CSF IgG is significantly reduced, for example, by steroids [83]. The CNS IgG synthesis rate remains roughly stable over several months [6]. When steroids are used to reduce the IgG index, pretreatment values are recovered in a few weeks or months [83]. Intrathecal steroids rarely obliterate OCB for more than 1 month [71], but this modification can be corrected when equal amounts of CSF Ig are applied in IEF.

Unfortunately, OCBs provide basic information and the future development of microarrays may provide more precise insight into the intimate evolution of clonality. For example, the involution of the antibody response against heat shock protein (HSP) in serum is a central modification in the immune response during the transition from RR to the progressive form [84], but the outcome of this immune signature in CSF is unknown.

The persistence of OCB suggests a local IgG production by long-lived plasma cells residing inside the CNS, suggesting that the B-cell fostering properties of the CNS deserve consideration [85]. On the other hand, minor changes in OCB pattern are in accordance with competition between plasma cells for a limited number of survival niches, as observed in the bone marrow. It seems unlikely that such a discrepancy between brain volume and the small number of CNS plasma cells can be explained only by the B-cell fostering properties of the CNS. Moreover, the intrathecal IgG synthesis rate is roughly stable over time, even though persistent local inflammation would be expected to induce a gradual increase in synthesis rate. These data suggest that the number of CNS niches is limited and that they are quickly saturated. Therefore, the putative role of CNS tertiary lymphoid organs (TLOs) deserves further consideration.

4.3. None of the available MS drugs deplete intrathecal Ig synthesis

In a complete review of the literature, we demonstrated that none of the available (approved or experimental) treatment proved to abate intrathecal Ig synthesis (review in reference [86]). A null or minimal (<20%) impact on intrathecal IgG synthesis was observed after the administration of azathioprine, β-interferons, cytarabine (intravenous or intrathecal), lomustine, 5-fluorouracil, CNS irradiation, mitoxantrone, methotrexate, cyclophosphamide, cyclosporin A, cladribine, alemtuzumab, daclizumab, fingolimod, or stem cell transplantation following myeloablation.

Steroid infusion decreases blood Ig levels in a few days [87]. However, high-dose steroid infusions have little effect on IgG index and OCB number [88–90], irrespective of the dosage or the mode of administration (intramuscular, intravenous, and intrathecal) [91]. Even if steroids can transiently lower the IgG index in most but not all patients, the decrease in the range of CSF IgG synthesis is low [90, 92]. The mean antibody reactivity and the mean number of targeted antigens in CSF are decreased in the 2 months following steroids [93].

Rituximab depletes CSF B-cells but fails to significantly decrease intrathecal IgG synthesis (<-20%) [45, 94], possibly because ITS may partly depend on plasma cells (CD20-), which are constitutively resistant. This failure to lower intrathecal IgG secretion was predictable from the absence of the effect of blood-infused rituximab upon serum IgG and IgA levels, contrary to a minor effect upon IgM levels [45, 95]. No data are available on intrathecal IgM synthesis after rituximab treatment.

Given the low diffusion of rituximab to CSF (<0.2%) and the growing body of evidence demonstrating the safe use of intrathecally infused rituximab, a rationale to infuse intrathecal rituximab in progressive MS recently emerged (review in reference [96]). Data obtained from a single patient receiving intrathecal rituximab (10 mg per month for 2 months) showed a major effect upon CSF cytokine levels although intrathecal IgG synthesis was unchanged [97, 98] (unpublished).

An unexpected partial repression of intrathecal IgG synthesis was obtained with natalizumab treatment in some series [99–101] but results were null or lower in two others [102, 103]. These findings need to be replicated in another large cohort. Three non-mutually exclusive explanations may be put forward. First, α4β1-integrin is expressed by B-cells (CD19+ and CD138+) at higher levels than CD3+ T-cells, and natalizumab impedes B-cell trafficking to the brain and renewal of the CNS plasmablast pool. Second, apart from cytokines, T-cells also play a supportive survival role in the survival niches of plasma cells [104]. Third, natalizumab inhibits the CNS migration of dendritic cells, which in turn may affect the maintenance of CNS lymphoid tissue [105], and dendritic cell counts in MS brains were lower than expected [106]. Of note, a significant decrease in IgM (≈-45%) (and less significantly in IgG1≈-18 to 36%) plasma levels also occurs during natalizumab treatment but is not correlated with treatment duration, suggesting that it effectively perturbs the IgG synthesis pathway [103, 107]. Future experiments should examine the kinetics of intrathecal IgG secretion after withdrawal of natalizumab. Data obtained from a single patient devoid of OCB under natalizumab and discontinuing treatment for progressive multifocal leukoencephalopathy (PML) showed that OCB returned shortly with a slightly modified pattern [101], whereas a sustained negativation was observed at 6 months in two other patients [99]. However, in a series of 23 patients, no increase of ITS or OCB was observed at 14 months after natalizumab discontinuation [108], suggesting that the impact of natalizumab on ITS is probably low.

A single patient treated by EBV-specific adoptive immunotherapy (autologous CD8+ T-cells activated against EBV) regained a normal level of IgG index at month 4 [109]. This single case needs to be replicated.

4.4. Prognostic value of ITS

Although the prognostic value of OCB positivity is not consensual, ITS is consistently associated with a worse outcome. In CIS patients, none of the IgG, IgA, or IgM indexes are predictive of clinical conversion to MS [110]. On the other hand, OCB positivity in CIS increases the risk of having a second attack irrespective of magnetic resonance imaging (MRI) results [111] and the number of OCB is an independent risk factor for relapses [112], whereas their absence is associated with a lower clinical conversion at 5 years and with a better clinical outcome [113]. Interestingly, double OCB positivity (IgG and IgM) is associated with an odds ratio (OR) of second relapses higher than fulfilling of Barkhof's criteria (OR 55.7 vs 3.5) [114]. The MRZ pattern is also an independent risk factor of clinical conversion [115] and all CIS patients displaying OCB targeting lipid antigens relapse in the first year [113].

In clinically defined MS patients, the IgG synthesis rate correlates with MRI burden and the IgG1 index correlates with expanded disability status scale (EDSS). Free light chains in CSF are predictive of impairment [116]. CSF IgM and IgM OCB are associated with a poorer clinical outcome [73, 117] and a lower brain volume [118, 119]. IgM OCBs reacting against myelin lipids are associated with a higher relapse rate, lower efficiency of IFNβ, and a faster EDSS increase [120, 121]. Time and probability to reach EDSS 3 and 4 are strongly correlated with the presence of IgM in CSF [122, 123]. The IgM index in CSF at onset is strongly correlated with a higher last follow-up EDSS [117, 124]. The time to conversion to the secondary progressive phase is shorter in the presence of IgM BOC or an elevated IgM index [73, 123, 124]. These attractive findings concerning IgM were established in a single group of patients. Stauch et al. [13] did not find any influence of IgM OCB on the evolution of MS in a pediatric group and raised some technical concerns about the IgM tests used previously, which may invalidate the results. Another group claimed negative results but they also obtained a shorter, albeit nonsignificant, time to relapse after CIS in OCB-IgM+ patients [125]. In a large retrospective study, disease severity appeared to be identical between OCB-positive and -negative patients [126], whereas in a study including 1800 MS patients, the number of OCB was considered to correlate with the course of the disease [127]. The mean number of OCB in the group of benign patients was 2.9 ± 3.6 compared to 5.7 ± 4.9 in the severe group ($p < 0.06$) [127]. Therefore, the evidence points to a poorer clinical prognosis in MS patients in association with ITS. On the other hand, OCB negativity correlates with a better outcome in many studies [70, 127–131], even after demographic adjustment [132].

5. Intrathecal Ig synthesis in animal models—technical limitations

IgG synthesis level in CSF is highly correlated with CD19+CD138+ plasmablast levels [133], but although ITS is commonly thought to be associated with CSF floating cells, this minute cell number may account for less than 0.1% of the whole ITS, meaning that the bulk of IgG synthesis is provided by resident IgG-secreting cells, residing either in the meninges or in the perivascular areas [134]. In experimental allergic encephalomyelitis (EAE) models, the parenchymal level of B-cell infiltration increases from null to 134 B-cell/cm^2 [135] and the whole number of infiltrating B-cells is in the range of 10^3–10^5 cells per mouse or rat brain [136, 137]. In MS, B-cells remain a minor proportion of the infiltrating lymphocytes (<5%), are virtually absent from the parenchyma, and are mostly observed around the small veins and meninges (4.6–6 cells/mm^2)[1, 138]. Plasma cells are occasionally found in demyelinated areas. No data are available regarding a possible role of meningeal B-cell aggregates in ITS.

IT Ig synthesis in animal models has received little attention since the very small volume of CSF does not facilitate sampling. Although older experiments based on low-sensitivity techniques failed to demonstrate any ITS during EAE, optimal techniques (IEF followed by anti-IgG staining) have subsequently confirmed the local synthesis of OCB and/or an elevated IgG index [139–142]. In viral models of demyelination (i.e., measles or JHM strain of coronavirus infection), a mirror pattern of OCB is common but local OCBs are always revealed by immunoblot against viral antigens [21, 143]. We are not aware of any EAE experiments aimed at demonstrating the nonspecific pattern of ITS observed in MS, especially the animal counterpart of the human MRZ pattern using common animal viruses or vaccines. From a theoretical point of view, animals receiving intrathecal vaccination with foreign antigens such as albumin are able to mount a strong intrathecal response [144–146]. In a unique case challenged intrathecally with ovalbumin (OVA), an increase in AI-herpes was also obtained apart from the expected increase in AI-ovalbumin, suggesting that animal models are promising for future studies of nonspecific ITS [145].

6. Non-IgG ITS

6.1. General background

The IgG class accounts for the bulk of locally synthesized Igs in MS and most knowledge to date concerns this class. All Ig classes may give rise to ITS. IgG, IgM, and IgA are, respectively, present in 100, 20–36, and 6–9% of MS patients [69, 78]. The relative absence of IgE is commonly interpreted as a clue to type I immunity [147].

6.2. IgM chains

Intrathecal IgM synthesis is always higher in MS than in controls [110]. IgM OCB may occur in about 20–75% of MS patients [78, 113, 118] and in 74% of CIS [125]. CD19+CD5+ lymphocytes are the predominant population of B-cells in CSF and are characterized by the T-cell independent secretion of IgM natural antibodies directed against phylogenetically conserved structures that target non-proteic epitopes. In a series of 53 CIS/relapsing-remitting multiple sclerosis (RRMS), 46 of them had oligoclonal IgM-recognizing lipid antigens, 30 targeted phosphatidylcholine (PC) alone, seven targeted PC and had additional reactivity against other myelin lipids (phosphatidylethanolamine, phosphatidylinositol, and sphingomyelin), and nine targeted myelin glycolipids, mostly sphingomyelin [113]. IgM OCB against lipids may be restricted to the RR and SP phases since they were not observed in PP patients [27]. Pentameric IgM strongly activates the complement cascade and is involved in the lesions of plaques (pattern II).

6.3. IgA

The IgA index is elevated in at least 9% of MS patients [54, 78, 148] and the mean intrathecal IgA index is modestly but significantly higher in patients than in controls [110]. Local synthesis of IgA may be the only clue to local Ig synthesis in some MS patients devoid of local synthesis of IgG [31]. About a quarter of Ig-secreting cells are IgA in choroid plexuses [149]. IgA cells are also common in plaques (3–9%) and demonstrate a high clonality (up to 80%) [149]. IgAs are mainly mucosal secretory antibodies but could be a major component of CNS immune responses in certain viral infections [148, 150]. OCB IgAs were reported to have a low frequency (2/33) in the earlier CSF studies [71, 150]. In a post-mortem analysis of plaques extracted from four MS brains, IgA+ plasma cells were recovered in 18/24 plaques and sometimes predominated on Ig+ plasma cells [148]. Clonality assessment in the plaques of two patients demonstrated a low diversity of clones and a clonal restriction confined to plaques [148]. The somatic mutations were highly concentrated in the complementary determining region (CDR) and FR3, which are considered critical for antigenic specificities, suggesting an antigen-driven maturation of affinity as observed for IgG. The locally synthesized IgA were demonstrated to target injured axons [148].

6.4. Free light chains

Light chains are normally synthesized more than heavy chains, with an FLCκ/λ ratio of 2:1 in normal blood. Serum circulating levels of FLC are about 1000-fold lower than Ig levels owing to rapid renal clearance (serum half-life of 2–6 h), whereas the rate of clearance from CSF is similar with Ig [151]. Therefore, the level of κFLC in MS is equal or higher in CSF than in serum. Although the absolute value of CSF FLC is variable among studies, the FLC level is always higher in MS than in controls, and the κFLC/protein ratio is even higher [152]. The κFLC index is more sensitive (Se 95%, Sp 91%) than the IgG index and OCB [153]. Since elevated CSF FLC is predictive of impairment [116], it has even been proposed as a therapeutic target [47].

7. Clues suggesting an antigen-driven maturation of the intrathecal clonal population of B-cells

The IgG1 subclass is significantly elevated in most MS CSF although some authors recovered rare higher CSF IgG2 or IgG3 indexes [110, 154]. The Ig repertoire uses 51 functional germline genes and the normal repertoire of naïve peripheral blood CD19+ cells closely approximates the frequency of the VH family gene segments within the germline. On the other hand, over-representation of a single VH family is common in MS plaques and CSF but not in blood [155]. The VH4 family is observed in more than 35–95% of CD19+ or CD138+ cells. However, the VH1 family, which represents 20% of the functional germline, is nearly absent from CSF in MS [156, 157]. As observed for IgG, the VH4 germline predominates in CSF IgM [158]. This bias precedes the onset of OCB [155] and is typical of MS whereas different biases are observed in other CNS disorders [155]. The clonal expansion of a single ancestor gene was robustly demonstrated by the analysis of clonal diversification from an ancestor gene accumulating substitutions [156]. In CIS patients, the presence of a VH2-VH4 CSF bias either in CD19 or in CD138 cells, which is observed in 7/10 patients, was highly correlated with a clinical conversion to MS in the following 6 months. By contrast, none of the CIS patients without the repertoire bias had developed MS at 2 years of follow-up.

Somatic hypermutation (SHM) drives the maturation of the variable regions of the Ig genes under the control of activation-induced cytidine deaminase (AID), with a preference to the hotspot regions (RGYW/WRCY motifs) of the CDR. The antigen-driven affinity maturation process positively selects replacement mutations occurring in the CDR, which are in contact with the antigen, whereas silent mutations predominate in the framework regions. Therefore, the R/S ratio, which is lower than 2.9 before antigen-driven maturation, is expected to be higher in CDR and the same or lower in the framework regions. In MS, the R/S ratio in the CDR of Ig genes was unchanged in blood B-cells but elevated in CSF B-cells [149, 158]. This ratio is elevated for both IgG- and IgM-producing CSF B-cells and occurs to the same extent in CSF, whereas the blood IgM ratio is about half of the IgG ratio [158]. The extent of SHM is in the expected range in CSF naïve B-cells, whereas its level increases in switched memory B-cells and plasma cells [159].

It is widely admitted that AID expression is a stage-specific hallmark of germinal center B-cells undergoing SHM and gene conversion. However, an aberrant expression of AID was demonstrated in CSF B-cells producing IgG and IgM [158].

A signature score of hot/cold spots of higher/lower frequency replacement was established with six key positions, mostly situated in the CDR [160]. The signature score was 4.5 in the CSF of non-MS patients, 2.0 in the blood of MS patients, and 10.9 ± 2.0 (7.6–11.9) in the CSF of MS patients (cutoff predictive of clinically defined MS $\geq$6.8). This technique was applied to B-cells extracted from the autopsied brains of four MS patients. The scores ranged from 10 to

14.5, so B-cells from plaques and CSF share the bias [161]. Unfortunately, these bench results cannot be translated into common practice. Various clones displaying the same amino acid sequences but encoded by different nucleotides reinforce the hypothesis of antigen-driven affinity maturation [158].

In summary, B-cells in CSF demonstrate the cardinal features of an antigen-driven humoral immune response: clonal expansion and somatically hypermutated VH family sequences [155]. This suggests that these lineage cells were expanded by antigen and have undergone a germinal center reaction [162]. Moreover, there is evidence that the maturation process takes place at least partly in the CNS compartment [163].

8. Maturating B-cells undergo bidirectional exchanges across the BBB

Authors are often reluctant to localize the SHM process inside the CNS and prefer models that posit peripheral antigenic stimulation followed by CNS migration, although evidence is accumulating in favor of a local maturation process. High-throughput sequencing techniques allow the analysis of clonal B-cell populations on both sides of the BBB. A common finding is the demonstration of IgG cell lineages either restricted to one compartment (CNS, blood, and lymph node) or overlapping multiple compartments. In a study pairing CNS and cervical lymph node (CLN) B-cells, about 6–15% of the IgG B-cell sequences in plaques were recovered

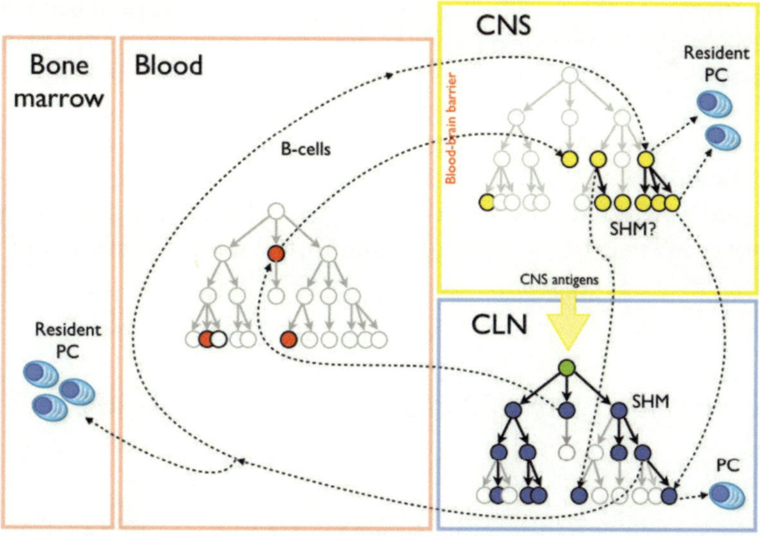

Figure 4. Schematic B-cell lineage tree and putative migration routes. Lineage founding B-cell is postulated in the CLN (green), which drains antigens and B-cells coming from the CNS. Immunoglobulins are subjected to somatic hypermutation (SHM) and proliferation in cervical lymph nodes (CLN). Migrating B-cell clones are sometimes encountered in blood on their way to the CNS. B-cell proliferation occurs both in CLN and in CNS. Evidence is growing that SHM may also occur inside the intrathecal compartment, possibly in meningeal tertiary lymphoid organs (TLOs). In such a model, rounds of B-cell maturation and proliferation may occur in a recursive way both in CNS and in CLN [14, 149]. Long-lived plasma cell (PC) differentiation occurs in the different compartments.

in the CLN [149]. Cell lineage analysis demonstrated that most of the founder cells originated in the CLN [149]. A tentative interpretation is that antigen-driven affinity maturation of B-cells takes place in the CLN, which drains CNS antigens [164], then B-cells migrate to colonies populating the CNS and continue to traffic between the CNS and the periphery, notwithstanding the possibility that a bidirectional traffic occurs in association with clonal expansion in both compartments (**Figure 4**) [149]. Clonal populations of CSF IgM- and IgG-secreting B-cells do not overlap and seem to have matured independently from each other [158]. This has been interpreted as a failure of IgM switching to IgG despite aberrant AID activity. However, only a partial overlapping of IgG and IgM populations has been demonstrated in various studies but it now needs to be replicated.

Naïve B-cells are probably not randomly recruited in the inflammatory CNS since the VH family is biased [159]. Although the fate of naïve B-cells emigrating to the CNS is still not clear, local maturation in the TLO structures and/or emigration to CLN are both probable (see below).

Most of the Ig peptides recovered from OCB by mass spectrometry match Ig-secreting CSF B-cells [14]. Moreover, clusters of related B-cells present in the CSF are also sometimes recovered from blood, the largest bi-compartmental proportion being observed in association with a recent relapse [14]. This observation may explain the existence of OCB "mirror" patterns 3 and 4 with overlapping B-cell lineage on both sides of the BBB.

8.1. Local synthesis also occurs in the eye

Inflammatory lesions are observed in the eye in association with MS and perivenous lymphocyte cuffings (i.e., periphlebitis) are commonly observed, reminiscent of lymphoid aggregates [165]. Therefore, besides the classical intrathecal Ig synthesis, local intraocular synthesis may also affect the eyes and glands. The MRZ reaction occurs with single specificity in up to 76% of cases and with ≥2 specificities in 82% [166, 167], but the ratio of F_s between Fuchs heterochromic uveitis syndrome (FHUS) and MS is about 40-fold, which is in the same range of ITS ratios as observed between MS and viral encephalitis. OCBs are always found in the CSF and aqueous humor of MS patients. Importantly, both OCB and MRZ patterns mismatch in most cases.

9. Meningeal tertiary lymphoid organs may play a role in B-cell traffic and maturation

Meningeal TLOs are ectopic follicles with germinal centers aggregating a reticulum of CD35+ and CXCL13+ stromal/dendritic follicular cells, proliferating CD20+/Ki67+ B-cells, Ig+ plasma/plasmablast cells, and CD138+ plasma cells [168]. The mantle zone is often lacking, whereas CD4+ and CD8+ T-cells infiltrate follicles [169]. CXCL13 immunoreactivity is confined to dendritiform cells inside intra-meningeal B-cell follicles [163]. The abundance of plasma cells is variable and proliferating cells in B-cell follicles, mostly CD20+ cells, are observed at rates varying from 0 to 43% [163]. CCL21 and adhesion molecule peripheral node addressin (PNAd), which selectively binds to naïve T and B lymphocytes and allows their homing to secondary lymphoid organs, are absent [163], suggesting that the homing is dependent on various markers specific to brain tissues (see reference [170]). TLO demonstration is associated with higher CSF cytokines (TNFα and IFNγ) [171] but further studies are needed. The functions of TLO have been well described in various models of peripheral inflammation. TLOs are able to mount a T-cell memory response in connection with the other lymphoid compartments [172]. In these models, the amount of Ig synthesis occurring in TLO is completely uncoupled from the blood response, meaning that local Ig-secreting cells are highly specific, although a nonspecific response is associated [173, 174]. In fact, TLOs commonly occur during EAE; AID is locally expressed in association with SHM and B-cell switching occurs [175–177]. The incidence of TLO in response to age insults is genetically determined in mice by two genes [178], but data are lacking in human and in EAE models.

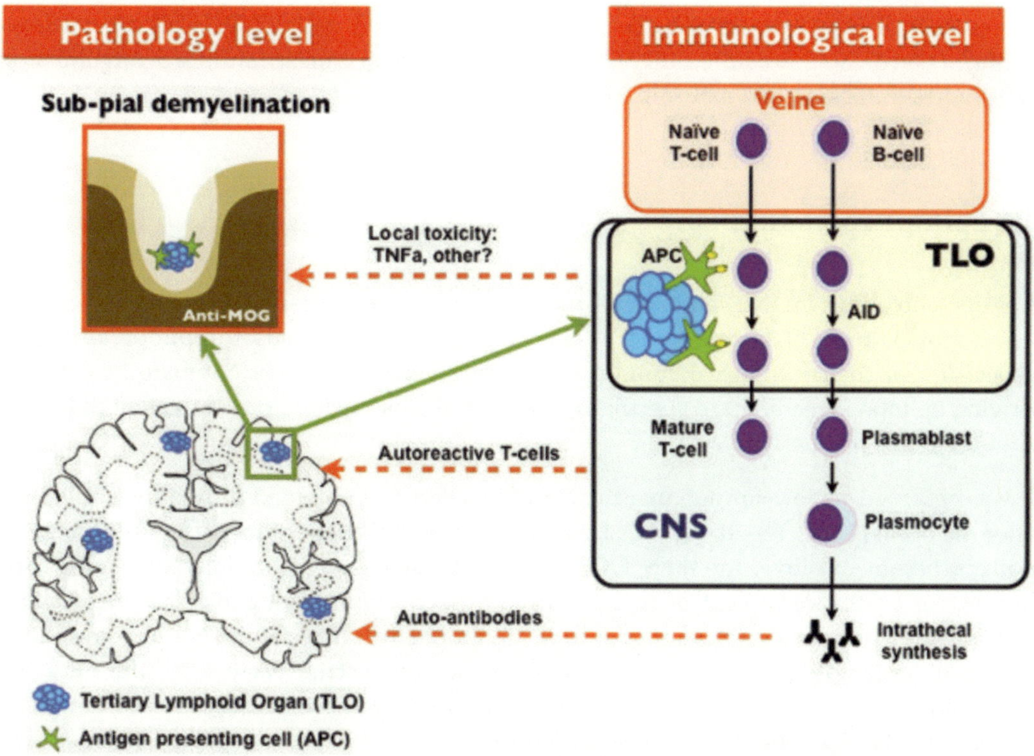

Figure 5. Schematic drawing of tertiary lymphoid organs (TLOs). A few TLOs are disseminated on the leptomeninges. At pathologic level, leptomeningeal TLOs are surrounded by subpial lesions (cell and myelin loss). The toxic mechanism is less certain and might involve TNFα secretion. At the immunological level, TLOs recruit naïve T- and B-cells that undergo antigen presentation, AID expression, affinity maturation, and proliferation of B-cells. Local Ig synthesis depends on plasmablasts/plasma cells and remains the only easily accessible bedside parameter indirectly informing about the presence of TLO (adapted from reference [179]).

In MS, the presence of TLO is associated with a more intense subpial demyelination (cortical lesions type III) and cell loss [169]. A strong topographical relationship is observed between TLO and subpial inflammation and an incidental observation showed that acute subpial lesions are associated with active local neurodegeneration (**Figure 5**) [180]. Owing to their small size and low number (about six follicles in positive blocks [168]), TLOs are probably largely underestimated by the sampling process of pathological examinations. Nevertheless, it was recently demonstrated that late post-contrast FLAIR sequences on 3T-MRI sequences might sample few leptomeningeal lesions (one lesion in 65% of patients, ≤6 in all of them) in a third of progressive patients [181], and this prevalence could be higher with 7T-MRI. Pathological examination of one of them confirmed the congruence of the MRI lesion with TLO. Given the massive underestimation of TLO lesions, the practical consequences of this technique are currently being examined for their predictive clinical value. The longitudinal evolution of these structures and the effect of immunosuppressive therapies on them are unknown. Up to now, TLO could only be examined in the removed CNS structures including brain and leptomeninges but excluding skull and dura mater. Therefore, the recently discovered dura mater lymphatic network, which drains CSF to CLN, has never been examined in the context of MS. Since lymphatics are closely associated with TLO in all other tissues, confirmation of these structures might open up unexpected avenues in studies of inflammatory cell studies trafficking and maturation [182].

10. Epitope spreading

Epitope spreading in EAE and MS is mainly documented for T-cells where it occurs in association with TLO formation [176]. The contribution of B-cells to epitope spreading, especially for their intrathecal counterpart, is less well known. The intimate mechanisms driving epitope spreading are speculative and it remains unclear to what extent SHM contributes to this process.

It was observed some years ago that the ITS of IgG becomes enriched during the early phase after MS onset [27, 42, 68–70, 74]. The frequency of the MRZ pattern increases, OCB-negative patients become positive, and more OCBs occur in the few patients initially displaying a low number of OCB. Assessment of IgG synthesis with multiplex antigen arrays now allows epitope spreading against CNS antigens to be monitored over time. Serum studies have shown that both intramolecular and intermolecular spreading occurs early after the very first demyelinating index event in children but only in patients demonstrating a further clinical MS conversion [42]. By contrast, pediatric patients remaining monophasic fail to diversify their antigenic response. A failure to regulate the aberrant autoimmune response is tentatively thought to explain this observation. Studies on early harvested CSF would give rewarding clues about CNS B-cell epitope spreading. A longitudinal description of the network of interactions in B- and T-cell epitopes (functional immunomics) at both serum and CSF level, and their interaction with HLA polymorphisms, might shed light on the pathophysiology of MS [183].

11. The problem of Ig directed against nonspecific targets

11.1. The "MRZ pattern"

ITS may occur in supposedly healthy patients or in those suffering from nonimmune CNS disorders, but in such cases, synthesis is always directed against a former healed CNS infection such as Lyme disease, VZV, or HSV [22].

The long-known "MRZ pattern" is an ITS of Ig directed against measles, rubella, and varicella zoster virus, the herpes virus sometimes being included ("MRZH"). Although the IgG fraction that belongs to this specific response in the CSF is estimated to represent less than 2% of the total amount of CSF IgG [78, 184, 185] and only a minor fraction of total OCB [77, 186, 187], the reaction is considered to be highly specific of MS. None of the MS patients in whom the MRZ pattern has been reported suffered from a history of clinical encephalitis involving these viruses. The proportion of MS patients with an elevated antibody index against ≥1 of these viruses increases over time and MS evolution [78]. This MRZ reaction is sometimes present in OCB-negative MS patients and in CIS patients who will convert and it becomes more pronounced over time, as demonstrated by follow-up LP [39, 188, 189].

ITS is polyspecific in a quarter of MS patients (against 2, 3, or 4 AI in 17, 4, and 2%), but remains monospecific (one elevated AI against M, R, Z, or H) in 22% [39]. The number of elevated AI strongly correlates with both age at spinal tap and disease duration and slightly changes over time [39, 190]. Moreover, there is a trend to a higher proportion of elevated AI in SP-MS than in RR-MS patients [191]. Immunosuppressive treatments including natalizumab are ineffective to prevent the persistence of the MRZ pattern [38, 103, 189]. Unlike in controls, no decline in AI levels occurs with age in MS patients considering either serum or CSF titers, and there is even a slight increase [192, 193].

11.2. Broadening the "MRZ pattern" to all encountered infectious agents?

A more comprehensive analysis of ITS with a larger range of infectious agents demonstrated that the MRZ pattern is an interesting concept that could be broadened. In fact, ITS against many other infectious agents has been confirmed in MS: rotavirus, HHV6 (20–30%), mumps, influenza, parainfluenza, adenovirus, respiratory syncytial virus, distemper virus, Coxsackie virus B4, vaccinia, JC virus (3%), CMV, poliovirus, toxoplasmosis (10%), *Borrelia burgdorferi* (26%), and mycoplasma (complete review in reference [194]). A previous silent CNS infection can be ruled out since the seroprevalence for each infection was the same in both MS and controls, whereas the latter had no specific reaction. Moreover, an ITS against tetanus and diphtheria toxoids was also demonstrated in vaccinated patients whose CNS was never exposed to native toxins [195, 196]. In a study of ITS against 17 infectious agents, 57% of MS patients had ITS against ≥5 infectious agents, with an increasing number over time [197], and virtually all patients demonstrated a reaction against at least one of nine viruses [198].

The pattern of reaction mirrors the individual's history of previous infections and the immunization level of the population: reaction against rubella is more observed in MS from Germany than in Cuban patients (lower incidence and immunization campaign in Cuban females) [199].

The rate of intrathecal reaction against a given infectious agent correlates with the rate of seroprevalence of this agent in the population.

Some major consequences can be drawn from these findings as follows:

1. ITS against an infectious agent in MS considered in isolation should not be considered as a clue for a chronic infection in MS, since the coexistence of reaction against many infectious agents is the rule in MS.

2. The concept of "MRZ pattern" should be extended to a "polyspecific infectious pattern."

3. The hypothesis of the antigenic mimicry of a single infectious agent should always be considered in the light of a broad reaction against various infectious agents, whose presence depends mostly on epidemiological variations.

Polyspecific ITS against all infectious agents is just a component of polyspecific ITS, which is thought to be characteristic of MS, and could throw light on the pathophysiology of MS.

11.3. Nonspecific synthesis against infectious agents is lower in MS than in CNS infections

The fraction of a specific antibody response against an infectious agent within the complete intrathecal IgG response is called the specific fraction (F_s) [200]. For example, an F_s value for measles of 2% means that 2% of the total intrathecal IgG response is directed against measles. Neuroinfections are thought to be associated with very high F_s against viruses: F_s are 8–45% for viral encephalitis (HSV, measles, VZV, subacute sclerosing panencephalitis). In other words, about 55–92% of the intrathecal Ig in infectious pathologies are directed against non-causative antigens [184, 200, 201], that is, a nonspecific ITS is very common even in neuroinfections. In MS, each specificity in the MRZH reaction typically retains a very low median F_s of 0.2–1.3% (ranging from 0.03 to 5.3) [200, 202, 203] and comparable results are obtained for F_s anti-EBV [203]. These specific F_s results are about 40-fold lower in MS patients than those found in neuroinfections without overlap.

The amount of intrathecally secreted specific antibodies should be proportional to the number of intrathecal plasma cells. If one considers that circulating plasma cells are nonspecifically and randomly selected from blood to home to CNS TLO, the relative proportion of each specific IgG synthesis in CSF should grossly parallel to their proportion in blood [197]. The ranking of specific antibody concentrations in blood and CSF differs in 67% of MS patients, confirming that CSF IgG secretion does not simply mirror blood secretion. ITS of the specific antibodies occurs independently from each other [200]. We propose two non-mutually exclusive explanations. A first hypothesis involves the differential intrathecal proliferation of specific B-cells after being recruited from blood but before being committed to terminal differentiation into plasma cells, owing to a favorable intrathecal lymphoid environment. A second hypothesis posits a nonrandom brain homing of circulating plasmablasts. It seems unlikely that plasmablast homing is driven by IgG specificity. Rather, the critical intensity of plasmablast/plasma cell recruitment to the brain owing to the intensity of the peripheral immune response to infection could be involved.

11.4. The paradox of low intrathecal anti-EBV reaction

Seroprevalence for EBV is virtually complete in MS patients, so the probability of ITS should be at least equal to or higher than other nonspecific viruses. However, anti-EBV intrathecal values have shown that an unexpectedly small proportion of patients have ITS (in the range of <20%) [203–211]. Comparing CSF OCB against HHV6 and EBV, OCB occurred twice more frequently against HHV6 than against EBV [211]. Moreover, AI against EBV is sometimes twofold lower than AI against each MRZ component [207]. A difference in seroprevalence can be ruled out. Measles and rubella seroprevalence resulting from either natural infection or vaccination exceed 90% in most populations and vaccination campaigns started decades before [39]. Furthermore, varicella seroprevalence exceeds 90% in all European populations and EBV seroprevalence is virtually complete in MS patients.

The lower-than-expected intrathecal response against EBV is not consistent with the strong correlation linking high serum anti-EBV levels and MS activity. In the light of this finding, such an extreme discrepancy can be interpreted as a strong clue for EBV infection preceding MS clinical onset [203]. Possible pathophysiological explanations have been developed elsewhere in the light of TLO [194]. The peculiar relationship between EBV and MS pathology is reinforced by the demonstration of a high intrathecal EBV-specific CD8+ cytotoxic activity only early in MS patients, without recruitment of CD8+ cells against different targets (CMV-specific CD8+ cells) [212] and the clearance of ITS in a case receiving autologous CD8+ T-cells activated against EBV [109].

11.5. Nonspecific synthesis may be a simple property of meningeal tertiary lymphoid organs

Chronic nonspecific synthesis is constant in MS, but may not strictly indicate a bystanding reaction since they are almost absent in other mostly acute CNS inflammations [194]. These unspecific reactions rather indicate a dedicated specific function suggestive of the persistence of TLO in CNS. During immune activation in the periphery, naïve B-cells undergo hypermutation of the Ig genes driven by germinal centers in the spleen and ganglia, and surviving cells are committed to plasmablasts released in the blood for a few days on their way to survival niches, where they differentiate into long-lived plasma cells. Most of the niches are situated in the bone marrow but they are also to be found in secondary and tertiary lymphoid organs, where they display the ability to retain the newly formed plasma cells. Cultures of synovial fragments (containing TLO) from rheumatoid arthritis retain the ability to secrete non-disease-specific antibodies, such as anti-tetanus toxin IgG [213]. Three weeks after, lupus-prone mice were vaccinated against OVA, and the same number of antibody-secreting cells against OVA was recovered in inflamed kidneys as in the bone marrow [214]. Therefore, nonspecific homing of plasma cells may be a common feature of inflammatory tissues and lead to local nonspecific synthesis.

The prolonged survival of retained plasma cells necessitates an anti-apoptotic environment provided by cell niches. For example, CXCL12, which is a major determinant of PC retention in niches, is elevated in MS CSF, expressed by astrocytes and in the vicinity of lymphoid infiltrates [215]. Therefore, we previously suggested that nonspecific Ig synthesis in MS might simply be a common function of TLO harvesting Ig-secreting cells, as is observed in most inflammatory disorders [194, 213]. An experimental demonstration was given by a series of MS patients who developed CSF IgG against TT after tetanus toxoid vaccination [196]. According to this assumption, the recruitment of intrathecal antibody-secreting cells should be progressive and the complete MRZ pattern might take years or even decades to achieve. This was observed in clinical studies where the mean age at spinal tap and disease duration correlated with the number of elevated antibody indices [39]. Half of the patients having fewer than 5 years of disease duration had no elevated AI (MRZ), whereas 70% of those with more than 10 years duration had AI ≥2 [39]. A similar trend was observed in a study based on 17 antigens [197].

12. Deciphering a potentially disease-related IgG ITS

12.1. MS-specific targets? A puzzling problem

From an historical point of view, the quest for an Ig target in MS has followed the methodology successfully used to solve the paradigmatic problem of subacute sclerosing panencephalitis (SSPE), where it was demonstrated that the majority of intrathecal IgG was virus-specific. Unfortunately, MS CSF demonstrated weak and inconsistent interaction with CNS antigens in numerous earlier studies. It was thereafter proposed that IgG production in MS may be due to nonsense antibodies [71]. These over-hasty conclusions should now be mitigated.

CSF Igs constitute a private repertoire that may harbor toxic properties [216]. Functional electrophysiological modifications of neurotransmission after CSF application were observed long ago. Patterns of demyelinating lesions containing Ig and complement deposition in and around macrophages are typical of pattern 2 observed in MS [148, 217, 218]. The application of CSF to cultured cells (rat cerebellar granule neurons) significantly labels the axonal surface with IgM dots [118] and purified antibodies against myelin/oligodendrocyte glycoprotein (MOG) from MS serum bind to intact myelin in rat [219]. Various recombinant antibodies (rAb) synthesized from CD138+ CSF B-cells of MS patients stain most of the glial components [220, 221] and many specific antibodies have been shown to react against cultured oligodendrocytes or human CNS tissue [222]. In animal models, anti-MOG antibodies purified from human MS serum strongly enhance lesions without increasing inflammation [219, 223]. In a model of focal implantation of hybridoma cells secreting Ig against myelin in rat spinal cord, demyelination occurred around the implantation site [224]. Moreover, the implantation of anti-GalC hybridoma cells may inhibit myelination in a complement-dependent pathway both in vivo and in vitro [225, 226]. These latter models elegantly combine focal IgG synthesis with focal anatomical lesions and are reminiscent of the infiltration by plasma cells inside non-remyelinated plaques.

In conclusion, the hypothesis that CSF Ig could play an active role in brain dysfunction, both at functional and at anatomical levels, is largely justified.

12.2. Does the microheterogeneity of ITS translate into disease heterogeneity?

Although the bulk of ITS targets unknown antigens, some of the antibody clones are thought to play an active biological role that could be either deleterious or beneficial. For example, occasional cases of MS may display anti-N-methyl-D-aspartate receptor (NMDAR) (<1%) or anti-MOG (12%) antibodies, which are associated with cognitive and demyelinating features [227]. However, until now and unlike the anti-aquaporin4 (AQP4) observed in neuromyelitis optica, none of the hundred or so identified antibodies has definitely been associated with the clinical (i.e., epilepsy, amnesia) or pathological distinctive features of MS (i.e., ability to remyelinate). The pathogenicity of these antibodies may be characterized in vitro by the extent of the demyelination or axonal loss obtained in myelinated cultures [216], by specific cell losses such as oligodendrocyte progenitors [228] or by functional alteration of synaptic transmission [89, 228]. For example, IgGs directed against MOG or sulfatide produce a complete myelin loss whereas the axons are preserved. On the other hand, IgG against neurofascine produces both myelin loss and loss of 15–40% of axons [216]. Therefore, at the global level, subsets of patients harbor variable toxicity against myelin or axons owing to one or more different antibody specificities against the targets. In the seminal work of Elliott et al. [216], a third of patients' sera were able to destroy myelin and only 6% targeted axons, but this was probably massively underestimated owing to the limited number of targets examined, fewer than 10. Heterogeneity is also present at the clonal level since different IgG clones targeting the same antigens may display different pathogenicity ranging from null to high. This clonal microheterogeneity is driven by the ability of each clone to fix complement, and, for example, among the many MOG-specific clones generated in EAE, only some of them also recognize the myelin sheath, and their pathogenicity is driven by complement fixation [187]. On the other end of the Ig spectrum, anti-MBP IgMs are associated with a more benign course. Interestingly, these Ig target a shared epitope antigen between MBP and the extracellular loop of CD64, which is one of the IgG Fc receptors responsible for the immunologic properties of macrophages [229].

Microarrays using a small subset of autoantigens discriminated immune signatures in the sera of RR, SP, and PP MS patients [84]. Interestingly, immune signatures based on 13 IgG and one IgM also discriminated pathologic patterns I and II. These results assign a main role to Ig patterns in the pathophysiology of axonal loss, and replication in the CSF may be even more informative since paired serum and CSF samples display different patterns [93]. The large-scale collection of targeted antigens would help to define the functional state of the intrathecal immune system. Moreover, the availability of techniques able to profile ITS IgG diversity and pathogenicity might help to decipher the crucial problem of predicting the severity of MS.

12.3. Putative target antigens—what do OCBs target inside the brain?

The targets are often considered to be largely unknown [230] and studies have yielded contradictory results. CSF antibodies were often considered to be nonspecific owing to their lack of specificity against the three major myelin proteins, but this does not preclude any other specificity and studies devoid of a priori may reveal unknown specificities against other membrane proteins, lipids, or glycolipids. The failure to find a major antigen for intra-BBB-synthesized Ig may not relate to a nonsense antibody production but instead may reflect the molecular complexity of the CNS and the presumed antigenic target [71]. By analogy with infectious diseases where the antigenic response is driven by pathogen antigenicity, most strategies have concentrated upon the identification of relevant antigenic targets. Paradoxically, from these efforts emerged the unexpected problem of the immense multiplicity and variability of targets.

12.3.1. A priori methods

In the last 30 years, the paradigmatic representation came by analogy with EAE models triggered by a single antigen vaccination, in line with Koch's postulates. Therefore, it was initially thought that ITS was directed against a (single) putative antigen. Unfortunately, intensive investigations of a wide range of potential targets were based on this misleading conception and failed to demonstrate any definitive association apart from more than 100 protein targets [231–233] and roughly 300 epitopes (6% being non-peptidic) [234]. Unlike in many other autoimmune disorders (e.g., myasthenia gravis), no study has succeeded in demonstrating any single antibody specificity for MS but few candidate epitopes (i.e., GAGA4) are still awaiting confirmation of their specificity by replication studies and the availability of commercial kits. Similar results have been obtained in SLE where large-scale clusters of antibodies capture significant information regarding diagnosis and prognosis, whereas limited information is obtained from routinely measured antibodies [235].

12.3.2. Non-a priori methods

12.3.2.1. Phage display

The phage display random peptide library was used to try to characterize unknown epitopes. Phagotopes identified from a CSF test pool of 10 MS patients were not recognized by the CSF of 55 other MS patients [76], which was interpreted as the demonstration that isolated phagotopes are patient- but not disease-specific epitopes [76]. In a study using a similar design, 6 clones were selected from a CSF of 4 CIS, but panning to 187 MS patients found 0–22% positivity depending on the clone and MS type [236]. In the seminal work by Yu et al. [72], one dominant peptide was isolated from each of five MS CSF. Each peptide was patient-specific, and in a given CSF, multiple OCBs (but not all) reacted against the peptide under study, confirming a restricted clonal IgG expression in CSF [72]. The specificity of CSF Ig against peptides was 10-fold higher than from serum, suggesting a local affinity maturation of antibodies.

12.3.2.2. Generation of recombinant antibodies (rAbs) from clonally expanded plasma cells from CSF

The major advantages of this technique are as follows: (a) absence of a priori knowledge of the putative targets, (b) revelation of the most representative targeted peptides, and (c) precise identification of the candidate protein. Its main drawbacks are that it samples very few clones from each CSF. The generated rAbs clones bound to neuronal or astrocyte targets but myelin array failed to identify any precise target in most of them [237]. Interestingly, the aligned protein candidates identified among the multiple CSF analysis from the different groups did not overlap, thus suggesting a broad range of specificities [72, 238].

12.3.2.3. CSF analysis with protein microarrays

Basically, protein microarray chips are high-throughput parallelized enzyme-linked immunosorbent assay (ELISA) enabling extensive analysis of the breadth of antibody response. Sera from 17 RR-MS patients were compared to those from 15 controls on a protein microarray printed with more than 3101 candidate antigens that represented multiple antigen families [231]. Although numerous candidate proteins were identified, no clue was obtained about individual pattern variability. A larger microarray displaying 37,000 tagged proteins was created in which patterns of immunoreactivity differed between individual patients [232]. The main drawback of this screening method is the biased antibody profiling approach, since the technique does not account for posttranslational modifications of proteins and non-proteic targets.

12.4. Screening new targets associated with chronic CNS inflammation

Comparison of CSF Ig recognition patterns against normal or MS brain tissue lysates revealed a profile of 16 bands highly predictive of MS, suggesting that new antigens are specifically expressed in inflamed brain [239]. Chronic inflammation was associated with the aberrant expression of carbohydrate markers, which were associated with a high level of specific antibodies in CSF [240].

Development of microarrays targeting myelin proteome or brain lipids allowed the confirmation of a diverse polyclonal reaction against these non-protidic targets both in humans and in EAE [84, 113, 241, 242]. Unconventional lipid targeting may be common since the proportion of CSF B-cells targeting lipids was as high as 27% in a study based on rAb [243] and injection of anti-sulfatid monoclonal antibody causes more severe EAE [241]. Unfortunately, only a limited number of potential targets were printed on these pioneering microarrays and only a minute number of rAb clones were obtained from a single patient.

Sugar moieties are an integral part of normal glycoproteins and glycolipids. Glycosylation occurs in the intracellular compartment where the first added sugar moieties are further masked in the mature-released glycoprotein. Such "cryptic" carbohydrate structures are potentially immunogenic as demonstrated in human immunodeficiency virus (HIV)-1 and cancer models [240]. Finally, an antigen microarray platform was constructed to display a wide range of autoantigens (proteins of the myelin sheath, liposomes of varying lipid composition, and cryptic glycan epitopes) and confirmed that CSF antibodies directed against various non-proteinic structures are common in EAE and MS [240]. Although simultaneously targeting a limited number of structures, these pioneering studies opened perspectives for subsequent work based on larger microarrays [244, 245], thereby acknowledging the necessity to include various natural targets such as peptides, lipids, and glycans of both human and foreign origin and their posttranslational modifications. Interestingly, microbe-derived polysaccharides are targeted by the host immune response and may share cross-reactivity with normal human glycan structures [245]. In-depth screening of foreign antigens including viral particles might be fruitful for deciphering a potential complex network of cross-reactivity (**Figure 6**).

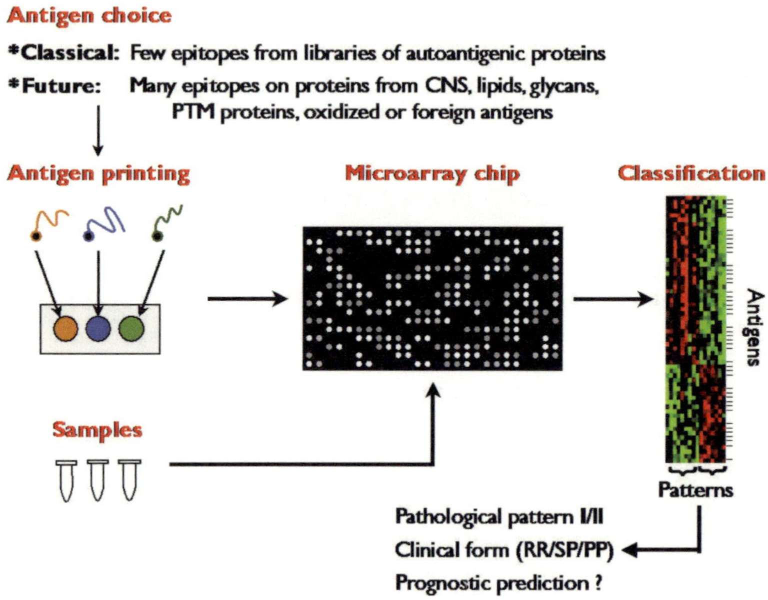

Figure 6. Overview of antigen microarray principles. Interesting antigens are selected from libraries of autoantigen peptides or foreign peptides (i.e., EBV proteins), but post-translationaly modified proteins, lipids, or glycans are suitable. Dense arrays of antigens are spotted on prepared glass slides. Patient samples (serum, CSF) are dropped on the chip, relevant antibodies hybridize to target antigens, and fluorescent-labeled antibodies are applied for detection. The specific antibody signature results in a pattern informative of disease (MS vs other) and stages (RR vs SP) and reveals the early dynamics of the antibody response [42, 93]. Future chips may include a large variety of antigens including atypical (i.e., lipids, glycans, oxidized) and foreign antigens (i.e., viral proteins).

12.5. Posttranslational modifications

About 200 posttranslational modifications for proteins and sharing common properties have been described to date: PTMs target protein hotspots, mostly exposed on the protein surface, they may occur in physiologic life or in reaction to pathology, and protein modifications are irreversible. Although PTM-targeting antibodies occurring in vivo have been rarely described until now in autoimmune disorders, they are being increasingly recognized and all of them might exist since most PTMs are targeted by commercially available monoclonal antibodies raised for research purposes. "Normal" antigens may be masked by PTM and may generate new self-antigens. A growing body of evidence suggests that PTM may play a central role in some inflammatory pathologies such as rheumatoid arthritis [246], and in inflammatory bowel diseases, type I diabetes, and atherosclerosis. Tolerance to self-antigens may be broken when self-antigens undergo protein modifications, whereby they are recognized by antibodies and T-cells as foreign antigens. This kind of molecular (self-)mimicry might trigger inflammation. Therefore, PTM may also be key players for specific autoantibody recognition in MS. This major hypothesis could account for the failure to uncover specific targets of the intrathecally synthesized antibodies screened using native protein microarrays. Screening of libraries of synthetically posttranslational-modified peptides mimicking antigenic epitopes may allow the characterization of new targets.

Citrullination is increased during EAE and MS and the targeted proteins are catabolized faster. Antibodies in rheumatoid arthritis mainly target citrullinated peptides. Methylation of arginine and lysine residues occurs in EAE brains and these PTMs are targeted in lupus erythematosus. Acetylation of intracellular proteins increases as MS evolves and acetylated MBP produces an immunodominant T-cell epitope in mice that may trigger EAE [247].

Enzymatic glycosylation of protein is a common PTM and polymorphism of N-glycan-branching enzyme (MGAT5) is associated with the risk of MS and spontaneous EAE. The MOG fragment (aa30-50) bears an N-glycosylated asparagine at position 31 that is responsible for its antigenic properties and this PTM peptide is mimicked by the synthetic peptide CSF114(Glc) [248]. Another interesting candidate is the glucose-based antigen GAGA4 [Glc(α1,4)Glc(α)] [249]. Both peptides are associated with specific serum antibodies in many MS patients.

Oxidization generates a large range of by-products since reactive oxygen species (ROS) are able to oxidize nearly all the biological components according to their oxidation potential as follows:

1. Oxidized proteins. Nitration of tyrosine residues, which normally occurs during brain aging and neurodegenerative processes, is specifically targeted by antibodies already identified during rheumatoid arthritis [246]. Malondialdehyde-acetaldehyde adducts (MAA) are generated by the reaction of products of ROS-mediated lipid peroxidation with peptidyl-lysine. MAA adducts are immunogenic in the absence of adjuvant, abundant in synovial lesions of RA, and anti-MAAs are elevated in rheumatoid arthritis and atherosclerosis patients [250]. Antibodies directed against oxidized proteins were demonstrated in the sera of EAE and SP-MS patients [251].

2. Oxidized sugars may form a stable advanced glycation end product that dramatically affects protein antigenicity since antibodies against the native form are usually non-cross reactive with the PTM form [246].

3. Oxidization of lipids may also create autoreactive antibodies. A high level of oxidation could be a distinctive feature of MS pathology in models of CNS inflammation and may be targeted by antibodies. Anti-oxidized-low-density lipoprotein (LDL) antibodies have been described in the serum of MS patients. Oxidized phosphatidylcholine is more abundant in MS brain extracts and anti-oxPCs are synthesized in the CSF of MS patients and EAE mice [252]. These results were confirmed in human MS and mice EAE with various lipid targets [241, 253]. The level of oxidative protein products in CSF does not influence the ITS level [254].

Considering the wide range of possibilities to modify self-antigens by oxidation, this process is an attractive candidate to initiate an "oxidative PTM intolerance" [255].

12.6. Designing microarrays of PTM proteins for multiplex screening with antibodies from CSF of MS patients

Most of the PTM described above are induced by enzymatic catalysis or a chemical reaction occurring under stringent conditions, and their biologic synthesis is not facilitated by the large range of parameters involved. The question is whether it is possible to print large microarrays of antigens able to express all or most of the possible combinations of PTM. Technical considerations and successful experimentation on a small scale suggest that various PTMs may be successfully applied on immobilized proteins [255, 256] and that the development of commercial PTM protein microarrays holds much promise for the future.

13. Conclusion

A distinctive feature of MS is a long-lasting intrathecal inflammatory response, unlike chronic CNS infections in which intrathecal inflammation abates after antibiotherapy. The next step will be to decipher the factors promoting the sustainment of the intrathecal inflammatory response and to identify specific antibody targets. Understanding the role of long-lived plasma cells that produce OCB during the chronic CNS surge could open up new prospects for progressive MS therapies. As Tourtellotte stated long ago, one of the goals of an effective MS treatment could be the eradication of ITS. Therapies targeting CNS B-cells to disrupt B-cell traffic on both sides of the BBB are under development and eradication of resident CNS plasma cells remains an ultimate goal.

14. Abbreviations

AI, activity index.

AID, activation-induced cytidine deaminase enzyme

BBB, blood-brain barrier

CDR, complementary-determining region

CIS, clinically isolated syndrome

CLN, cervical lymph node

CMV, cytomegalovirus

CNS, central nervous system

CSF, cerebrospinal fluid

EAE, experimental allergic encephalomyelitis

EBV, Epstein-Barr virus

http://dx.doi.org/10.5772/63201

EDSS, expanded disability status scale

FLC, free light chain

HSV, herpes simplex virus

IEF, isoelectric focusing

Ig, immunoglobulin

ITS, intrathecal (Ig) synthesis

MS, multiple sclerosis

OCB, oligoclonal bands

PP, primary progressive MS

PTM, posttranslational modification

rAb, recombinant antibodies

RR, relapsing-remitting MS

SHM, somatic hypermutation

SP, secondary progressive MS

TLO, tertiary lymphoid organs

VZV, varicella zoster virus.

Acknowledgements

We are indebted to R. Cooke for copyediting and to Christel Baigts and Aurora Medevielle for bibliographical assistance.

Author details

Mickael Bonnan

Address all correspondence to: mickael.bonnan@ch-pau.fr

Neurology and Neurovascular Unit, General Hospital, Pau, France

References

[1] Androdias G, Reynolds R, Chanal M, *et al.* Meningeal T cells associate with diffuse axonal loss in multiple sclerosis spinal cords. Ann Neurol 2010; 68(4): 465–76.

[2] Anthony IC, Crawford DH, Bell JE. B lymphocytes in the normal brain: contrasts with HIV-associated lymphoid infiltrates and lymphomas. Brain 2003; 126(Pt 5): 1058–67.

[3] Doyle KP, Quach LN, Sole M, *et al.* B-lymphocyte-mediated delayed cognitive impairment following stroke. J Neurosci 2015; 35(5): 2133–45.

[4] Felgenhauer K. Protein size and cerebrospinal fluid composition. Klin Wochenschr 1974; 52(24): 1158–64.

[5] Reiber H. Dynamics of brain-derived proteins in cerebrospinal fluid. Clin Chim Acta 2001; 310(2): 173–86.

[6] Tourtellotte WW, Potvin AR, Fleming JO, *et al.* Multiple sclerosis: measurement and validation of central nervous system IgG synthesis rate. Neurology 1980; 30(3): 240–4.

[7] Reiber H, Teut M, Pohl D, *et al.* Paediatric and adult multiple sclerosis: age-related differences and time course of the neuroimmunological response in cerebrospinal fluid. Mult Scler 2009; 15(12): 1466–80.

[8] Reiber H, Felgenhauer K. Protein transfer at the blood cerebrospinal fluid barrier and the quantitation of the humoral immune response within the central nervous system. Clin Chim Acta 1987; 163(3): 319–28.

[9] Reiber H. Flow rate of cerebrospinal fluid (CSF)—a concept common to normal blood-CSF barrier function and to dysfunction in neurological diseases. J Neurol Sci 1994; 122(2): 189–203.

[10] Reiber H, Lange P. Quantification of virus-specific antibodies in cerebrospinal fluid and serum: sensitive and specific detection of antibody synthesis in brain. Clin Chem 1991; 37(7): 1153–60.

[11] Castillo-Gomez E, Kastner A, Steiner J, *et al.* The brain as 'immunoprecipitator' of serum autoantibodies against NMDAR1. Ann Neurol 2016; 79(1):144–51

[12] Rand KH, Houck H. Improved methods for the application of random peptide phage libraries to the study of the oligoclonal bands in cerebrospinal fluid of patients with multiple sclerosis. J Neurosci Methods 2000; 101(2): 131–9.

[13] Stauch C, Reiber H, Rauchenzauner M, *et al.* Intrathecal IgM synthesis in pediatric MS is not a negative prognostic marker of disease progression: quantitative versus qualitative IgM analysis. Mult Scler 2011; 17(3): 327–34.

[14] Bankoti J, Apeltsin L, Hauser SL, *et al.* In multiple sclerosis, oligoclonal bands connect to peripheral B-cell responses. Ann Neurol 2014; 75(2): 266–76.

[15] Obermeier B, Mentele R, Malotka J, *et al.* Matching of oligoclonal immunoglobulin transcriptomes and proteomes of cerebrospinal fluid in multiple sclerosis. Nat Med 2008; 14(6): 688–93.

[16] Siden A, Kjellin KG. Isoelectric focusing of CSF and serum proteins in neurological disorders combined with benign and malignant proliferations of reticulocytes, lymphocytes and plasmocytes. J Neurol 1977; 216(4): 251–64.

[17] Tourtellotte WW, Shapshak P, Staugaitis SM, *et al.* Hypothesis: multiple sclerosis cerebrospinal fluid IgG multiple bands are derived from one or a few IgG secretor cell clones. Prog Clin Biol Res 1984; 146(371-8).

[18] Fasulo L, Fulgosi B, Colombatto S, *et al.* Uptake of polyamines by human lymphocytes. Ital J Biochem 1989; 38(4): 295A–6A.

[19] Jefferis R. Glycosylation of recombinant antibody therapeutics. Biotechnol Prog 2005; 21(1): 11–6.

[20] Halbgebauer S, Haussmann U, Klafki H, *et al.* Capillary isoelectric focusing immunoassay as a new nanoscale approach for the detection of oligoclonal bands. Electrophoresis 2015; 36(2): 355–62.

[21] Dorries R, Watanabe R, Wege H, *et al.* Analysis of the intrathecal humoral immune response in Brown Norway (BN) rats, infected with the murine coronavirus JHM. J Neuroimmunol 1987; 14(3): 305–16.

[22] Rostrom B, Link H, Laurenzi MA, *et al.* Viral antibody activity of oligoclonal and polyclonal immunoglobulins synthesized within the central nervous system in multiple sclerosis. Ann Neurol 1981; 9(6): 569–74.

[23] Cruz M, Olsson T, Ernerudh J, *et al.* Immunoblot detection of oligoclonal anti-myelin basic protein IgG antibodies in cerebrospinal fluid in multiple sclerosis. Neurology 1987; 37(9): 1515–9.

[24] Bourahoui A, De Seze J, Guttierez R, *et al.* CSF isoelectrofocusing in a large cohort of MS and other neurological diseases. Eur J Neurol 2004; 11(8): 525–9.

[25] Davies G, Keir G, Thompson E, *et al.* The clinical significance of an intrathecal monoclonal immunoglobulin band: a follow-up study. Neurology 2003; 60:1163–6.

[26] Freedman MS, Thompson EJ, Deisenhammer F, *et al.* Recommended standard of cerebrospinal fluid analysis in the diagnosis of multiple sclerosis: a consensus statement. Arch Neurol 2005; 62(6): 865–70.

[27] Villar LM, Masterman T, Casanova B, *et al.* CSF oligoclonal band patterns reveal disease heterogeneity in multiple sclerosis. J Neuroimmunol 2009; 211(1–2): 101–4.

[28] Andersson M, Alvarez-Cermeno J, Bernardi G, *et al.* Cerebrospinal fluid in the diagnosis of multiple sclerosis: a consensus report. J Neurol Neurosurg Psychiatr 1994; 57(8): 897–902.

[29] Jarius S, Eichhorn P, Wildemann B, *et al.* Usefulness of antibody index assessment in cerebrospinal fluid from patients negative for total-IgG oligoclonal bands. Fluids Barriers CNS 2012; 9(1): 14.

[30] Lolli F, Halawa I, Link H. Intrathecal synthesis of IgG, IgA, IgM and IgD in untreated multiple sclerosis and controls. Acta Neurol Scand 1989; 80(3): 238–47.

[31] Sena A, Rosado P, Ferret-Sena V, *et al.* Multiple sclerosis and intrathecal IgA synthesis. Acta Neurol Belg 1997; 97(1): 36–8.

[32] Kaplan B, Aizenbud BM, Golderman S, *et al.* Free light chain monomers in the diagnosis of multiple sclerosis. J Neuroimmunol 2010; 229(1–2): 263–71.

[33] Sindic CJ, Laterre EC. Oligoclonal free kappa and lambda bands in the cerebrospinal fluid of patients with multiple sclerosis and other neurological diseases. An immunoaffinity-mediated capillary blot study. J Neuroimmunol 1991; 33(1): 63–72.

[34] Goffette S, Schluep M, Henry H, *et al.* Detection of oligoclonal free kappa chains in the absence of oligoclonal IgG in the CSF of patients with suspected multiple sclerosis. J Neurol Neurosurg Psychiatr 2004; 75(2): 308–10.

[35] Presslauer S, Milosavljevic D, Huebl W, *et al.* Validation of kappa free light chains as a diagnostic biomarker in multiple sclerosis and clinically isolated syndrome: a multicenter study. Mult Scler 2015;22(4):502-10.

[36] Stich O, Kluge J, Speck J, *et al.* Oligoclonal restriction of antiviral immunoreaction in oligoclonal band-negative MS patients. Acta Neurol Scand. 2015; 131(6):381-8.

[37] Bednárová J, Stourac P, Adam P. Relevance of immunological variables in neuroborreliosis and multiple sclerosis. Acta Neurol Scand 2005; 112(2): 97–102.

[38] Jarius S, Franciotta D, Bergamaschi R, *et al.* Polyspecific, antiviral immune response distinguishes multiple sclerosis and neuromyelitis optica. J Neurol Neurosurg Psychiatr 2008; 79(10): 1134–6.

[39] Brecht I, Weissbrich B, Braun J, *et al.* Intrathecal, polyspecific antiviral immune response in oligoclonal band negative multiple sclerosis. PLoS One 2012; 7(7): e40431.

[40] Frederiksen JL, Sindic CJ. Intrathecal synthesis of virus-specific oligoclonal IgG, and of free kappa and free lambda oligoclonal bands in acute monosymptomatic optic neuritis. Comparison with brain MRI. Mult Scler 1998; 4(1): 22–6.

[41] Stich O, Kluge J, Speck J, *et al.* Detection of virus-specific (measles, rubella, zoster) oligoclonal IgG-bands in CSF from multiple sclerosis patients without oligoclonal bands of total IgG. Mult Scler 2009; 15(S86).

[42] Quintana FJ, Patel B, Yeste A, *et al.* Epitope spreading as an early pathogenic event in pediatric multiple sclerosis. Neurology 2014; 83(24): 2219–26.

[43] Cabre P, Heinzlef O, Merle H, *et al.* MS and neuromyelitis optica in Martinique (French West Indies). Neurology 2001; 56(4): 507–14.

[44] Yoshimura S, Isobe N, Matsushita T, *et al.* Genetic and infectious profiles influence cerebrospinal fluid IgG abnormality in Japanese multiple sclerosis patients. PLoS One 2014; 9(4): e95367.

[45] Cross AH, Stark JL, Lauber J, *et al.* Rituximab reduces B cells and T cells in cerebrospinal fluid of multiple sclerosis patients. J Neuroimmunol 2006; 180(1–2): 63–70.

[46] Izquierdo G, Angulo S, Garcia-Moreno JM, *et al.* Intrathecal IgG synthesis: marker of progression in multiple sclerosis patients. Acta Neurol Scand 2002; 105(3): 158–63.

[47] Rudick RA, Medendorp SV, Namey M, *et al.* Multiple sclerosis progression in a natural history study: predictive value of cerebrospinal fluid free kappa light chains. Mult Scler 1995; 1(3): 150–5.

[48] da Gama PD, Machado Ldos R, Livramento JA, *et al.* Oligoclonal bands in cerebrospinal fluid of black patients with multiple sclerosis. Biomed Res Int 2015; 2015(217961).

[49] Rinker JR, 2nd, Trinkaus K, Naismith RT, *et al.* Higher IgG index found in African Americans versus Caucasians with multiple sclerosis. Neurology 2007; 69(1): 68–72.

[50] Chang KH, Lyu RK, Chen CM, *et al.* Clinical characteristics of multiple sclerosis in Taiwan: a cross-sectional study. Mult Scler 2006; 12(4): 501–6.

[51] Kim SH, Huh SY, Kim W, *et al.* Clinical characteristics and outcome of multiple sclerosis in Korea: does multiple sclerosis in Korea really differ from that in the Caucasian populations? Mult Scler 2013; 19(11): 1493–8.

[52] Li B, Dong H, Zhang J, *et al.* Cerebrospinal fluid IgG profiles and oligoclonal bands in Chinese patients with multiple sclerosis. Acta Neurol Scand 2007; 115(5): 319–24.

[53] Niino M, Sato S, Fukazawa T, *et al.* Latitude and HLA-DRB1 alleles independently affect the emergence of cerebrospinal fluid IgG abnormality in multiple sclerosis. Mult Scler 2015; 21(9): 1112–20.

[54] Sellebjerg F, Jensen J, Madsen HO, *et al.* HLA DRB1*1501 and intrathecal inflammation in multiple sclerosis. Tissue Antigens 2000; 55(4): 312–8.

[55] Gama PD, Machado Ldos R, Livramento JA, *et al.* Study of oligoclonal bands restricted to the cerebrospinal fluid in multiple sclerosis patients in the city of Sao Paulo. Arq Neuropsiquiatr 2009; 67(4): 1017–22.

[56] Leone MA, Barizzone N, Esposito F, *et al.* Association of genetic markers with CSF oligoclonal bands in multiple sclerosis patients. PLoS One 2013; 8(6): e64408.

[57] Mero IL, Gustavsen MW, Saether HS, *et al.* Oligoclonal band status in Scandinavian multiple sclerosis patients is associated with specific genetic risk alleles. PLoS One 2013; 8(3): e58352.

[58] Pandey JP, Li Z. The forgotten tale of immunoglobulin allotypes in cancer risk and treatment. Exp Hematol Oncol 2013; 2(1): 6.

[59] Raposo B, Dobritzsch D, Ge C, *et al.* Epitope-specific antibody response is controlled by immunoglobulin V(H) polymorphisms. J Exp Med 2014; 211(3): 405–11.

[60] Lefranc MP, Lefranc G. Human Gm, Km, and Am allotypes and their molecular characterization: a remarkable demonstration of polymorphism. Methods Mol Biol 2012; 882:635–80.

[61] Raknes G, Fernandes Filho JA, Pandey JP, *et al.* IgG allotypes and subclasses in Norwegian patients with multiple sclerosis. J Neurol Sci 2000; 175(2): 111–5.

[62] Sandberg-Wollheim M, Baird LG, Schanfield MS, *et al.* Association of CSF IgG concentration and immunoglobulin allotype in multiple sclerosis and optic neuritis. Clin Immunol Immunopathol 1984; 31(2): 212–21.

[63] Goris A, Pauwels I, Gustavsen MW, *et al.* Genetic variants are major determinants of CSF antibody levels in multiple sclerosis. Brain 2015; 138(Pt 3): 632–43.

[64] Persson L, Longhi S, Enarsson J, *et al.* Elevated antibody reactivity to measles virus NCORE protein among patients with multiple sclerosis and their healthy siblings with intrathecal oligoclonal immunoglobulin G production. J Clin Virol 2014; 61(1):107–12.

[65] Poser CM. Multiple sclerosis trait: the premorbid stage of multiple sclerosis. A hypothesis. Acta Neurol Scand 2004; 109(4): 239–43.

[66] Duquette P, Charest L. Cerebrospinal fluid findings in healthy siblings of multiple sclerosis patients. Neurology 1986; 36(5): 727–9.

[67] Haghighi S, Andersen O, Rosengren L, *et al.* Incidence of CSF abnormalities in siblings of multiple sclerosis patients and unrelated controls. J Neurol 2000; 247(8): 616–22.

[68] Ghezzi A, Pozzilli C, Liguori M, *et al.* Prospective study of multiple sclerosis with early onset. Mult Scler 2002; 8(2): 115–8.

[69] Pohl D, Rostasy K, Reiber H, *et al.* CSF characteristics in early-onset multiple sclerosis. Neurology 2004; 63(10): 1966–7.

[70] Zeman AZ, Kidd D, McLean BN, *et al.* A study of oligoclonal band negative multiple sclerosis. J Neurol Neurosurg Psychiatr 1996; 60(1): 27–30.

[71] Walsh MJ, Tourtellotte WW. Temporal invariance and clonal uniformity of brain and cerebrospinal IgG, IgA, and IgM in multiple sclerosis. J Exp Med 1986; 163(1): 41–53.

[72] Yu X, Burgoon M, Green M, *et al.* Intrathecally synthesized IgG in multiple sclerosis cerebrospinal fluid recognizes identical epitopes over time. J Neuroimmunol 2011; 240–241: 129–36.

[73] Villar LM, Masjuan J, González-Porqué P, *et al.* Intrathecal IgM synthesis is a prognostic factor in multiple sclerosis. Ann Neurol 2003; 53(2): 222–6.

[74] Owens GP, Ritchie AM, Burgoon MP, *et al.* Single-cell repertoire analysis demonstrates that clonal expansion is a prominent feature of the B cell response in multiple sclerosis cerebrospinal fluid. J Immunol 2003; 171(5): 2725–33.

[75] Colombo M, Dono M, Gazzola P, *et al.* Maintenance of B lymphocyte-related clones in the cerebrospinal fluid of multiple sclerosis patients. Eur J Immunol 2003; 33(12): 3433–8.

[76] Cortese I, Capone S, Luchetti S, *et al.* CSF-enriched antibodies do not share specificities among MS patients. Mult Scler 1998; 4(3): 118–23.

[77] Derfuss T, Gurkov R, Then Bergh F, *et al.* Intrathecal antibody production against *Chlamydia pneumoniae* in multiple sclerosis is part of a polyspecific immune response. Brain 2001; 124(Pt 7): 1325–35.

[78] Reiber H, Ungefehr S, Jacobi C. The intrathecal, polyspecific and oligoclonal immune response in multiple sclerosis. Mult Scler 1998; 4(3): 111–7.

[79] Kuenz B, Lutterotti A, Ehling R, *et al.* Cerebrospinal fluid B cells correlate with early brain inflammation in multiple sclerosis. PLoS ONE 2008; 3(7):e2559

[80] Lamers KJ, de Reus HP, Jongen PJ. Myelin basic protein in CSF as indicator of disease activity in multiple sclerosis. Mult Scler 1998; 4(3): 124–6.

[81] Lamers KJ, Uitdehaag BM, Hommes OR, *et al.* The short-term effect of an immunosuppressive treatment on CSF myelin basic protein in chronic progressive multiple sclerosis. J Neurol Neurosurg Psychiatr 1988; 51(10): 1334–7.

[82] Confavreux C, Chapuis-Cellier C, Arnaud P, *et al.* Oligoclonal "fingerprint" of CSF IgG in multiple sclerosis patients is not modified following intrathecal administration of natural beta-interferon. J Neurol Neurosurg Psychiatr 1986; 49(11): 1308–12.

[83] Tourtellotte WW, Baumhefner RW, Syndulko K, *et al.* The long march of the cerebrospinal fluid profile indicative of clinical definite multiple sclerosis; and still marching. J Neuroimmunol 1988; 20(2–3): 217–27.

[84] Quintana FJ, Farez MF, Viglietta V, *et al.* Antigen microarrays identify unique serum autoantibody signatures in clinical and pathologic subtypes of multiple sclerosis. Proc Natl Acad Sci U S A 2008; 105(48): 18889–94.

[85] Meinl E, Krumbholz M, Derfuss T, *et al.* Compartmentalization of inflammation in the CNS: a major mechanism driving progressive multiple sclerosis. J Neurol Sci 2008; 274(1–2): 42–4.

[86] Bonnan M. Intrathecal IgG synthesis: a resistant and valuable target for future multiple sclerosis treatments. Mult Scler Int 2014; 2015:296184.

[87] Butler WT, Rossen RD. Effects of corticosteroids on immunity in man. I. Decreased serum IgG concentration caused by 3 or 5 days of high doses of methylprednisolone. J Clin Invest 1973; 52(10): 2629–40.

[88] Baumhefner RW, Booe MM, Tourtellotte WW. Modulation of de novo CNS IgG synthesis with preservation of oligoclonal IgG in multiple sclerosis. Neurology 1979; 29(4):549.

[89] Frequin ST, Barkhof F, Lamers KJ, *et al.* CSF myelin basic protein, IgG and IgM levels in 101 MS patients before and after treatment with high-dose intravenous methylprednisolone. Acta Neurol Scand 1992; 86(3): 291–7.

[90] Trotter JL, Garvey WF. Prolonged effects of large-dose methylprednisolone infusion in multiple sclerosis. Neurology 1980; 30(7 Pt 1): 702–8.

[91] Tourtellotte WW, Baumhefner RW, Potvin AR, *et al.* Multiple sclerosis de novo CNS IgG synthesis: effect of ACTH and corticosteroids. Neurology 1980; 30(11): 1155–62.

[92] Miro J, Aguayo F, Garrido JC, *et al.* Intrathecal immunoglobulin synthesis in multiple sclerosis: effect of corticosteroids and azathioprine. Eur Neurol 1992; 32(6): 349–53.

[93] Quintana F, Rahbari R, Magalhaes S, *et al.* Specific Serum Antibody Patterns Detected with Antigen Arrays Are Associated to the Development of MS in Pediatric Patients (S60.006). Neurology 2012; 78(Meeting Abstracts 1): S60.006–S60.

[94] Piccio L, Naismith RT, Trinkaus K, *et al.* Changes in B- and T-lymphocyte and chemokine levels with rituximab treatment in multiple sclerosis. Arch Neurol 2010; 67(6): 707–14.

[95] Hawker K, O'Connor P, Freedman MS, *et al.* Rituximab in patients with primary progressive multiple sclerosis: results of a randomized double-blind placebo-controlled multicenter trial. Ann Neurol 2009; 66(4): 460–71.

[96] Bonnan M, Ferrari S, Bertandeau E, *et al.* Intrathecal rituximab therapy in multiple sclerosis: review of evidence supporting the need for future trials. Curr Drugs Targets 2014; 15(13): 1205–14.

[97] Rossi S, Motta C, Studer V, *et al.* Tumor necrosis factor is elevated in progressive multiple sclerosis and causes excitotoxic neurodegeneration. Mult Scler 2014; 20(3): 304–12.

[98] Studer V, Rossi S, Motta C, *et al.* Peripheral B cell depletion and central proinflammatory cytokine reduction following repeated intrathecal administration of rituximab in progressive multiple sclerosis. J Neuroimmunol 2014;276(1-2):229-31.

[99] Harrer A, Tumani H, Niendorf S, *et al.* Cerebrospinal fluid parameters of B cell-related activity in patients with active disease during natalizumab therapy. Mult Scler 2013; 19(9): 1209–12.

[100] Mancuso R, Franciotta D, Rovaris M, *et al.* Effects of natalizumab on oligoclonal bands in the cerebrospinal fluid of multiple sclerosis patients: a longitudinal study. Mult Scler 2014;20(14):1900-3.

[101] von Glehn F, Farias AS, de Oliveira AC, *et al.* Disappearance of cerebrospinal fluid oligoclonal bands after natalizumab treatment of multiple sclerosis patients. Mult Scler 2012; 18(7): 1038–41.

[102] Romme Christensen J, Ratzer R, Bornsen L, *et al.* Natalizumab in progressive MS: results of an open-label, phase 2A, proof-of-concept trial. Neurology 2014; 82(17): 1499–507.

[103] Warnke C, Stettner M, Lehmensiek V, *et al.* Natalizumab exerts a suppressive effect on surrogates of B cell function in blood and CSF. Mult Scler 2014;21(8):1036-44.

[104] Withers DR, Fiorini C, Fischer RT, *et al.* T cell-dependent survival of CD20+ and CD20- plasma cells in human secondary lymphoid tissue. Blood 2007; 109(11): 4856–64.

[105] de Andres C, Teijeiro R, Alonso B, *et al.* Long-term decrease in VLA-4 expression and functional impairment of dendritic cells during natalizumab therapy in patients with multiple sclerosis. PLoS One 2012; 7(4): e34103.

[106] Martin M, Cravens PD, Winger R, *et al.* Decrease in the numbers of dendritic cells and CD4+ T cells in cerebral perivascular spaces due to natalizumab. Arch Neurol 2008; 65(12): 1596–603.

[107] Selter RC, Biberacher V, Grummel V, *et al.* Natalizumab treatment decreases serum IgM and IgG levels in multiple sclerosis patients. Mult Scler 2013; 19(11): 1454–61.

[108] Stuve O, Cravens PD, Frohman EM, *et al.* Immunologic, clinical, and radiologic status 14 months after cessation of natalizumab therapy. Neurology 2009; 72(5): 396–401.

[109] Pender MP, Csurhes PA, Smith C, *et al.* Epstein-Barr virus-specific adoptive immunotherapy for progressive multiple sclerosis. Mult Scler 2014;20(11):1541-4.

[110] Di Pauli F, Gredler V, Kuenz B, *et al.* Features of intrathecal immunoglobulins in patients with multiple sclerosis. J Neurol Sci 2010; 288(1–2): 147–50.

[111] Tintore M, Rovira A, Rio J, *et al.* Do oligoclonal bands add information to MRI in first attacks of multiple sclerosis? Neurology 2008; 70(13 Pt 2): 1079–83.

[112] Dalla Costa G, Passerini G, Messina MJ, *et al.* Clinical significance of the number of oligoclonal bands in patients with clinically isolated syndromes. J Neuroimmunol. 2015; 289:62-7.

[113] Villar LM, Sadaba MC, Roldan E, *et al.* Intrathecal synthesis of oligoclonal IgM against myelin lipids predicts an aggressive disease course in MS. J Clin Invest 2005; 115(1): 187–94.

[114] Boscá I, Magraner MJ, Coret F, *et al.* The risk of relapse after a clinically isolated syndrome is related to the pattern of oligoclonal bands. J Neuroimmunol 2010; 226(1–2): 143–6.

[115] Tumani H, Tourtellotte WW, Peter JB, *et al.* Acute optic neuritis: combined immunological markers and magnetic resonance imaging predict subsequent development of multiple sclerosis. The Optic Neuritis Study Group. J Neurol Sci 1998; 155(1): 44–9.

[116] Rinker JR, 2nd, Trinkaus K, Cross AH. Elevated CSF free kappa light chains correlate with disability prognosis in multiple sclerosis. Neurology 2006; 67(7): 1288–90.

[117] Villar LM, Masjuan J, Gonzalez-Porque P, *et al.* Intrathecal IgM synthesis in neurologic diseases: relationship with disability in MS. Neurology 2002; 58(5): 824–6.

[118] Beltrán E, Hernández A, Lafuente EM, *et al.* Neuronal antigens recognized by cerebrospinal fluid IgM in multiple sclerosis. J Neuroimmunol 2012; 247(1–2): 63–9.

[119] Magraner MJ, Bosca I, Simó-Castelló M, *et al.* Brain atrophy and lesion load are related to CSF lipid-specific IgM oligoclonal bands in clinically isolated syndromes. Neuroradiology 2012; 54(1): 5–12.

[120] Bosca I, Villar LM, Coret F, *et al.* Response to interferon in multiple sclerosis is related to lipid-specific oligoclonal IgM bands. Mult Scler (Houndmills, Basingstoke, England) 2010; 16(7): 810–5.

[121] Garcia-Barragan N, Villar LM, Espino M, *et al.* Multiple sclerosis patients with antilipid oligoclonal IgM show early favourable response to immunomodulatory treatment. Eur J Neurol 2009; 16(3): 380–5.

[122] Mandrioli J, Sola P, Bedin R, *et al.* A multifactorial prognostic index in multiple sclerosis. Cerebrospinal fluid IgM oligoclonal bands and clinical features to predict the evolution of the disease. J Neurol 2008; 255(7): 1023–31.

[123] Thangarajh M, Gomez-Rial J, Hedstrom AK, *et al.* Lipid-specific immunoglobulin M in CSF predicts adverse long-term outcome in multiple sclerosis. Mult Scler 2008; 14(9): 1208–13.

[124] Perini P, Ranzato F, Calabrese M, *et al.* Intrathecal IgM production at clinical onset correlates with a more severe disease course in multiple sclerosis. J Neurol Neurosurg Psychiatr 2006; 77(8): 953–5.

[125] Schneider R, Euler B, Rauer S. Intrathecal IgM-synthesis does not correlate with the risk of relapse in patients with a primary demyelinating event. Eur J Neurol 2007; 14(8): 907–11.

[126] Imrell K, Landtblom A-M, Hillert J, *et al.* Multiple sclerosis with and without CSF bands: clinically indistinguishable but immunogenetically distinct. Neurology 2006; 67(6): 1062–4.

[127] Avasarala JR, Cross AH, Trotter JL. Oligoclonal band number as a marker for prognosis in multiple sclerosis. Arch Neurol 2001; 58(12): 2044–5.

[128] Annunziata P, Giorgio A, De Santi L, *et al.* Absence of cerebrospinal fluid oligoclonal bands is associated with delayed disability progression in relapsing-remitting MS patients treated with interferon-beta. J Neurol Sci 2006; 244(1–2): 97–102.

[129] Lechner-Scott J, Spencer B, de Malmanche T, *et al.* The frequency of CSF oligoclonal banding in multiple sclerosis increases with latitude. Mult Scler 2012; 18(7): 974–82.

[130] Rojas JI, Tizio S, Patrucco L, *et al.* Oligoclonal bands in multiple sclerosis patients: worse prognosis? Neurol Res 2012; 34(9): 889–92.

[131] Siritho S, Freedman MS. The prognostic significance of cerebrospinal fluid in multiple sclerosis. J Neurol Sci 2009; 279(1–2): 21–5.

[132] Joseph FG, Hirst CL, Pickersgill TP, *et al.* CSF oligoclonal band status informs prognosis in multiple sclerosis: a case control study of 100 patients. J Neurol Neurosurg Psychiatr 2009; 80(3): 292–6.

[133] Cepok S, Rosche B, Grummel V, *et al.* Short-lived plasma blasts are the main B cell effector subset during the course of multiple sclerosis. Brain 2005; 128(Pt 7): 1667–76.

[134] Bonnan M, Barroso B, Demasles S, *et al.* Compartmentalized intrathecal immunoglobulin synthesis during HIV infection: a model of chronic CNS inflammation? J Neuroimmunol 2015; 285:41-52.

[135] Bernheimer H, Lassmann H, Suchanek G. Dynamics of IgG+, IgA+, and IgM+ plasma cells in the central nervous system of guinea pigs with chronic relapsing experimental allergic encephalomyelitis. Neuropathol Appl Neurobiol 1988; 14(2): 157–67.

[136] Dorries R, Schwender S, Imrich H, *et al.* Population dynamics of lymphocyte subsets in the central nervous system of rats with different susceptibility to coronavirus-induced demyelinating encephalitis. Immunology 1991; 74(3): 539–45.

[137] Rainey-Barger EK, Rumble JM, Lalor SJ, *et al.* The lymphoid chemokine, CXCL13, is dispensable for the initial recruitment of B cells to the acutely inflamed central nervous system. Brain Behav Immun 2011; 25(5): 922–31.

[138] Choi SR, Howell OW, Carassiti D, *et al.* Meningeal inflammation plays a role in the pathology of primary progressive multiple sclerosis. Brain 2012; 135(Pt 10): 2925–37.

[139] Iivanainen M, Driscoll B, Richert J, *et al.* Oligoclonal IgG in the cerebrospinal fluid of guinea pigs with experimental allergic encephalomyelitis. Proc Soc Exp Biol Med 1982; 171(3): 272–5.

[140] Mehta PD, Lassmann H, Wisniewski HM. Immunologic studies of chronic relapsing EAE in guinea pigs: similarities to multiple sclerosis. J Immunol 1981; 127(1): 334–8.

[141] Pachner AR, Li L, Lagunoff D. Plasma cells in the central nervous system in the Theiler's virus model of multiple sclerosis. J Neuroimmunol 2011; 232(1–2): 35–40.

[142] Walls AF, Suckling AJ, Rumsby MG. The origin and specificity of intrathecal IgG in chronic relapsing experimental allergic encephalomyelitis. Autoimmunity 1989; 2(2): 123–32.

[143] Dorries R, Liebert UG, ter Meulen V. Comparative analysis of virus-specific antibodies and immunoglobulins in serum and cerebrospinal fluid of subacute measles virus-induced encephalomyelitis (SAME) in rats and subacute sclerosing panencephalitis (SSPE). J Neuroimmunol 1988; 19(4): 339–52.

[144] Cserr HF, DePasquale M, Harling-Berg CJ, *et al.* Afferent and efferent arms of the humoral immune response to CSF-administered albumins in a rat model with normal blood-brain barrier permeability. J Neuroimmunol 1992; 41(2): 195–202.

[145] Furr M. Humoral immune responses in the horse after intrathecal challenge with ovalbumin. J Vet Intern Med 2007; 21(4): 806–11.

[146] Gordon LB, Knopf PM, Cserr HF. Ovalbumin is more immunogenic when introduced into brain or cerebrospinal fluid than into extracerebral sites. J Neuroimmunol 1992; 40(1): 81–7.

[147] Greve B, Magnusson CG, Melms A, *et al.* Immunoglobulin isotypes reveal a predominant role of type 1 immunity in multiple sclerosis. J Neuroimmunol 2001; 121(1–2): 120–5.

[148] Zhang Y, Da R-R, Hilgenberg LG, *et al.* Clonal expansion of IgA-positive plasma cells and axon-reactive antibodies in MS lesions. J Neuroimmunol 2005; 167(1–2): 120–30.

[149] Stern JN, Yaari G, Vander Heiden JA, *et al.* B cells populating the multiple sclerosis brain mature in the draining cervical lymph nodes. Sci Transl Med 2014; 6(248): 248ra107.

[150] Sindic CJ, Monteyne P, Bigaignon G, *et al.* Polyclonal and oligoclonal IgA synthesis in the cerebrospinal fluid of neurological patients: an immunoaffinity-mediated capillary blot study. J Neuroimmunol 1994; 49(1–2): 109–14.

[151] Nakano T, Matsui M, Inoue I, *et al.* Free immunoglobulin light chain: its biology and implications in diseases. Clin Chim Acta 2011; 412(11–12): 843–9.

[152] Hassan-Smith G, Durant L, Tsentemeidou A, *et al.* High sensitivity and specificity of elevated cerebrospinal fluid kappa free light chains in suspected multiple sclerosis. J Neuroimmunol 2014; 276(1–2): 175–9.

[153] Duranti F, Pieri M, Centonze D, *et al.* Determination of kappaFLC and kappa Index in cerebrospinal fluid: a valid alternative to assess intrathecal immunoglobulin synthesis. J Neuroimmunol 2013; 263(1–2): 116–20.

[154] Mehta PD. Quantitation of IgG subclasses in cerebrospinal fluid of patients with multiple sclerosis. Ann N Y Acad Sci 1988; 540:261–3.

[155] Bennett JL, Haubold K, Ritchie AM, *et al.* CSF IgG heavy-chain bias in patients at the time of a clinically isolated syndrome. J Neuroimmunol 2008; 199(1–2): 126–32.

[156] Colombo M, Dono M, Gazzola P, *et al.* Accumulation of clonally related B lymphocytes in the cerebrospinal fluid of multiple sclerosis patients. J Immunol 2000; 164(5): 2782–9.

[157] Owens GP, Winges KM, Ritchie AM, *et al.* VH4 gene segments dominate the intrathecal humoral immune response in multiple sclerosis. J Immunol 2007; 179(9): 6343–51.

[158] Beltran E, Obermeier B, Moser M, *et al.* Intrathecal somatic hypermutation of IgM in multiple sclerosis and neuroinflammation. Brain 2014; 137(Pt 10): 2703–14.

[159] Palanichamy A, Apeltsin L, Kuo TC, *et al.* Immunoglobulin class-switched B cells form an active immune axis between CNS and periphery in multiple sclerosis. Sci Transl Med 2014; 6(248): 248ra106.

[160] Cameron EM, Spencer S, Lazarini J, *et al.* Potential of a unique antibody gene signature to predict conversion to clinically definite multiple sclerosis. J Neuroimmunol 2009; 213(1–2): 123–30.

[161] Ligocki AJ, Lovato L, Xiang D, *et al.* A unique antibody gene signature is prevalent in the central nervous system of patients with multiple sclerosis. J Neuroimmunol 2010; 226(1–2): 192–3.

[162] Meinl E, Krumbholz M, Hohlfeld R. B lineage cells in the inflammatory central nervous system environment: migration, maintenance, local antibody production, and therapeutic modulation. Ann Neurol 2006; 59(6): 880–92.

[163] Serafini B, Rosicarelli B, Magliozzi R, *et al.* Detection of ectopic B-cell follicles with germinal centers in the meninges of patients with secondary progressive multiple sclerosis. Brain Pathol (Zurich, Switzerland) 2004; 14(2): 164–74.

[164] Walter BA, Valera VA, Takahashi S, *et al.* Evidence of antibody production in the rat cervical lymph nodes after antigen administration into the cerebrospinal fluid. Arch Histol Cytol 2006; 69(1): 37–47.

[165] Arnold AC, Pepose JS, Hepler RS, *et al.* Retinal periphlebitis and retinitis in multiple sclerosis. I. Pathologic characteristics. Ophthalmology 1984; 91(3): 255–62.

[166] Quentin CD, Reiber H. Fuchs heterochromic cyclitis: rubella virus antibodies and genome in aqueous humor. Am J Ophthalmol 2004; 138(1): 46–54.

[167] Reiber H, Kruse-Sauter H, Quentin CD. Antibody patterns vary arbitrarily between cerebrospinal fluid and aqueous humor of the individual multiple sclerosis patient: specificity-independent pathological B cell function. J Neuroimmunol 2015; 278:247–54).

[168] Magliozzi R, Howell O, Vora A, *et al.* Meningeal B-cell follicles in secondary progressive multiple sclerosis associate with early onset of disease and severe cortical pathology. Brain 2007; 130(Pt 4): 1089–104.

[169] Magliozzi R, Howell OW, Reeves C, *et al.* A gradient of neuronal loss and meningeal inflammation in multiple sclerosis. Ann Neurol 2010; 68(4): 477–93.

[170] Chaitanya GV, Omura S, Sato F, *et al.* Inflammation induces neuro-lymphatic protein expression in multiple sclerosis brain neurovasculature. J Neuroinflammation 2013; 10(1): 125.

[171] Gardner C, Magliozzi R, Durrenberger PF, *et al.* Cortical grey matter demyelination can be induced by elevated pro-inflammatory cytokines in the subarachnoid space of MOG-immunized rats. Brain 2013; 136(Pt 12): 3596–608.

[172] Nasr IW, Reel M, Oberbarnscheidt MH, *et al.* Tertiary lymphoid tissues generate effector and memory T cells that lead to allograft rejection. Am J Transplant 2007; 7(5): 1071–9.

[173] Thaunat O, Patey N, Caligiuri G, *et al.* Chronic rejection triggers the development of an aggressive intragraft immune response through recapitulation of lymphoid organogenesis. J Immunol 2010; 185(1): 717–28.

[174] Thaunat O, Patey N, Morelon E, *et al.* Lymphoid neogenesis in chronic rejection: the murderer is in the house. Curr Opin Immunol 2006; 18(5): 576–9.

[175] Columba-Cabezas S, Griguoli M, Rosicarelli B, *et al.* Suppression of established experimental autoimmune encephalomyelitis and formation of meningeal lymphoid follicles by lymphotoxin β receptor-Ig fusion protein. J Neuroimmunol 2006; 179(1–2): 76–86.

[176] Kuerten S, Schickel A, Kerkloh C, *et al.* Tertiary lymphoid organ development coincides with determinant spreading of the myelin-specific T cell response. Acta Neuropathol 2012; 124(6): 861–73.

[177] Peters A, Pitcher LA, Sullivan JM, *et al.* Th17 cells induce ectopic lymphoid follicles in central nervous system tissue inflammation. Immunity 2011; 35(6): 986–96.

[178] Huang Y, Caputo CR, Noordmans GA, *et al.* Identification of novel genes associated with renal tertiary lymphoid organ formation in aging mice. PLoS One 2014; 9(3): e91850.

[179] Bonnan M. Meningeal tertiary organs: Major actors in intrathecal autoimmunity. Rev Neurol (Paris) 2014; 171(1): 65–74.

[180] Lucchinetti CF, Popescu BF, Bunyan RF, *et al.* Inflammatory cortical demyelination in early multiple sclerosis. N Engl J Med 2011; 365(23): 2188–97.

[181] Absinta M, Vuolo L, Rao A, *et al.* Gadolinium-based MRI characterization of leptomeningeal inflammation in multiple sclerosis. Neurology 2015; 85(1): 18–28.

[182] Aspelund A, Antila S, Proulx ST, *et al.* A dural lymphatic vascular system that drains brain interstitial fluid and macromolecules. J Exp Med 2015; 212(7): 991–9.

[183] Braga-Neto UM, Marques ET, Jr. From functional genomics to functional immunomics: new challenges, old problems, big rewards. PLoS Comput Biol 2006; 2(7): e81.

[184] Reiber H. Cerebrospinal fluid—physiology, analysis and interpretation of protein patterns for diagnosis of neurological diseases. Mult Scler 1998; 4(3): 99–107.

[185] Rostasy K, Reiber H, Pohl D, *et al.* Chlamydia pneumoniae in children with MS: frequency and quantity of intrathecal antibodies. Neurology 2003; 61(1): 125–8.

[186] Franciotta D, Di Stefano AL, Jarius S, *et al.* Cerebrospinal BAFF and Epstein-Barr virus-specific oligoclonal bands in multiple sclerosis and other inflammatory demyelinating neurological diseases. J Neuroimmunol 2011; 230(1–2): 160–3.

[187] Owens GP, Burgoon MP, Devlin ME, *et al.* Extraction and purification of active IgG from SSPE and MS brain. J Virol Methods 1997; 68(2): 119–25.

[188] Brettschneider J, Tumani H, Kiechle U, *et al.* IgG antibodies against measles, rubella, and varicella zoster virus predict conversion to multiple sclerosis in clinically isolated syndrome. PloS One 2009; 4(11): e7638.

[189] Petereit HF, Reske D. Expansion of antibody reactivity in the cerebrospinal fluid of multiple sclerosis patients – follow-up and clinical implications. Cerebrospinal Fluid Res 2005; 2:3.

[190] Sandberg-Wollheim M, Vandvik B, Nadj C, *et al.* The intrathecal immune response in the early stage of multiple sclerosis. J Neurol Sci 1987; 81(1): 45–53.

[191] Fainardi E, Castellazzi M, Tamborino C, *et al.* Chlamydia pneumoniae-specific intrathecal oligoclonal antibody response is predominantly detected in a subset of multiple sclerosis patients with progressive forms. J Neurovirol 2009; 15(5–6): 425–33.

[192] Ahlgren C, Oden A, Bergstrom T, *et al.* Serum and CSF measles antibody levels increase over time in patients with multiple sclerosis or clinically isolated syndrome. J Neuroimmunol 2012; 247(1–2): 70–4.

[193] Ahlgren C, Oden A, Haghighi S, *et al.* The effect of live, attenuated measles vaccine and measles infection on measles antibody levels in serum and CSF of patients with multiple sclerosis or clinically isolated syndrome. J Neuroimmunol 2011; 235(1–2): 98–103.

[194] Bonnan M. Does disease-irrelevant intrathecal synthesis in multiple sclerosis make sense in the light of tertiary lymphoid organs? Front Neurol 2014; 5:27.

[195] Salmi A, Viljanen M, Reunanen M. Intrathecal synthesis of antibodies to diphtheria and tetanus toxoids in multiple sclerosis patients. J Neuroimmunol 1981; 1(3): 333–41.

[196] Sandberg-Wollheim M, Zweiman B, Levinson AI, *et al.* Humoral immune responses within the human central nervous system following systemic immunization. J Neuroimmunol 1986; 11(3): 205–14.

[197] Salmi A, Reunanen M, Ilonen J, *et al.* Intrathecal antibody synthesis to virus antigens in multiple sclerosis. Clin Exp Immunol 1983; 52(2): 241–9.

[198] Arnadottir T, Reunanen M, Salmi A. Intrathecal synthesis of virus antibodies in multiple sclerosis patients. Infect Immun 1982; 38(2): 399–407.

[199] Robinson-Agramonte M, Reiber H, Cabrera-Gomez JA, *et al.* Intrathecal polyspecific immune response to neurotropic viruses in multiple sclerosis: a comparative report from Cuban patients. Acta Neurol Scand 2007; 115(5): 312–8.

[200] Jacobi C, Lange P, Reiber H. Quantitation of intrathecal antibodies in cerebrospinal fluid of subacute sclerosing panencephalitis, herpes simplex encephalitis and multiple sclerosis: discrimination between microorganism-driven and polyspecific immune response. J Neuroimmunol 2007; 187(1–2): 139–46.

[201] Conrad AJ, Chiang EY, Andeen LE, *et al.* Quantitation of intrathecal measles virus IgG antibody synthesis rate: subacute sclerosing panencephalitis and multiple sclerosis. J Neuroimmunol 1994; 54(1–2): 99–108.

[202] Otto C, Hofmann J, Finke C, *et al.* The fraction of varicella zoster virus-specific antibodies among all intrathecally-produced antibodies discriminates between patients with varicella zoster virus reactivation and multiple sclerosis. Fluids Barriers CNS 2014; 11(1): 3.

[203] Otto C, Oltmann A, Stein A, *et al.* Intrathecal EBV antibodies are part of the polyspecific immune response in multiple sclerosis. Neurology 2011; 76(15): 1316–21.

[204] Castellazzi M, Contini C, Tamborino C, *et al.* Epstein-Barr virus-specific intrathecal oligoclonal IgG production in relapsing-remitting multiple sclerosis is limited to a subset of patients and is composed of low-affinity antibodies. J Neuroinflammation 2014; 11:188.

[205] Castellazzi M, Tamborino C, Cani A, *et al.* Epstein-Barr virus-specific antibody response in cerebrospinal fluid and serum of patients with multiple sclerosis. Mult Scler 2010; 16(7): 883–7.

[206] Nociti V, Frisullo G, Marti A, *et al.* Epstein-Barr virus antibodies in serum and cerebrospinal fluid from multiple sclerosis, chronic inflammatory demyelinating polyradiculoneuropathy and amyotrophic lateral sclerosis. J Neuroimmunol 2010; 225(1–2): 149–52.

[207] Pohl D, Rostasy K, Jacobi C, *et al.* Intrathecal antibody production against Epstein-Barr and other neurotropic viruses in pediatric and adult onset multiple sclerosis. J Neurol 2010; 257(2): 212–6.

[208] Rand KH, Houck H, Denslow ND, *et al.* Epstein-Barr virus nuclear antigen-1 (EBNA-1) associated oligoclonal bands in patients with multiple sclerosis. J Neurol Sci 2000; 173(1): 32–9.

[209] Sargsyan SA, Shearer AJ, Ritchie AM, *et al.* Absence of Epstein-Barr virus in the brain and CSF of patients with multiple sclerosis. Neurology 2010; 74(14): 1127–35.

[210] Villegas E, Santiago O, Carrillo JA, *et al.* Low intrathecal immune response of anti-EBNA-1 antibodies and EBV DNA from multiple sclerosis patients. Diagn Microbiol Infect Dis 2011; 70(1): 85–90.

[211] Virtanen JO, Wohler J, Fenton K, *et al.* Oligoclonal bands in multiple sclerosis reactive against two herpesviruses and association with magnetic resonance imaging findings. Mult Scler 2014; 20(1): 27–34.

[212] Jaquiery E, Jilek S, Schluep M, *et al.* Intrathecal immune responses to EBV in early MS. Eur J Immunol 2010; 40(3): 878–87.

[213] Rosengren S, Wei N, Kalunian KC, *et al.* Elevated autoantibody content in rheumatoid arthritis synovia with lymphoid aggregates and the effect of rituximab. Arthr Res Ther 2008; 10(5): R105.

[214] Cassese G, Lindenau S, de Boer B, *et al.* Inflamed kidneys of NZB/W mice are a major site for the homeostasis of plasma cells. Eur J Immunol 2001; 31(9): 2726–32.

[215] Corcione A, Casazza S, Ferretti E, *et al.* Recapitulation of B cell differentiation in the central nervous system of patients with multiple sclerosis. Proc Natl Acad Sci U S A 2004; 101(30): 11064–9.

[216] Elliott C, Lindner M, Arthur A, *et al.* Functional identification of pathogenic autoantibody responses in patients with multiple sclerosis. Brain 2012; 135(Pt 6): 1819–33.

[217] Breij ECW, Brink BP, Veerhuis R, *et al.* Homogeneity of active demyelinating lesions in established multiple sclerosis. Ann Neurol 2008; 63(1): 16–25.

[218] Sadaba MC, Tzartos J, Paino C, *et al.* Axonal and oligodendrocyte-localized IgM and IgG deposits in MS lesions. J Neuroimmunol 2012; 247(1–2): 86–94.

[219] Zhou D, Srivastava R, Nessler S, *et al.* Identification of a pathogenic antibody response to native myelin oligodendrocyte glycoprotein in multiple sclerosis. Proc Natl Acad Sci U S A 2006; 103(50): 19057–62.

[220] von Budingen HC, Harrer MD, Kuenzle S, *et al.* Clonally expanded plasma cells in the cerebrospinal fluid of MS patients produce myelin-specific antibodies. Eur J Immunol 2008; 38(7): 2014–23.

[221] Zhang Y, Da R-R, Guo W, *et al.* Axon reactive B cells clonally expanded in the cerebrospinal fluid of patients with multiple sclerosis. J Clin Immunol 2005; 25(3): 254–64.

[222] Pandey S, Alcaro MC, Scrima M, *et al.* Designed glucopeptides mimetics of myelin protein epitopes as synthetic probes for the detection of autoantibodies, biomarkers of multiple sclerosis. J Med Chem 2012; 55(23): 10437–47.

[223] Linington C, Lassmann H. Antibody responses in chronic relapsing experimental allergic encephalomyelitis: correlation of serum demyelinating activity with antibody titre to the myelin/oligodendrocyte glycoprotein (MOG). J Neuroimmunol 1987; 17(1): 61–9.

[224] Rosenbluth J, Schiff R, Liang W-L, *et al.* Antibody-mediated CNS demyelination II. Focal spinal cord lesions induced by implantation of an IgM antisulfatide-secreting hybridoma. J Neurocytol 2003; 32(3): 265–76.

[225] Blauth K, Soltys J, Matschulat A, *et al.* Antibodies produced by clonally expanded plasma cells in multiple sclerosis cerebrospinal fluid cause demyelination of spinal cord explants. Acta Neuropathol 2015; 130(6): 765–81.

[226] Keirstead HS, Pataky DM, McGraw J, *et al.* In vivo immunological suppression of spinal cord myelin development. Brain Res Bull 1997; 44(6): 727–34.

[227] Ramberger M, Bsteh G, Schanda K, *et al.* NMDA receptor antibodies: a rare association in inflammatory demyelinating diseases. Neurol Neuroimmunol Neuroinflamm 2015; 2(5): e141.

[228] Niehaus A, Shi J, Grzenkowski M, *et al.* Patients with active relapsing-remitting multiple sclerosis synthesize antibodies recognizing oligodendrocyte progenitor cell surface protein: implications for remyelination. Ann Neurol 2000; 48(3): 362–71.

[229] Annunziata P, Cioni C, Cantalupo L, *et al.* Immunosuppressive monoclonal antibody to CD64 from patients with long-term stable multiple sclerosis. J Neuroimmunol 2013; 256(1–2): 62–70.

[230] Gredler V, Reindl M. B cells accumulate in the cerebrospinal fluid in inflammatory neurological diseases. J Cytol Histol 2012; S1(001): 1–7.

[231] Beyer NH, Lueking A, Kowald A, *et al.* Investigation of autoantibody profiles for cerebrospinal fluid biomarker discovery in patients with relapsing-remitting multiple sclerosis. J Neuroimmunol 2012; 242(1–2): 26–32.

[232] Cepok S, Zhou D, Srivastava R, *et al.* Identification of Epstein-Barr virus proteins as putative targets of the immune response in multiple sclerosis. J Clin Invest 2005; 115(5): 1352–60.

[233] Fraussen J, Claes N, deBock L, *et al.* Targets of the humoral autoimmune response in multiple sclerosis. Autoimmun Rev 2014; Nov;13(11):1126-37

[234] Vaughan K, Peters B, O'Connor KC, *et al.* A molecular view of multiple sclerosis and experimental autoimmune encephalitis: what can we learn from the epitope data? J Neuroimmunol 2014; 267(1–2): 73–85.

[235] Sherer Y, Gorstein A, Fritzler MJ, *et al.* Autoantibody explosion in systemic lupus erythematosus: more than 100 different antibodies found in SLE patients. Semin Arthr Rheum 2004; 34(2): 501–37.

[236] Rouwette M, Somers K, Govarts C, *et al.* Novel cerebrospinal fluid and serum autoantibody targets for clinically isolated syndrome. J Neurochem 2012; 123(4): 568–77.

[237] Ligocki AJ, Rivas JR, Rounds WH, *et al.* A distinct class of antibodies may be an indicator of gray matter autoimmunity in early and established relapsing remitting multiple sclerosis patients. ASN Neuro 2015; 7:5.

[238] Somers V, Govarts C, Somers K, *et al.* Autoantibody profiling in multiple sclerosis reveals novel antigenic candidates. J Immunol (Baltimore, MD: 1950) 2008; 180(6): 3957–63.

[239] Lefranc D, Almeras L, Dubucquoi S, *et al.* Distortion of the self-reactive IgG antibody repertoire in multiple sclerosis as a new diagnostic tool. J Immunol 2004; 172(1): 669–78.

[240] Wang D, Bhat R, Sobel RA, *et al.* Uncovering cryptic glycan markers in multiple sclerosis (MS) and experimental autoimmune encephalomyelitis (EAE). Drug Dev Res 2014; 75(3): 172–88.

[241] Kanter JL, Narayana S, Ho PP, *et al.* Lipid microarrays identify key mediators of autoimmune brain inflammation. Nat Med 2006; 12(1): 138–43.

[242] Robinson WH, Fontoura P, Lee BJ, *et al.* Protein microarrays guide tolerizing DNA vaccine treatment of autoimmune encephalomyelitis. Nat Biotechnol 2003; 21(9): 1033–9.

[243] Brennan KM, Galban-Horcajo F, Rinaldi S, *et al.* Lipid arrays identify myelin-derived lipids and lipid complexes as prominent targets for oligoclonal band antibodies in multiple sclerosis. J Neuroimmunol 2011; 238(1–2): 87–95.

[244] Hecker M, Lorenz P, Steinbeck F, *et al.* Computational analysis of high-density peptide microarray data with application from systemic sclerosis to multiple sclerosis. Autoimmun Rev 2012; 11(3): 180–90.

[245] Wang D, Liu S, Trummer BJ, *et al.* Carbohydrate microarrays for the recognition of cross-reactive molecular markers of microbes and host cells. Nat Biotechnol 2002; 20(3): 275–81.

[246] Burska AN, Hunt L, Boissinot M, *et al.* Autoantibodies to posttranslational modifications in rheumatoid arthritis. Mediators Inflamm 2014; 2014:492873.

[247] Zamvil SS, Mitchell DJ, Moore AC, *et al.* T-cell epitope of the autoantigen myelin basic protein that induces encephalomyelitis. Nature 1986; 324(6094): 258–60.

[248] Papini AM. The use of post-translationally modified peptides for detection of biomarkers of immune-mediated diseases. J Pept Sci 2009; 15(10): 621–8.

[249] Brettschneider J, Jaskowski TD, Tumani H, *et al.* Serum anti-GAGA4 IgM antibodies differentiate relapsing remitting and secondary progressive multiple sclerosis from primary progressive multiple sclerosis and other neurological diseases. J Neuroimmunol 2009; 217(1–2): 95–101.

[250] Thiele GM, Duryee MJ, Anderson DR, *et al.* Malondialdehyde-acetaldehyde adducts and anti-malondialdehyde-acetaldehyde antibodies in rheumatoid arthritis. Arthr Rheumatol 2015; 67(3): 645–55.

[251] Boullerne AI, Rodriguez JJ, Touil T, *et al.* Anti-S-nitrosocysteine antibodies are a predictive marker for demyelination in experimental autoimmune encephalomyelitis: implications for multiple sclerosis. J Neurosci 2002; 22(1): 123–32.

[252] Qin J, Goswami R, Balabanov R, *et al.* Oxidized phosphatidylcholine is a marker for neuroinflammation in multiple sclerosis brain. J Neurosci Res 2007; 85(5): 977–84.

[253] Ho PP, Kanter JL, Johnson AM, *et al.* Identification of naturally occurring fatty acids of the myelin sheath that resolve neuroinflammation. Sci Transl Med 2012; 4(137): 137ra73.

[254] Pasquali L, Pecori C, Chico L, *et al.* Relation between plasmatic and cerebrospinal fluid oxidative stress biomarkers and intrathecal Ig synthesis in multiple sclerosis patients. J Neuroimmunol 2015; 283:39–42).

[255] Eggleton P, Nissim A, Ryan BJ, *et al.* Detection and isolation of human serum autoantibodies that recognize oxidatively modified autoantigens. Free Radic Biol Med 2013; 57:79–91.

[256] Merbl Y, Kirschner MW. Protein microarrays for genome-wide posttranslational modification analysis. Wiley Interdiscip Rev Syst Biol Med 2011; 3(3): 347–56.

Chapter 4

Autoimmune Processes in Multiple Sclerosis: Production of Harmful Catalytic Antibodies Associated with Significant Changes in the Hematopoietic Stem Cell Differentiation and Proliferation

Georgy A. Nevinsky

Additional information is available at the end of the chapter

http://dx.doi.org/10.5772/63824

Abstract

Multiple sclerosis (MS) is a chronic demyelinating disease of the central nervous system. MS pathogenesis is not clear. Destruction of myelin by inflammation caused by autoimmune reactions has been proposed. Interestingly, healthy humans usually do not develop abzymes (Abzs). It was shown that DNase and MBP-hydrolyzing Abzs are easily detectable at the beginning of autoimmune diseases (ADs) including MS, when concentrations of antibodies to autoantigens are not yet significantly increased and correspond to levels in healthy donors. In addition, the relative enzymatic activity of antibodies from cerebrospinal fluid (CSF) is ~50-fold higher than that from the sera of the same MS patients. Experimental autoimmune encephalomyelitis (EAE) in C57BL/6 mice, a model mimicking relevant aspects of human MS was used. During development of spontaneous and MOG35-55-induced EAE in C57BL/6 mice, a specific reorganization of the immune system of mice was observed. It leads to a condition which was associated with the generation of catalytically active IgGs-hydrolyzing DNA, myelin basic protein (MBP), and MOG. Production of Abzs was associated with increased proteinuria, leading changes in differentiation of mice bone marrow hematopoietic stem cells (HSCs) and an increase in proliferation of lymphocytes in bone marrow, spleen, and thymus as well as a significant suppression of cell apoptosis in these organs. Treatment of control non-autoimmune CBA mice with MOG led to the different differentiation and proliferation of HSCs comparing with EAE C57BL/6 mice. The treatment of EAE mice with cuprizone inducing demyelination lead to a significant decrease in the size of the brain corpus callosum, but do not significantly change the differentiation profile of HSCs differentiation when compared with untreated mice. It indicates that cuprizone treatment is associated with demyelination, but not autoimmune reactivity. The possible differences in immune system reorganizations during preclinical phases of the disease, acute and late EAE, leading to production of different autoantibodies and Abzs as well other changes are discussed.

Keywords: catalytic antibodies, autoimmunity, hematopoietic stem cells, multiple sclerosis, cell differentiation, cell proliferation

1. Introduction

Classically, antibodies (Abs) have been characterized as proteins produced by the immune system, which have the sole function of binding other molecules, called antigens, and eliciting an immune response. In this classical conception, Abs act similarly to enzymes in specific binding to other molecules. However, in contrast to enzymes, they do not have the ability to catalyze chemical conversions of their bound partners. For the vast majority of Abs, this observation is correct. However, it was shown that antibodies against chemically stable analogues of the transition states of chemical reaction can possess different enzymatic activities [1–8]. These artificial catalytic Abs were termed "abzymes" (derived from antibody enzymes). Abzymes (Abzs) catalyzing more than 100 distinct chemical reactions are novel biological catalysts that attracted interest in recent years reviewed repeatedly [1–8].

The first example of natural Abzs was an IgG found in bronchial asthma patients, which hydrolyzed intestinal vasoactive peptide [9], the second Abz was an IgG with DNase activity in a systemic lupus erythematosus (SLE) patient [10], and the third was an IgG with RNase activity in an SLE patient [11]. Later, catalytic IgGs and/or IgAs, IgMs hydrolyzing different oligopeptides, proteins, DNA, RNA, nucleotides, and polysaccharides were detected in the sera of patients with several autoimmune diseases (ADs) and some viral pathologies (for review see [8, 12–21] and refs therein).

Some Abs and auto-Abs with different catalytic activities may be induced spontaneously by primary antigens and can have characteristics of the primary antigen, including the catalytic activity of idiotypic and/or anti-idiotypic Abs [8, 12–21]. Healthy humans usually do not develop catalytic Abs or their activities are very low. Detection of Abzs was shown to be the earliest indicator of development of different ADs [8, 12–21]. At the early stages of ADs, the repertoire of Abzs is usually relatively narrow, but it greatly expands with the progress of the disease, leading to the generation of catalytically diverse Abs with various activities and functions [8, 12–21]. Some Abzs are cytotoxic and can play an important negative role in the pathogenesis of different ADs, while positive roles have been also proposed for other Abzs [8, 12–21]. Abzs activities increase in association with a specific reorganization of the immune system, such as differentiation and proliferation of bone marrow hematopoietic stem cells and lymphocyte proliferation in various organs of SLE mice [22–24]. Different mechanisms of Abzs production exist in healthy externally immunized animals and of autoimmune mammals during the development of pathological reactions were revealed ([8, 12–24], see below).

Catalysis by auto-Abzs is potentially applicable in many different fields, including efficient catalysts, the generation of new drugs, and evaluation of the functional roles of Abzs in innate and adaptive immunity, the understanding of self-tolerance and of destructive responses in ADs [25–27]. Abzs can be employed for the development of new of drugs, some of which may be useful for therapy.

In this review, Abzs with different catalytic activities in multiple sclerosis (MS) are compared with other Abzs in ADs. In addition, a role of defects of immune systems leading to changes in differentiation of mice bone marrow hematopoietic stem cells (HSCs) and an increase in proliferation of lymphocytes in bone marrow, spleen, and thymus as well as a significant suppression of cell apoptosis in these organs associated with the production of Abzs is discussed.

2. Features of the immune status of patients with multiple sclerosis

The development of ADs is characterized by spontaneous generation of primary Abs to proteins, nucleic acids and their complexes, polysaccharides, nucleotides, etc. [8, 16–21, 28–32]. The origin of natural Abzs is complex. On the one hand, they are similar to artificial Abzs may be directed against analogues of transitional states of catalytic reagents or even against substrates of enzymes acting as haptens. Some antigens may change conformation when they associate with other proteins, and their structure in such complexes could mimic that of a transitional state of the antigenic reaction. On the other hand, later in ADs anti-idiotypic Abs can be induced by a primary antigen and may show some of the characteristics of catalytic activity [8, 33, 34].

MS is known as a chronic demyelinating disease of the central nervous system. Its etiology to date is unclear, and the most widely accepted theory of MS pathogenesis assigns the main role in the destruction of myelin to the inflammation related to autoimmune (AI) reactions [32]. Activated CD4+ myelin-reactive T cells are generally considered as major mediators of MS. Several recent findings imply an important role of B cells and auto-Abs against myelin autoantigens in the pathogenesis of MS [32, 33, 35, 36]. Different studies suggest that a crucial role in MS immunopathogenesis can belong to auto-Abs against myelin autoantigens exercising Ab-mediated demyelination [36]. Auto-antibodies against oligodendrocyte progenitor cell surface protein could block remyelination by eliminating or incapacitating these cells [37]. An important dual role of auto-Abs is suggested: They may be harmful in lesion formation but also potentially beneficial in the repair [35]. It is appropriate to mention here that the main targets of both above-mentioned auto-Abs are glycoproteins: myelin oligodendrocyte glycoprotein that is expressed preferentially on the surface of the myelin sheath [38] and progenitor cell-specific surface glycoprotein AN2 [37], respectively. Elevated level of oligoclonal IgGs in the cerebrospinal fluid (CSF) and B cell accumulation in the CSF and in lesions of MS patients provide evidence for antibody involvement in demyelination [39].

After cloning, the IgG repertoire directly from active plaques and periplaque regions in MS brain and from B cells recovered from the cerebrospinal fluid of a patient with MS with subacute disease for understanding MS pathogenesis new keys have been proposed [40]. It was shown that in the MS patients' high-affinity anti-DNA Abs are the major components of intrathecal IgG response. Furthermore, DNA-specific monoclonal Abs obtained from patients with MS and DNA-specific Ab derived from a SLE patient bound efficiently to the oligodendrocytes and surface of neuronal cells. Cell-surface recognition of these Abs was DNA-dependent. The results obtained indicate that anti-DNA Abs may promote important neuropathological mechanisms in chronic inflammatory disorders, such as MS and SLE [40]. It should be mentioned that SLE and MS demonstrated some similarities in the development of the same medical, biochemical, and immunological indexes including anti-DNA antibodies. Relative levels of auto-Abs to native (nat) and denatured (den) DNA in the blood of 49 MS patients and healthy donors were compared [41, 42]. The levels of anti-nat-DNA and anti-den-DNA Abs in 18% and 53% of the patients, respectively, were significantly higher than in controls. The titters of Abs to den-DNA in MS patients are usually higher than to nat-DNA. The correlation coefficients between titters of Abs to nat-DNA and den-DNA for a complete group (0.88) and its subgroups with remission (0.81), primary progressing (0.88), and secondary chronic-progressive (0.89) state of the disease were estimated [41, 42]

Interestingly, the titters of Abs against human myelin basic protein (MBP) in SLE patients 2.2-fold higher than in healthy individuals, but 2.1-fold lower than in patients with MS [43, 44]. In the case of 49 patients with MS, a possible correlation between titters of Abs to DNA [41, 42] and to MBP [44] and 13 different standard clinical parameters including Poser criteria (indexes for evaluation of damage to functional systems: pyramidal functions; cerebellar functions; functions of brain stem; sensitive functions; functions of intestines and urinary bladder; visual functions; cerebral (psychical) functions and sum of these characteristics) [45] was carried out [21, 44]. High percent of MS patients showed significantly higher anti-MBP and anti-DNA Abs levels as compared to healthy subjects. For the whole group of MS patients, the absolute values of positive CCs between titters of anti-DNA or anti-MBP Abs and clinical Poser indexes were very low (between 0.01 and 0.19), absent (~0), or were negative (−0.02 to −0.07) and statistically insignificant. Several CCs become higher increasing values up to 0.1–0.55 and −0.04 to −0.47 after the cohort was divided into subgroups of patients with primary progressing, secondary progressing, and remitting course of the disease [44].

The groups of secondary progressing, primary progressing, and remitting course of MS patients were not "homogenous" in relation to the characteristics of the patients, and their further subdivision using cluster and factorial analysis showed high statistically significant correlation coefficients [44]. For example, a direct dependence between titters of anti-MBP and symptoms of damage of the pyramidal tract for one sub-subgroup of the remitting course subgroup was observed (CC = 0.92). In some cases, correlations of the opposite sign were found for the same pairs of analyzed parameters for the three subgroups with different MS courses and their sub-subgroups obtained by cluster analysis.

Interestingly, in the case of different MS subgroups, the level of anti-DNA Abs correlates with various clinical parameters, more often with the disturbance in the function of cerebrum, bladder, and intestines, and, to a less extent, cerebellum [41, 42]. In contrast to anti-DNA Abs, a positive correlation of anti-MBP titters with disturbed brain stem function was revealed in a relatively large fraction of patients (~37%), while a negative correlation was shown with pyramid function and with the rate of disease progression [42, 44]. The correlation between

Abs to DNA and to MBP in MS patients was also very weak. On overall, the correlation coefficients between the same two analyzed parameters can be either positive or negative in the case of whole group, different subgroups, and their sub-subgroups [41, 42, 44]. The absence of a definite dependence between titters of anti-DNA and anti-MBP Abs and these parameters with the standard clinical indices may be due to the several reasons. Taken together, during analysis of biochemical, immunological and clinical indices must taken into account the current phase of the disease. It should be mentioned; quite different characteristics of pathologic processes can be obtained in individual patients, as the disease progresses against the background of the continually changing immunoregulation including exhaustion of different compensatory and adaptive mechanisms and systemic metabolic changes. This causes the clinical course in individual MS patients hardly predictable [46, 47]. Since each patient can be characterized by an individual combination of genetic, environmental, chronic, inflammatory, autoimmune, demyelinating, neurodegenerative, and other factors [41, 42, 44], it is not surprising that we could not find statistically significant correlation of titters of antibodies to DNA and MBP with the standard clinical parameters in the whole group of 49 MS patients.

3. Catalytic antibodies of MS patients

Natural Abzs from the sera of patients with various diseases are usually polyclonal in origin and may be products of different immuno-competent cells ([13–24] and references cited here). Natural abzyme purification is one of the most complicated aspects of their study; it was discussed in detail in reviews [13, 19]. In study of Abzs with different activities from the sera and CSF of MS patients and healthy donors, electrophoretically and immunologically homogeneous Ab fraction (IgG+IgM + IgA) was first purified by affinity chromatography of the serum or CSF proteins on Protein A-Sepharose under conditions that remove nonspecifically bound proteins. Then IgMs were separated from IgAs and IgGs by FPLC gel filtration [48–56]. 150 kDa IgG, 170 kDa IgA, and ~900 kDa IgM did not contain any contaminating proteins detectable by silver staining under non-reducing and reducing conditions (e.g., **Figure 1**) [48–56].

The application of rigid criteria allowed the authors of the first article concerning natural Abzs [9] to conclude that vasoactive intestinal peptide-hydrolyzing activity is an intrinsic property of Abs from the sera of patients with asthma. Later several additional rigid criteria were proposed (for review see [13, 19]). We applied a set of strict criteria worked out previously [9, 13–21] for the analysis of DNase [52, 54–56], MBP-hydrolyzing [48–51, 53] and amylase [57, 58] activities as intrinsic properties of IgGs, IgAs, and IgMs from the sera and IgGs from the CSF of MS patients [52, 53]. They may be summarized as follows: (a) the IgGs, IgAs, and IgMs were electrophoretically homogeneous (e.g., **Figure 1**); (b) FPLC gel filtration of these Abs using conditions dissociating strong noncovalent complexes in an acidic buffer did not eliminate analyzed activities, and the peaks of the activities and intact Abs exactly coincided (**Figure 2A**); (c) immobilized polyclonal mouse IgGs against the light chains of human antibodies completely absorbed the activities; peaks of these activities coincided with the peak of IgGs (IgA or IgM) eluted with an acidic buffer (e.g., **Figure 2B**). (d) F(ab) and F(ab)2 fragments obtained using digestion by proteases of corresponding catalytic IgGs showed comparable levels of the activities comparing with intact Abs. The fulfillment of these criteria was observed for MS Abzs with all activities mentioned above.

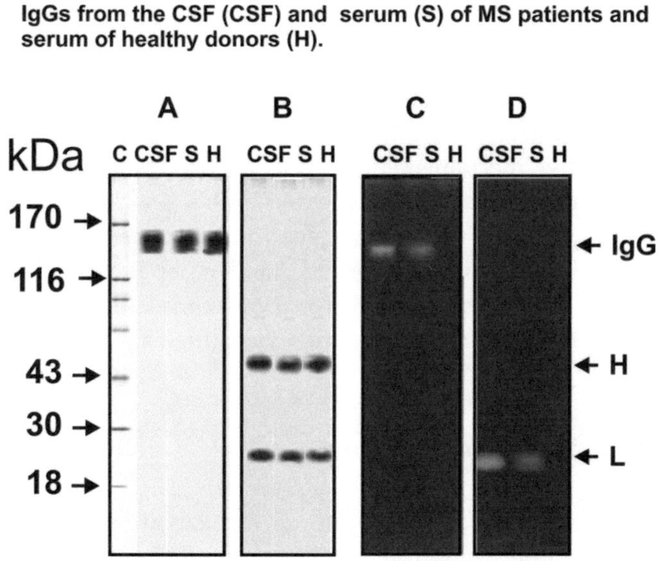

Figure 1. SDS-PAGE analysis of IgGmix (7 μg) corresponding to equimolar mixtures of 13 IgG preparations of CSFs and 13 IgGs from sera of MS patients, and 10 healthy donors in 3–16% gradient gel before (A) and after treatment with DTT (B) followed by silver staining [52, 54–56]. The arrows (lane C) indicate the positions of molecular mass markers. In situ gel assay of DNase activity of IgGmix (15 μg) corresponding to CSFs and to sera of MS patients, and healthy donors in a gel containing DNA before (C) and after treatment with DTT (D). DNase activity was revealed by ethidium bromide staining as a dark band on the fluorescent background. A part of the gel corresponding to Panels C and D was stained with Coumassie R250 to show the position of intact IgGs and separated light and heavy chains (the arrows of Panels C and D).

To exclude possible artifacts due to the hypothetical traces of contaminating enzymes, IgGs from sera and CSF were subjected to SDS-PAGE in a gel co-polymerized with calf thymus DNA, and their DNase activity was detected by incubating the gel in the standard reaction buffer (**Figure 1C** and **D**). Ethidium bromide staining of the gels after the electrophoresis and refolding of IgGs revealed sharp dark bands against a fluorescent background of DNA. In addition, after incubation of IgGs with DTT only light chains of MS csf-IgGmix and serum-IgGmix demonstrated DNase activity (**Figure 1D**). Since SDS dissociates all protein complexes, the revealing of the DNase activity in the gel zones of only to intact IgGs (Panel C) and separated light chains (Panel D) together with the absence of any other activity or protein bands (**Figure 1**), guaranty direct evidence that IgGs from sera and CSFs of MS patients cleavage DNA and they do not contain canonical DNases [52, 54–56].

MS IgGs and IgAs were separated by SDS-PAGE, respectively, under non-reducing and reducing conditions, and their MBP-hydrolyzing and amylase activities were detected after the extraction of Abs from excised gel slices (for example, **Figure 2C**) [44, 48–51, 53, 57, 58].

The detection of MBP-hydrolyzing and amylase activities in the gel region corresponding only to intact IgGs, together with the absence of any other bands of the activity or protein, provided direct evidence that IgG possesses MBP-hydrolyzing and amylase activities [44, 48–51, 57, 58]. Similar results were obtained for MS IgAs- and IgMs-hydrolyzing MBP [49]. In addition, it was shown that the fractions of IgGs (IgAs or IgMs) having affinity to MBP-Sepharose hydrolyze effectively only human and MBPs, but not other control proteins [48–50].

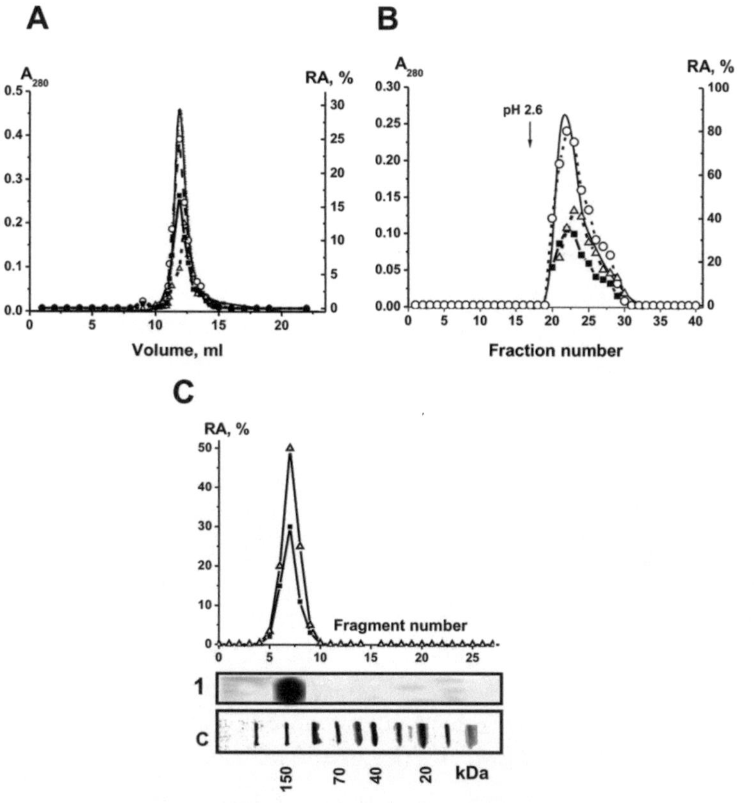

Figure 2. Analysis of strict criteria fulfilment to show that the enzymatic activities are intrinsic properties of IgGs from cerebrospinal fluid of MS patients. FPLC gel filtration of mixture of equal amounts of electrophoretically homogeneous IgGs from 15 preparations of CSF (csf-IgGmix) on a Superdex 200 column in an acidic buffer (pH 2.6) destroying immunocomplexes after Abs incubation in the same buffer (A) and csf-IgGmix affinity chromatography on Sepharose bearing mouse IgGs against human IgGs (B): (—), absorbance at 280 nm (A280); relative activity (RA) of IgGs in the hydrolysis of DNA (○), BMP (■), and maltoheptaose (Δ). In-gel assay of MBP-hydrolyzing (■) and amylase (Δ) activities of csf-IgGmix (15 μg) (C). The relative MBP-hydrolyzing and amylase activities (RA, %) were revealed using the extracts of 2–3-mm fragments of one longitudinal slice of the gel. The RA of IgGs corresponding to complete hydrolysis of the substrates was taken for 100%. The second control longitudinal slice of the same gel was stained with Coomassie Blue (Panel C, lane 1); lane C shows positions of protein markers. The average error in the initial rate determination from three experiments did not exceed 7–10%.

It is known that catalytic centers of nuclease and proteolytic Abzs are usually located on the light chain, while the heavy chain is more often responsible for specific antigen recognition and increased antigen affinity for Abs [13–21]. It was shown that catalytic centers of DNase, protease, and amylase Abzs from MS patients are located on the light chains of these Abs [48–53, 54, 56–58]. Intact proteins usually interact with both light and heavy chains of Abzs, thus ensuring the specificity of the target protein recognition and its cleavage. Overall, it is obvious that nuclease, amylase, and MBP-hydrolyzing activities are intrinsic properties of Abzs from sera and CSF of MS patients and do not due to the admixture of any possible canonical enzymes.

4. Comparison of the relative catalytic activity of Abs from different MS patients

4.1. Abzymes with DNase and RNase activities

Anti-DNA Abs are detectable even in the sera of healthy mammals, but their titters vary significantly [59]. In comparison with healthy donors, concentrations of anti-DNA antibodies are higher in patients with rheumatoid arthritis (7% of patients) [59], myasthenia gravis (6%), Sjogren's syndrome (18%), multiple sclerosis (17–18%), primary Hashimoto's thyroiditis (23%), and systemic lupus erythematosus (SLE, 36%). Anti-DNA Abs are directed against histone-DNA nucleosomal complexes appearing in the circulation from internucleosomal cleavage during apoptosis in many SLE patients [60].

Healthy humans do not develop Abzs with detectable DNase activity, their levels being usually on the borderline of sensitivity of the detection methods [13–21]. The RAs of Abs from the sera of MS patients vary markedly from patient to patient [54]. **Figure 3A** illustrates cleavage of plasmid DNA by Abs from sera of ten MS patients after 2 h of incubation. During this time, some Abs cause only single breaks in one strand of plasmid supercoiled DNA converting it to the relaxed form (lanes 1–3), whereas others cause multiple breaks causing DNA linearization (lanes 4–6). The most active Abs hydrolyze DNA into short- and medium-length oligonucleotides (lanes 7–10). Relative activity (RA) of different MS IgG preparations was first estimated using arbitrary units (a/u) from 0 to 10 a/u (**Figure 3A**).

IgGs from 53 of 55 MS patients (~96%) demonstrated detectable RAs from 1 to 10 a/u; the average values of IgG DNase activity were 5 ± 4 a/u. MS Abzs hydrolyze single- and double-stranded DNAs of different sequences and length [52, 54–56]. The affinity of Abzs with DNase activity for DNA is usually high (1–10 nM) and corresponds to the typical affinity of Abs for nucleic acids and ~104- and 105-fold higher than that for canonical DNases [54–56].

Recently, we have shown, for the first time, that average concentration of total proteins (132-fold), total IgGs (194-fold), and anti-DNA antibodies (1986-fold; **Figure 3B**) in the sera (average value 437 ± 311 A450 units) is significantly higher than that in the CSF (average value 0.22 ± 0.008 A450 units, **Figure 3B**) of fifteen MS patients [52]. In the sera and CSFs, the relative activities of total protein varied remarkably from patient to patient. Specific DNase activity of the total protein of CSF reparations were surprising approximately 198-fold higher than the serum ones. We present first evidence showing that IgGs from CSF not only bind but efficiently hydrolyze DNA and that average specific DNase activity of homogeneous antibodies from CSF (543.3 ± 239.7 pmole DNA/1 mg of Ab/1 h) is unpredictably ~49-fold higher than that from the sera (average value 11.2±4.3 pmole DNA/1 mg of Ab/1 h) of the same MS patients (**Figure 3C**) [52].

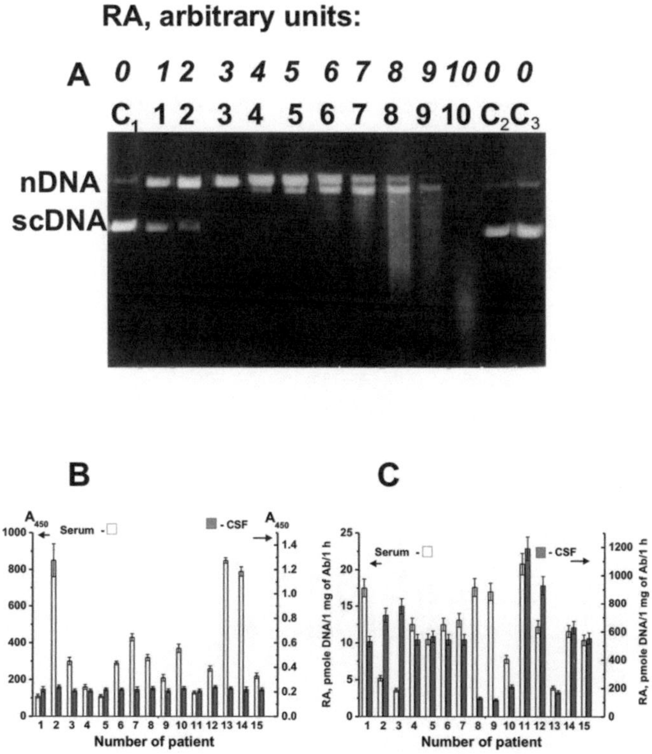

Figure 3. DNase activities of catalytic IgGs from sera of ten different patients with MS in the cleavage of supercoiled (sc) and nicked (n) plasmid DNA (A). Lanes 1–10, IgGs from the sera of 10 different patients; C1, scDNA incubated alone; C2 and C3, scDNA incubated with Ab from the sera of two healthy donors [54, 55]. Relative content (A450 units) of anti-DNA IgGs determined by ELISA in serum (the right hand axis) and in CSF (the left hand axis) preparations of fifteen MS patients (B) and RAs of polyclonal IgGs purified from these fifteen serum and CSF preparations in the hydrolysis of supercoiled DNA (C) [52].

4.2. Abzymes with protease activity

It was shown that IgGs from sera of healthy donors do not hydrolyze MBP [13–21]. We have compared the RAs of IgGs, IgAs, and IgMs from sera of 35 MS patients in the hydrolysis of MBP (**Figures 4A** and **B**) [48, 49]. Specific activities of IgGs from sera of any single patient were usually significantly lower than those of IgMs and sIgAs. Specific inhibitors of thiol and acidic proteases had a weak effect on protease activity of IgGs and IgMs. But, specific inhibitors of serine proteases (PMSF and AEBSF) significantly suppressed proteolytic activity of the Abzs. IgGs, IgMs, and IgAs hydrolyze specifically human MBP, but not many other tested proteins [48, 49].

The sera of healthy donors demonstrated ~four- and fivefold lower concentration of anti-MBP concentration (average value 0.08 ± 0.05 A450 units) than that for MS patients (average value 0.32 ± 0.08 A450 units) [43, 44]. We used ELISA to compare the relative levels of Abs against MBP in the sera and CSFs of 15 MS patients (**Figure 4C**) [53]. The average relative content of anti-MBP Abs in the sera of MS patients is approximately 230-fold higher than in the corresponding CSFs (**Figure 4C**). We present first evidence showing that IgGs from CSF efficiently hydrolyze MBP and that their average specific catalytic activity is unpredictably ~54-fold higher than that of Abs from sera of the same MS patients (**Figure 4D**) [53].

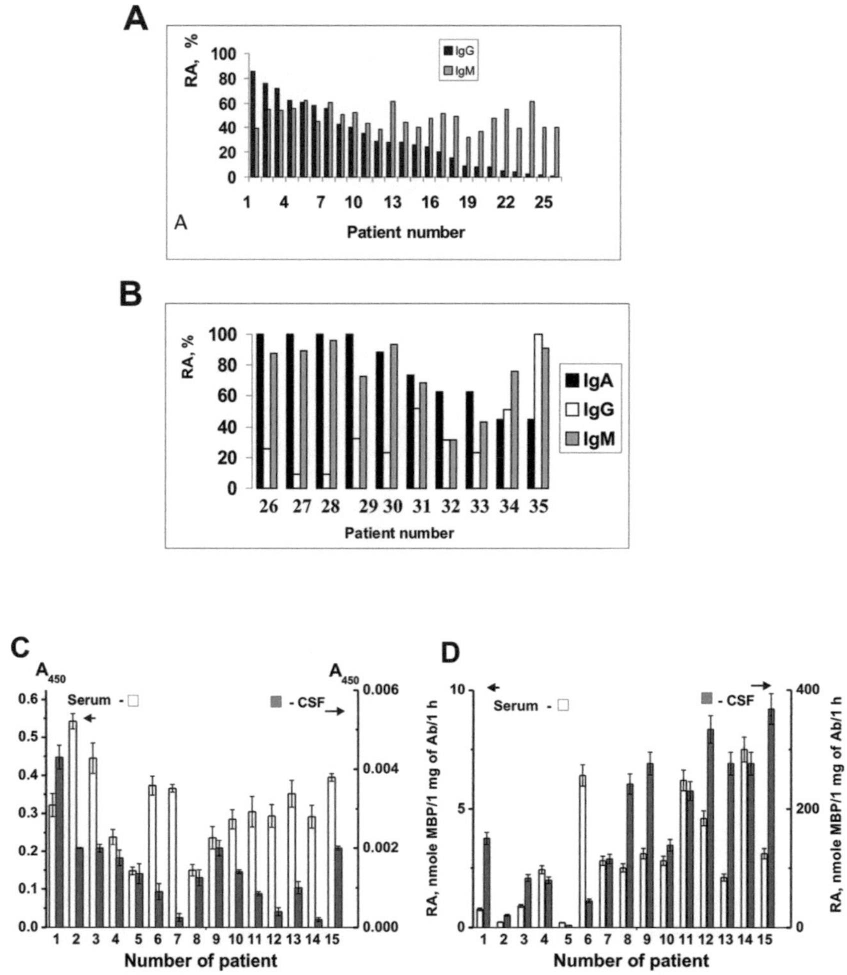

Figure 4. The relative activities (RA) of polyclonal IgGs and IgMs from the sera of 25 different MS patients (A) and of IgGs, IgMs, and IgAs from the sera of other 10 MS patients (B) in the hydrolysis of MBP. The RAs were determined from decrease of initial MBP; the relative intensity of the main bands of MBP incubated alone for 3 h was taken as 100% [49]. Relative content (A450 units) of anti-MBP IgGs determined by ELISA in serum (the right hand axis) and in CSF (the left hand axis) preparations of fifteen MS patients (C) and RAs of polyclonal IgGs purified from these fifteen preparations of biological fluids in the hydrolysis of supercoiled MBP (D) [53].

IgGs and sIgAs from breast milk demonstrated high ATPase activity [61]. It has recently been shown that during spontaneous development of a profound SLE-like pathology in MRL-lpr/lpr mice leads to a production of DNase, protease, ATPase, and amylase Abzs [22–24]. Interestingly, individual IgGs from sera and CSF of MS patients did not possess detectable ATPase activity [62].

IgGs and IgMs from sera of patients with several autoimmune diseases [57, 58, 63–66] and sIgAs from human breast milk [67] possess amylase activity; however, the maximal activity was observed for Abs from sera of patients with MS [57, 58, 63] and SLE [63, 65, 66]. Individual IgGs and IgMs isolated from patients with MS and SLE had approximately three orders of magnitude higher specific amylolytic activity than that for healthy donors [57, 58, 63–66].

The ability of the presence of MBP- and DNA-hydrolyzing antibodies in the cerebrospinal fluid of MS patients may be related to the fact that anti-MBP and anti-DNA Abs may play an important role in the pathogenesis of this disease. Anti-MBP Abzs can attack MBP of the myelin-proteolipid shell of axons [48–51]. In addition, DNase Abzs of MS patients [16, 21] similarly to SLE patients [68] are cytotoxic and induce cell apoptosis, which can play an important role in SLE and MS pathogenesis. At the same time, the involvement of antibodies with amylase activity in the pathogenesis of any autoimmune diseases has not yet been identified. We have recently shown the first unpredictable evidence showing that IgGs from CSF (average value 9.0 ± 4.9 μM/1 h/mg) possess amylase activity and efficiently hydrolyze maltoheptaose; their average specific Ab activity is ~30-fold higher than that of antibodies from sera (average value 0.30 ± 0.14 μM/1 h/mg) of the same MS patients [62]. Specific average RA for IgGs from healthy volunteers was approximately ~1000 lower than that for MS patients [57, 58]. It was shown that a relative RA of total proteins of CSF (including Abs) is ~15-fold lower than that for purified IgGs, while the RAs of the total sera protein is higher than that of sera IgGs by a factor of 1033. This result speaks in favor of the fact that amylolytic activity of CSF proteins is mainly caused by the activity of amylase Abzs. One cannot exclude that amylase Abzs of CSF can also play a, as yet unknown, role in the pathogenesis of MS.

As it was mentioned above, the correlation coefficients between titters of Abs to DNA and to MBP and 13 different standard clinical parameters, including Poser criteria in the case of 49 patients with MS, were very low [21, 44]. We have not revealed high correlation coefficients between different RAs characterizing IgGs of CSF and serum as well as RAs of these IgGs and total proteins corresponding CSF and serum. All CCs varied from −0.03 to +0.18 except unpredicted correlation of RAs for IgGs from serum and total protein corresponding to CSF (CC = 0.7). Similar situation was observed earlier for CCs between RAs of these IgGs and total proteins corresponding CSF and serum in the hydrolysis of DNA (CCs = −0.05 – +0.03) [52]. In addition, we calculated a possible correlation between RAs characterizing 15 IgGs in the hydrolysis of DNA [52], MBP [53], and oligosaccharide [62] (**Table 1**). All CCs were relatively low (−0.009 – +0.2) except some of them: IgG amylase activity of CSF correlates with MBP-hydrolyzing activity of serum (CC = +0.41) and CSF (CC = +0.45); DNase activity of serum IgGs correlates with MBP-hydrolyzing activity of serum (CC = +0.44) and CSF (CC = +0.61), as well as MBP-hydrolyzing activity of serum and CSF (CC = +0.59). However, all these correlation coefficients were very low or relatively low. Thus, an additional question is why there is no good correlation between various indexes, characterizing different MS patients. As mentioned above, each patient can be characterized by an individual combination of genetic, environmental, chronic, inflammatory, autoimmune, demyelinating, neurodegenerative, and other factors [46, 47]. This can be the main reason for the lack of a good correlation between the different indicators of MS development by various patients. However, taking all data together, it is reasonable to propose that MBP-, DNA-, and polysaccharide-hydrolyzing Abzs can probably cooperatively promote important neuropathological mechanisms in MS.

Number of patient	**Amylase activity of sera IgGs**	**Amylase activity of CSF IgGs**	**DNase activity of sera IgGs**	**DNase activity of CSF IgGs**	**MBP-hydrolyzing activity of plasma IgGs**	**MBP-hydrolyzing activity of CSF IgGs**
Parameter number	**1**	**2**	**3***	**4***	**5***	**6***
Correlation coefficient	1/2: 0.22	1/3: 0.03	1/4: - 0.009	1/5: - 0.13	1/6: 0.1	2/3: 0.22
	2/4: 0.03	2/5: 0.41	2/6: 0.45	3/4: 0.11	3/5: 0.44	3/6: 0.61
	4/5: 0.34	4/6: 0.11	5/6: 0.59	–	–	–

* Parameters 1 and 2 [62], 3 and 4 [52] and 5 and 6 [53]. Here the same 15 preparations of IgGs from the same MS patients were compared.

Table 1. Correlation coefficients between relative activities of 15 IgGs from sera and CSFs of MS patients in the hydrolysis of oligosaccharide, DNA, and MBP.

4.3. Extreme diversity of MS Abzs

The extreme diversity of RNase and DNase activity of IgG and/or IgM Abzs from the sera of autoimmune patients and also of MRL-lpr/lpr mice was observed [13–21, 69–76]. It was demonstrated that different patients (and animals) may have an extremely large a relatively small content of polyclonal nuclease Abzs containing different relative amounts of kappa and lambda light chains and demonstrating at various optimal pHs maximal activity, possessing a different net charge, dependent or not on different metal ions, and characterized by different substrate specificities.

Different auto-Abs, including Abs to DNA, and different DNA-dependent enzymes can interact with DNA [13–21, 77, 78]. DNase, RNase, and MBP-hydrolyzing IgGs from the sera of autoimmune patients are usually very heterogeneous in their affinity for these substrates and can be separated into many fractions by chromatography on DNA-cellulose and MBP-Sepharose ([13–21] and refs therein). MS Abs with DNase [54–56] and MBP-hydrolyzing [43] activities were distributed all over the profiles of chromatographies (e.g., **Figure 5A**). The affinity of abzyme fractions for these substrates (in terms of Km values) was increased gradually with the increase in eluting salts concentrations. In contrast to MS IgGs, Abzs from SLE patients are more sensitive to EDTA (**Figure 5B** and **C**) and less sensitive to specific inhibitors of serine-like proteases. Similar data of extreme diversity of DNase activity of IgGs were observed in the case of other autoimmune diseases and autoimmune mice [13–21, 75]. All these data are indicative of the extreme diversity of Abzs with different activities in their affinity for specific substrates and in their relative specific activities.

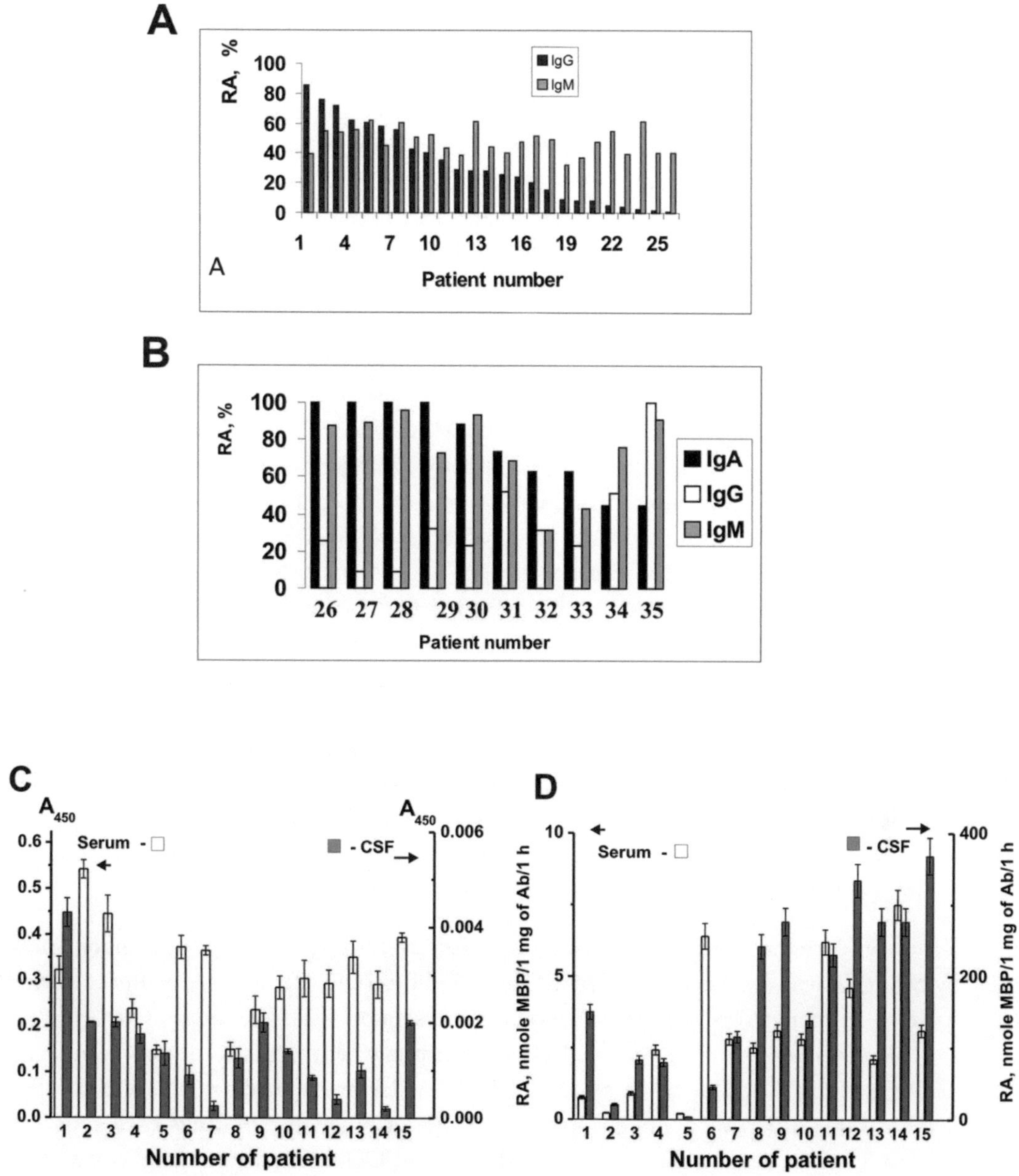

Figure 5. Affinity chromatography of MS IgGs on DNA cellulose: (–), absorbance at 280 nm; columns, relative DNase activity (A) [54, 56]. Affinity chromatography of mixtures of IgGs from sera of 15 SLE (B) and 15 MS (C) patients on MBP-Sepharose [43]: (—), absorbance at 280 nm; the relative catalytic activities (RA) of IgGs of different fractions in the absence (□) and in the presence of EDTA (■) was measured. Depending on the RA, the reaction mixtures were incubated for 0.3–16 h in the presence of 0.01–0.1 mg/ml IgGs and then the RAs were normalized to the standard conditions: the complete transition oligopeptide corresponding to MBP and DNA to their products was taken for 100%.

Theoretically, the human immune system can produce up to 106 specificities of Abs against one antigen. Affinity chromatography data (**Figure 5**) do not give possibility to estimate a possible number of monoclonal DNase antibodies that correspond to the polyclonal IgGs, eluting at various Ab peaks. For this evaluation, we have used the analysis of possible number of monoclonal Abs with DNase activity [79–81]. An immunoglobulin kappa light chain library from blood of SLE patients was cloned into a phagemid vector. Phage particles displaying recombinant monoclonal light chains (MLChs) capable of binding DNA were isolated by affinity chromatography on DNA cellulose. The phage particles containing MLChs bound with DNA-cellulose were distributed between eleven peaks (11 different fractions) eluted during chromatography, and all fractions obtained were active in the hydrolysis of DNA. The fraction eluted by 0.5 M NaCl (peak 7) and an acidic buffer (pH 2.6; peak 11) were used for preparation of individual monoclonal light chains (MLChs, ~28 kDa). Then, 45 of 451 and 33 of 687 individual colonies corresponding respectively to peaks 7 and 11 were randomly chosen for study of MLCh DNase activity [79–81]. Fourteen of 45 and nineteen of 33 clones, respectively, contained MLChs with DNase activity. Totally, all 33 of 78 purified MLChs (42%) containing no canonical DNases demonstrated various enzymatic properties including different k_{cat} values, one or two pH optima, were inactive after dialysis against EDTA, but could be activated by several externally added metal ions; the ratio of relative activity in the presence of Mn^{2+}, Ca^{2+}, Mg^{2+}, Ni^{2+}, Zn^{2+}, Cu^{2+}, and Co^{2+} was individual for each MLCh, with Mn^{2+}, Mg^{2+}, and Co^{2+} being among the best activators of their DNase activity [79–81]. In the presence of Mn^{2+} or Mg^{2+}, the DNase activity of some MLChs did not require K_+ or Na^+, while the others could be activated by KCl or NaCl at optimal concentrations from 1 to 100 mM. It should be mentioned that not only Abs from sera of patients with different ADs containing kappa, but also lambda light chains possess DNase activity [13–21]. In addition, we have analyzed MLChs corresponding only to two of eleven peaks obtained [79–81], while Abs of all 11 peaks were catalytically active. It means that the sera of SLE (and MS) patients in principle can contain some hundreds of catalytic DNase lambda- and kappa-IgGs with different catalytic properties.

In order to compare the substrate specificity of Abzs, the hydrolysis of various oligonucleotides by MS IgGs was analyzed [55]. The oligonucleotides (ODNs) cleavage patterns varied from patient to patient. Some Abs demonstrated sequence-independent hydrolysis of ODNs, while other produced in parallel both 5′-phosphate terminated products (similar to those of DNase I) or 3′-phosphate terminated ODNs, which are typical for DNase II. Several IgGs demonstrate sequence-dependent manner, while for other the products correspond to both 3′- and 5′-exonuclease activities. The hydrolysis of ODNs by different IgGs was also strongly dependent on the reaction conditions used including addition of MgCl2, EDTA, increase in NaCl or potassium phosphate concentration [55]. All the data obtained show that MS IgGs can demonstrate different combinations of endo- and exonuclease activities and properties of the MS DNase IgGs distinguished them from all known canonical DNases [55]. The extreme diversity of RNase and DNase IgG and/or IgM Abzs in their affinity to DNA (and in k_{cat} values) was also revealed for several other autoimmune diseases [13–21, 55, 68, 69, 76].

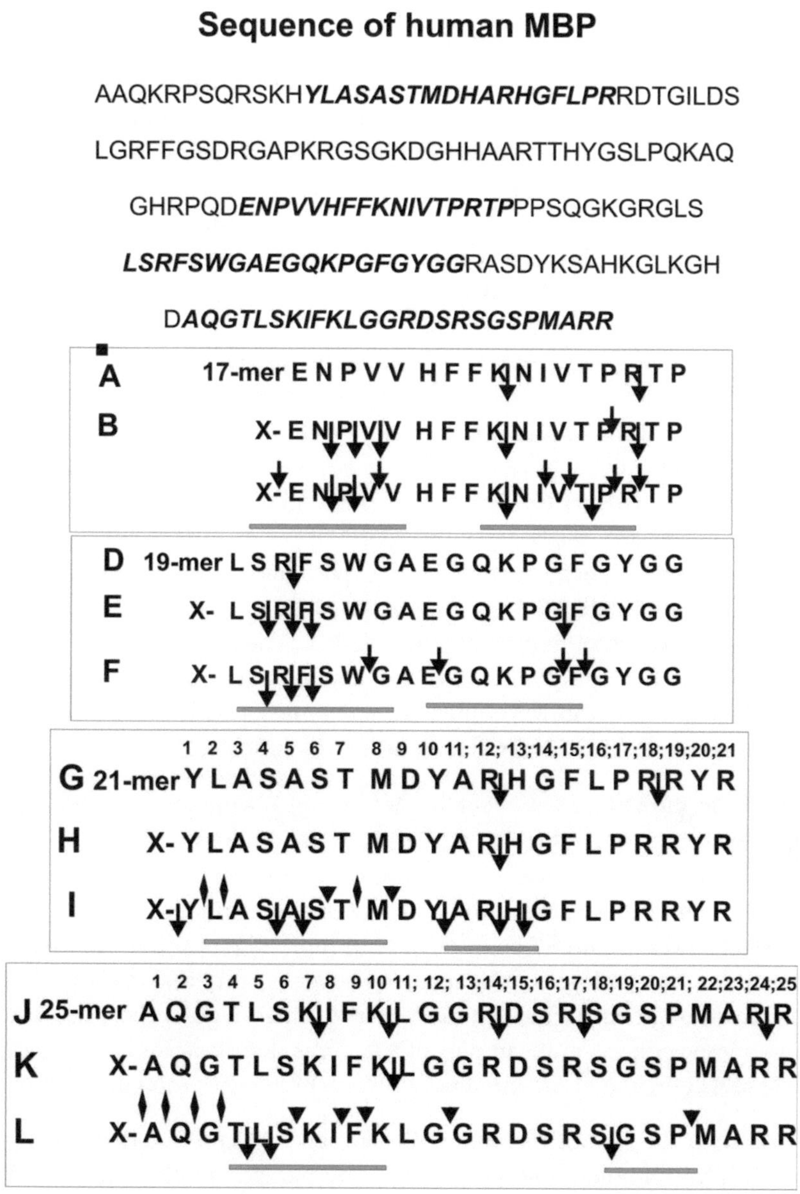

Figure 6. Complete sequence of human MBP (on the top); the positions of OP17, OP19, OP21, and OP25 sequences in the human MBP sequence are shown in bold. All sites of cleavage of X-OP17 (B–C) and X-OP19 (E–F) (X is fluorescent label of OPs), corresponding to detectable major and minor products of these OPs digestion after their mild (B and E) and deep (C and F) hydrolysis by equimolar mixture of 15 SLE IgGs are shown [80]. Panels A and D show the major cleavage sites, which were found previously in the case of hydrolysis of globular intact MBP by MS and SLE IgGs [43, 78]; trypsin hydrolyzes these OPs at the same sites. All sites of the OP21 (I) and OP25 (L) corresponding to major and moderate products of the cleavage are shown by long and short arrows respectively, while corresponding to minor ones by diamonds [81]. Panels G and J show all possible sites of these OPs cleavage by trypsin, while panels H and K demonstrate the major cleavage sites of MBP, which were found previously in the case of hydrolysis of globular intact MBP by MS and SLE IgGs [43, 78]. Clustered major and minor sites of cleavage are underlined.

Anti-MBP Abzs of MS patients' cleavage MBP at several sites corresponding to four known immunodominant regions of human MBP [82]. It was demonstrated that anti-MBP Abzs of SLE patients hydrolyze MBP at the same four immunodominant regions of MBP [43]. Four different encephalytogenic peptides corresponding to known antigenic determinants (AGDs) of MBP can play a negative role in the MS and SLE pathogenesis [82]. Therefore, it was interesting to study the specific sequences of MBP in more detail. Interestingly, MS and SLE anti-MBP IgGs hydrolyze nonspecific tri- and tetrapeptides with an extremely low efficiency and they cannot efficiently cleavage longer oligopeptides corresponding AGDs of HIV-1 integrase [83]. To identify all MBP cleavage sites corresponding to anti-MBP IgGs in the case of four AGDs of MBP, we have used a combination of MALDI mass spectrometry, reverse-phase chromatography, and thin layer chromatography for revealing of the cleavage products of four (17-, 19-, 21, and 25-mer) encephalytogenic oligopeptides corresponding to these AGDs [84, 85]. Several clustered major and minor sites of cleavage were revealed in the case of all oligopeptides (**Figure 6**). It was shown that the number of oligopeptide cleavage sites is greater than that of intact MBP. The active sites of anti-MBP Abzs are located on their light chains, while the heavy chains are responsible for Abs increased affinity for protein substrates. Interactions of both light and heavy chains of Abzs with intact globular proteins provide high affinity and specificity of intact MBP hydrolysis. The affinity of anti-MBP Abzs for oligopeptides was ~103-fold lower than that for the intact MBP. These data indicate that a relatively short oligopeptides interact mainly with the light chain of different monoclonal Abzs of total pool of IgGs, which possesses lower affinity for substrates, and therefore, depending on the oligopeptide sequences, their hydrolysis may be less specific [84, 85].

IgGs and IgMs from the sera of patients with MS and SLE were found to possess amylolytic activity hydrolyzing $\alpha-$(1-4)-glucosyl linkages of maltooligosaccharides, glycogen, and several synthetic substrates [57, 58, 63–67]. The specific amylolytic activity of individual IgGs and IgMs from MS patients was about three orders of magnitude higher than that of healthy donors [57, 58]. Fractions of auto-Abs from human milk [67] and from sera of patients with different autoimmune pathologies [57, 58 63–65] revealed different modes of action in the hydrolysis of maltooligosaccharides, p-nitrophenyl maltooligosaccharides, p-nitrophenyl, and α-D-glucopyranoside; several samples of MS Abzs demonstrated β-xylosidase activity, which is not observed in known mammalian polysaccharide-hydrolyzing enzymes.

Proteolytic Abs from the sera of patients with various autoimmune diseases [9, 86] casein-hydrolyzing Abzs from human milk [87], casein-, human serum albumin-, and HIV reverse transcriptase-hydrolyzing Abs from AIDS patients [88] are serine-like proteases, and their activity is most strongly reduced by specific serine protease inhibitors PMSF or AEBSF. Specific inhibitors of acidic and thiol proteases demonstrated a weak effect on proteolytic activity of MS polyclonal IgGs and IgMs [48–51]. However, specific inhibitors of serine proteases significantly inhibited proteolytic activity. In addition, MS polyclonal IgGs contained several chelated metals and the relative amount of which decreases in the order: $Fe^{2+} > Ca^{2+} > Cu^{2+} > Zn^{2+} > Mg^{2+} > Mn^{2+} > Co^{2+} > Ni^{2+}$ [50]. After removing of Mg^{2+} ions by dialysis against EDTA, MS IgGs have not completely lost proteolytic activity, which was increased after addition of different external Me^{2+} ions. After chromatography of MS IgGs on Chelex-100, a minor metal-dependent fraction did not cleavage MBP in the absence Mg^{2+} ions, but it was activated after addition of metal ions: $Ca^{2+} < Cu^{2+} < Mn^{2+} < Mg^{2+}$ [50]. Protease activities of several MS IgGs were also activated by other metal ions (Ni^{2+}, Fe^{2+}, Co^{2+}, Zn^{2+}, Pb^{2+}, and Co^{2+}) and especially Ni^{2+}. Observed properties of MS Abzs distinguish them from other known mammalian metalloproteases and demonstrate their pronounced catalytic diversity. Metal-dependent IgG from MS patients was the first example of Abzs with metal-dependent proteolytic activity [50]. Later, we have revealed an important metal-dependent casein-hydrolyzing sIgA from human milk [89] and MBP-hydrolyzing IgGs from SLE patients [43]. We have recently shown that anti-integrase IgGs and IgMs from AIDS patients can contain Abzs cleaving HIV integrase by small subfractions resembling thiol, serine, acidic, and metal-dependent proteases, the ratio of which may be individual for every HIV-infected patient [90, 91]. Since anti-MBP from sera of MS and SLE patients are very similar, we have analyzed in more details monoclonal Abzs from SLE patients [92, 93].

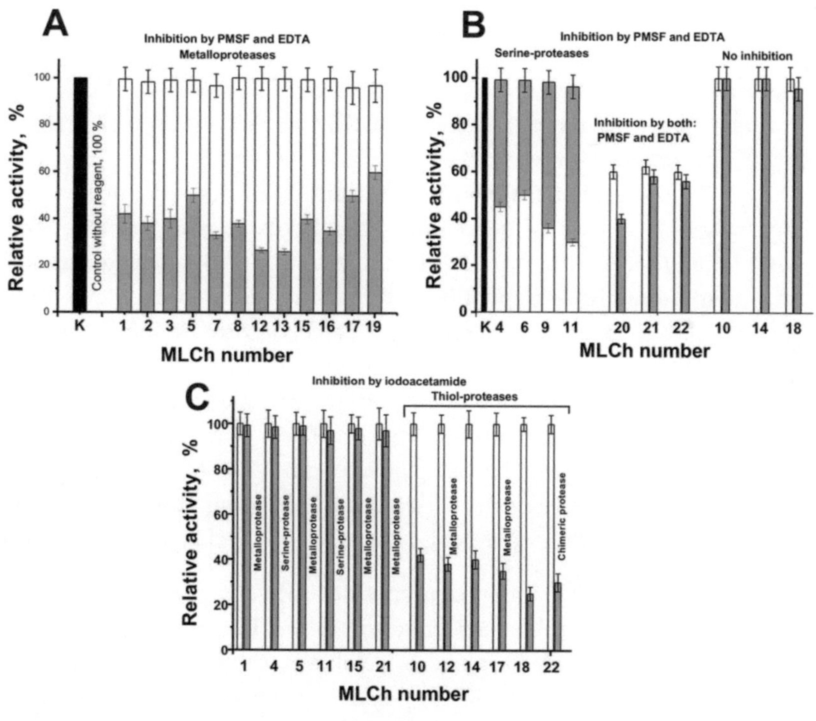

Figure 7. The relative MBP-hydrolyzing activity of 22 MLChs after their pre-incubation with specific inhibitors of different type proteases [92]. Various MLChs (0.1 mg/ml) were pre-incubated in the absence of other components (black bars, control—C), in the presence of 50 mM EDTA (gray bars) or 1 mM PMSF (white bars) and then added to standard reaction mixture containing MBP substrate (A and B). Panel C shows several examples of the relative activity of MLChs with metalloprotease activity (numbers: 1, 5, 12, 15, and 21) and serine-like activity (numbers: 4 and 11), which do not change their activity after pre-incubation with iodoacetamide; three MLChs (numbers: 10, 14, and 18) demonstrating negative response to PMSF and EDTA as well as chimeric MLCh-22 after their pre-incubation with iodoacetamide leading to a significant decrease in the activity. White and grey bars correspond respectively to the activity before (control) and after these MLChs pre-incubation with iodoacetamide (Panel C). The relative activity of all MLChs before their pre-incubation with different inhibitors was taken for 100% [92].

An immunoglobulin light chain phagemid library corresponding to peripheral blood of SLE patients lymphocytes was used [92, 93]. Small pools of phage particles displaying light chains with different affinity for MBP were obtained using affinity chromatography on MBP-Sepharose. For preparation of the individual monoclonal light chains (MLChs, 27–28 kDa), the fraction eluted with 0.5 M NaCl was used. Seventy two of 440 individual colonies were randomly chosen, expressed in E. coli in a soluble form, and individual MLChs were purified by metal chelating chromatography. 22 of 72 MLChs efficiently cleaved MBP showing various pH optima in a 5.7–9.0 range and different substrate specificity in the hydrolysis of four various MBP oligopeptides. Four light chains demonstrated serine-like, three MLChs—thiol protease-like activities, while eleven MLChs were metal-dependent (**Figure 7**). PMSF and EDTA inhibited by the activity of three chimeric MLChs, two other chains were supressed by EDTA and iodoacetamide, and one by PMSF, EDTA, and iodoacetamide. In the presence of Ca^{2+}, Mg^{2+}, Mn^{2+}, Ni^{2+}, Zn^{2+}, Cu^{2+}, and Co^{2+}, the ratio of relative activity was individual for each of 22 MLCh preparations [92, 93]. These observations suggest an extreme diversity of anti-MBP Abzs in SLE (and most probably MS) patients.

As it was mentioned above, iodoacetamide weakly (5–15%) suppress MBP-hydrolyzing activity of polyclonal Abs from sera of patients with MS and SLE [43, 48–51]. It was shown that the relative number of iodoacetamide-dependent MLChs is only approximately 27% of all MLChs analyzed, and several of them possess at the same time activity of serine- and metal-loproteases (**Figure 7**) [92, 93]. Thus, a relative contribution of thiol-like proteolytic activity to a total MBP-hydrolyzing activity of polyclonal Abzs pools in SLE and MS patients can be remarkably lower than that of antibodies with serine-like and metalloprotease activities and may be estimated for total IgGs depending on patients comparable to 5–15%, as found previously [43, 48–51]. Using different methods, it has been proven that recombinant monoclonal kappa light chain NGTA2-Me-pro-ChTr possess two different activities—trypsin-like and metalloprotease activities [93], while other with trypsin-like, metalloprotease and DNase activities (Timofeeva AM, personal communication). Thus, it reasonable to believe that the immune system of SLE and MS patients can produce anti-MBP Abzs not only with one type but also with a combined structure of the active center, carrying amino acid residues typical for different proteases with metal-dependent, serine-, thiol-, and acidic-like activities.

Mammalian blood DNase II and DNase I demonstrate only one pronounced pH optimum in hydrolysis of scDNA (pH 5.2 and 7.0, respectively) [94–96]. In contrast to all human DNases, all polyclonal MS IgGs demonstrated high or detectable activity at a wide range of pH values between 5.0 and 9.5 [56]. The heights of the peaks corresponding to various optima were different, and the ratios of RAs at these pH values were individual for each polyclonal IgG preparation. **Figure 8A** demonstrates typical data for two individual MS patients. Similar results were obtained for DNase IgGs and/or IgMs from patients with other autoimmune diseases [13–21].

It is well known that mammalian, bacterial, and plant canonical proteases, depending on their biological function, can have optimal pHs ranging from acidic (2.0) to neutral and alkaline (8–10) [97, 98]. We have measured the relative activity of polyclonal IgGs at pH from 2.6 to 10.5. In contrast to canonical proteases, the pH profile of each preparation of polyclonal IgGs from

MS [51] and SLE [43] patients was unique (**Figures 8C** and **8D**). In contrast to all human proteases having one pronounced pH optimum, catalytic MS and SLE polyclonal IgGs demonstrated high specific MBP-hydrolyzing activity within a wide range of pH values (2.6–10). Taking this into account, one cannot exclude that human immune system could, in principle, produce Abzs with very different proteolytic activities including similar to that of stomach acidic proteases. The above results clearly demonstrate that polyclonal IgGs from individual MS and SLE patients are very heterogeneous and can consist of different sets of catalytic IgG subfractions demonstrating quite distinct pH dependencies.

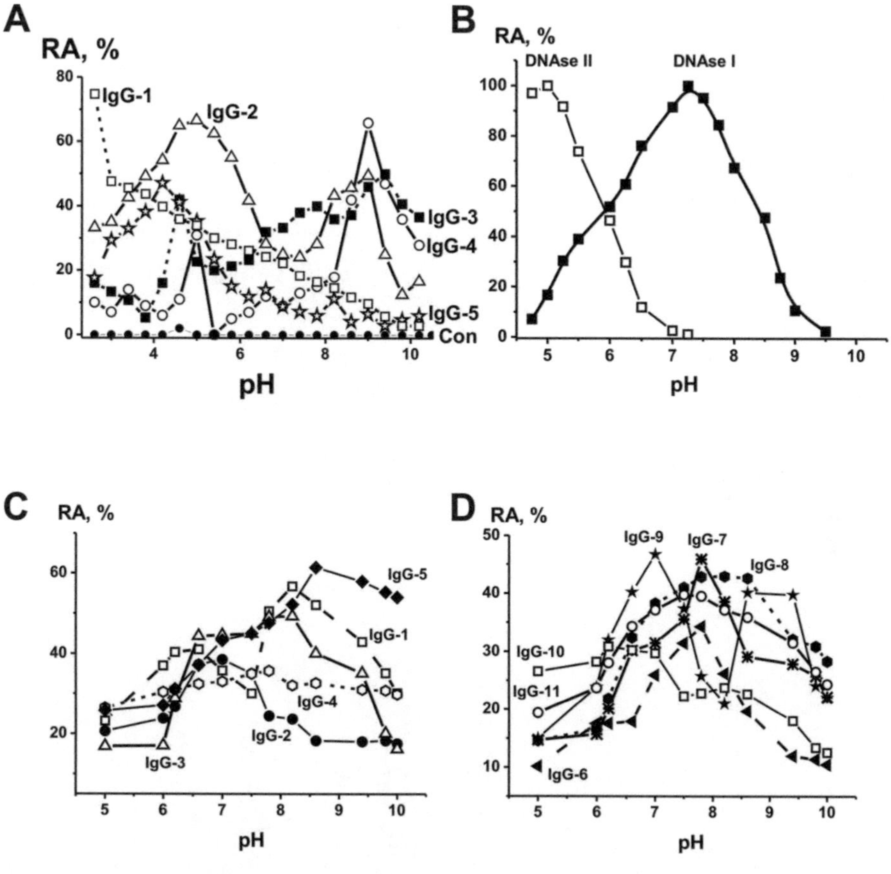

Figure 8. pH dependences of the RAs in the hydrolysis of plasmid DNA by five individual MS polyclonal IgGs (IgG-1–IgG-5) (A) and by canonical DNase I and DNase II (B) [56] as well as pH dependences of the relative MBP-hydrolyzing activity of five individual IgGs from the sera of five different MS (C) and six various SLE (D) patients [43, 51]. Hydrolysis of DNA incubated alone was used as control (A, "Con.") The relative DNase and protease activities corresponding to a complete transition of substrates to their shorter products as well as maximal activities of DNase I and DNase II were taken for 100%.

The next question concerning structural diversity of MS abzymes is related to a possibility of existence of catalytic Abs of different subclasses. It was interesting whether the cerebrospinal fluid similarly to serum of MS patients can contain IgG antibodies of all four subclasses. We have recently analyzed CSF and sera of MS patients, the average content of lambda- and kappa-IgGs as well as IgGs of four different subclasses (IgG1-IgG4) [53]. The average relative content of lambda-IgGs and kappa-IgGs in the case of CSFs (8.0 and 92.0%) and sera (12.3 and 87.7%) are comparable, while IgG1, IgG2, IgG3, and IgG4: CSF—40.4, 49.0, 8.2, and 2.5% of total IgGs, respectively, and the sera—53.6, 36.0, 5.6, and 4.8%, decreased in different order [53].

To analyze an "average" situation concerning a possible catalytic heterogeneity of MBP- and DNA-hydrolyzing IgGs from sera, we have prepared a mixture of equal amounts of IgGs from the sera of ten MS patients [51, 99]. The purity of IgGs of all types was confirmed by ELISA. It was shown that small fractions of IgGs of all four subclasses (IgG1–IgG4) are catalytically active in the DNA cleavage and their relative activity (nM supercoiled DNA/1 mg IgG/1 h) on average decreases in the order: IgG4 (4.1) < IgG3 (1.4) < IgG2 (0.94) < IgG1 (0.58), while their approximate relative contribution to the total activity of Abzs (taking into account their relative content in the sera) decreases in the order: IgG4 (65.6%) > IgG2 (18.2%) > IgG3 (9.3%) > IgG1 (6.9% [99]. In the hydrolysis of DNA on average, k-IgGs are several folds more active than λ-IgGs. By different physico-chemical methods of Abs analysis, it was shown that the immune systems of MS patients can generate a variety of different type of anti-DNA Abzs and with various catalytic properties, which can play an important role in MS pathogenesis.

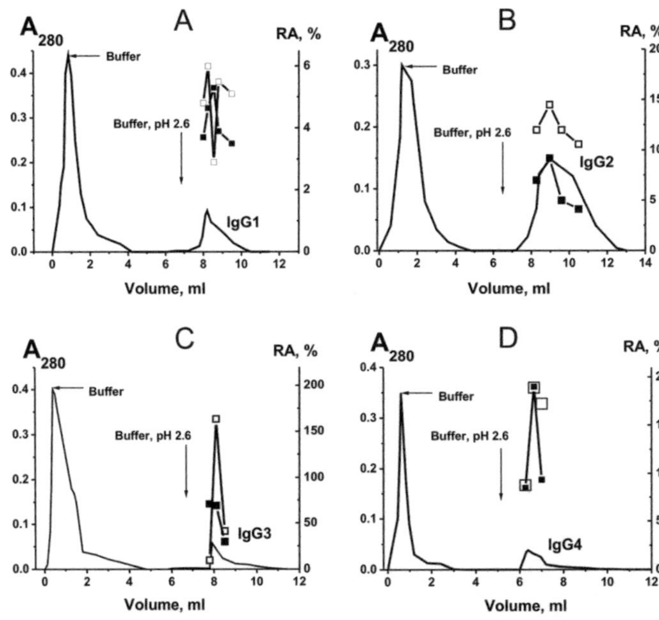

Figure 9. Affinity chromatography of polyclonal IgGs (mixture of 10 preparations from sera of MS patients) on anti-IgG1 (A), anti-IgG2 (B), anti-IgG3 (C), and anti-IgG4 (D) Sepharoses [84]: (—), absorbance at 280 nm, (□) and (■), relative catalytic activities (RA) in the hydrolysis of MBP and OP-19 corresponding to one of immunodominant region of MBP, respectively. Depending on the RA, the reaction mixtures were incubated for 0.3–16 h in the presence of 10–100 μg/ml IgGs and then the RAs were normalized to the standard conditions: the complete transition of 0.19 mg/ml MBP and 0.33 mM OP-19 to their hydrolyzed forms in the presence of 0.1 mg/ml IgGs after 1 h of incubation was taken for 100%. The average error in the initial rate determination from two experiments in each case did not exceed 7–10%.

It was shown that IgGs from sera of MS patients containing k- and λ-types of light chains demonstrated comparable relative activities in the hydrolysis of MBP [51]. IgGs of all four subclasses (IgG1–IgG4) demonstrate catalytic activity (**Figure 9**), their contribution to the total activity of Abzs in the hydrolysis of MBP and its 19-mer oligopeptide increasing in the order: IgG1 (1.5–2.1%) < IgG2 (4.9–12.8%) < IgG3 (14.7–25.0%) < IgG4 (71–78%). Interestingly, the RAs of DNase polyclonal IgGs from MS patients increased in the same order (IgG1 < IgG2 < IgG3 < IgG4 [99]) as the RAs of MBP-hydrolyzing IgGs from SLE patients [43]. These data provide the evidence that all types of human MS and SLE IgGs, IgG1–IgG4 can possess various catalytic activities, but differ in their RAs and contribution into the total activity of MBP- and DNA-hydrolyzing polyclonal Abzs.

4.4. Relative catalytic activity of MS abzymes

The catalysis mediated by artificial Abzs is usually characterized by relatively low k_{cat} values, which are 102- to 106-fold lower than those for canonical enzymes [1–8]. The known k_{cat} values for natural Abzs from AI patients vary in the range of 0.0001–40 min^{-1} [8–21]. The k_{cat} of polyclonal IgGs with various activities from sera of MS patients is in average varied in different ranges. Overall, the k_{cat} values characterizing hydrolysis of DNA, RNA, MBP, oligosaccharides in the reactions catalyzed by non-separated polyclonal MS IgGs and their subfractions separated by affinity chromatographies are comparable with or even higher than those for other known Abzs [8–21]. In addition, the RAs of DNase non-separated polyclonal Abs from patients with different diseases increase approximately in the order: diabetes [100] ≤ viral hepatitis [101] ≈ thick bone encephalitis [102] < polyarthritis ≤ Hashimoto's thyroiditis [71, 76, 103] ≤ schizophrenia [104] < AIDS [105] ≤ MS [54–56, 99] < SLE [10, 68–70]. At first glance, the k_{cat} values characterizing some polyclonal Abs may seem relatively low compared with those for canonical enzymes with the same enzymatic functions. At the same time, some DNA-dependent enzymes with very important functions, for example, repair enzymes and EcoRI endonuclease demonstrate the k_{cat} values comparable or even lower [106] than those for Abzs analyzed. In addition, the RAs of RNase IgGs and IgMs from the sera of patients with different autoimmune diseases including MS may be 10- to 1000-fold higher than those of DNase Abzs from the same patients. RNase activities of autoimmune Abzs were more often 0.1–20% of that of RNase A and of six known human sera RNases, while poly(A) was hydrolyzed by MS and other autoimmune Abs 2–10 times faster than by RNase A, one of the most active RNases known [11, 13–21, 54, 101]. The specific activity of IgGs of several MS patients was 40–400% of that of RNase A [101].

Notably, currently there are no methods that could efficiently separate Abzs from catalytically inactive antibodies against the same substrate (antigen). The specific activities were calculated using the total concentrations of polyclonal Abs, and affinity chromatography on DNA-cellulose or MBP-Sepharose leads only to partial enrichment of individual fractions with proteolytic and DNase activities. Thus, the specific substrate-hydrolyzing activities of the individual monoclonal Ab subfractions in pool of polyclonal Abs may be significantly higher than those of the non-fractionated or partially fractionated polyclonal IgGs, IgAs, and IgMs. In addition, it is impossible not to take into account catalytic activities of Abs from patients with MS and other autoimmune diseases in the analysis of their possible role in the pathogenesis of these pathologies, since some of them may be very harmful for people health.

5. Specific reorganization of immune system of SLE prone MRL-lpr/lpr mice

According to our data, the catalytic activity of nuclease and protease Abzs in sera of autoimmune patients is usually very easily detectable at the beginning of autoimmune diseases, when concentrations of Abs to DNA or other autoantigens are not yet significantly increased, and correspond to levels in healthy donors [13–21]. It was shown that detection of Abzs with different activities in human serum may be considered a good indicator of the onset or a significant progression of autoimmune reactions associated with several pathologies [13–21]. In this regard, is of great interest to understand what mechanisms underlie the development of autoimmune processes and how they associated with the production of catalytic antibodies. Some observations suggest that autoimmune diseases can be originated from defects in the hematopoietic stem cells (HSCs) [107]. Therefore, one can assume that in the development of different Ads, there may be some common objective laws. Taking this into account, it seems reasonable first to consider what regularities were found by us in the development of SLE in MRL-lpr/lpr mice. First, it was shown that IgGs from the sera of 2-month-old to 7-month-old control non-autoimmune BALB/c and (CBAxC57BL)F1 mice and conditionally healthy 2-month-old to3-month-old autoimmune prone MRL-lpr/lpr mice are catalytically inactive [22–24].

It is known that MRL-lpr/lpr mice spontaneously developing a lupus-like AI disorder are characterized by visual symptoms of the pathology (pink spots, baldness of head, and parts of the back, general health deterioration, etc.). The sera of these mice contain Abzs with DNase, amylase and ATPase activities [22–24, 108]. Appearance of proteinuria (≥3-mg/ml concentration of protein in urine) correlated well with pronounced visual symptoms [22–24]. The highest levels of anti-DNA Abs, catalytic activities of Abzs, visible markers of SLE and proteinuria were observed usually at 5–12 months of age, which agrees with previously reported data for typical period of signs of pathology appearance in MRL-lpr/lpr mice [109]. We have analyzed spontaneously diseased mice with all visible symptoms no older than 7 months. Although the state of "health" in the case of AI-prone mice should be considered very provisional, the mouse SLE pathology is nevertheless spontaneous and autoimmune reactions, leading to deep pathology develop gradually. To distinguish various levels of the pathology development, MRL-lpr/lpr mice demonstrating no typical SLE indices and Abzs activities (similar to healthy control non-autoimmune mice) were conditionally designated (independently of age) as healthy MRL-lpr/lpr mice, whereas the animals demonstrating no visual or biochemical SLE indices but having detectable abzyme activities were conditionally designated as pre-diseased mice.

A specific reorganization of immune system of these mice after spontaneous development of deep SLE-like pathology results in conditions associated with a production of Abs hydrolyzing

DNA, ATP, and polysaccharides with low catalytic activities (conditionally pre-diseased mice). A significant increase in amylase and especially DNase, ATPase relative activities was associated with a transition from pre-diseased to deep diseased mice correlating with additional changes in differentiation and proliferation of mouse bone marrow hematopoietic stem cells and lymphocyte proliferation in different organs. The highest increase in activities of all Abzs was revealed in 3-month healthy mice immunized with DNA, which are characterized by a different profile of HSC differentiation and by a significant suppression of cell apoptosis in comparison with pre-diseased and diseased mice. Overall, all mouse groups investigated were characterized by a specific relationship between abzyme activities, HSC differentiation profiles, levels of lymphocyte proliferation, and cell apoptosis in different organs [22–24]. We came to the conclusion that the appearance of ATPase and DNase activities in diseased mice [22–24] similarly to SLE and MS patients [13–21] may be considered as the earliest statistically significant marker of spontaneous SLE and a further significant increase in catalytic activities correlates with the appearance of SLE visible markers and with an increase in proteinuria and concentrations of anti-DNA Abs. Some differences in immune system reorganizations at pre-disease and deep disease leading to the production of different autoantibodies and Abzs comparing with healthy mice were revealed [22–24].

6. Change of some indexes characterizing development of EAE in C57BL/6 mice

We tried to compare several different indexes associated with development of ADs in autoimmune prone mice MRL-lpr/lpr and experimental autoimmune encephalomyelitis (EAE; C57BL/6) mice, the models of human SLE and MS, respectively. When for acceleration of SLE development in MRL-lpr/lpr DNA is usually used [22–24], the stimulation of EAE in C57BL/6mice is usually carried out using mouse myelin oligodendrocyte glycoprotein (MOG35-55), which is an antigen of the myelin sheath [112, 113].

In our study, we have used four experimental groups of C57BL/6 and (CBA × C57BL) F1 or CBA mice:

- untreated control EAE C57BL/6 mice [110],
- MOG-immunized C57BL/6 mice [110],
- control untreated non-autoimmune CBA mice [111],
- control MOG-immunized non-autoimmune CBA mice [111].

In MOG-induced EAE mice, first clinical symptoms appear at 5–7 days after immunization, while the maximum stage of the disease is usually manifested at 14–16 days after immunization [112, 113]. A possible change in the relative weight, different immunological and biochemical parameters at 3 months of age (zero time; control) as well as MOG-treated C57BL/6 and CBA mice during consecutive 40 days was analyzed. After 6 days but not at later stages an average decrease in weight of EAE mice was observed in MOG treated compared to untreated control mice (**Figure 10A**), but the weight of CBA mice increase slower, than untreated mice during 40 days (**Figure 10B**). In other models of autoimmunity including MRL-lpr/lpr, the appearance of pronounced visual symptoms usually correlates well with proteinuria (≥3 mg/ml concentration of protein in urine) [22–24]. Control non-autoimmune CBA mice at 7 months demonstrated no proteinuria (<2 mg/ml) [22–24]. At the same time, EAE C57BL/6 mice at three months of age are usually characterized by a significantly higher level of proteinuria (up to 10–12 mg/ml) [114]. We have analyzed the time-dependent change in proteinuria for immunized and untreated C57BL/6 mice (**Figure 10C**) and control CBA mice (**Figure 10D**). In seven mice of the EAE control group, the average proteinuria was 7.2 ± 0.8 mg/ml at time zero (3 months of age) and was nearly the same until day 20, but increased to 12 ± 0.8 mg/ml at 40 days (**Figure 10C**). For control CBA untreated mice, there was no remarkable change in concentration of urine proteins during 40 days (**Figure 10D**). In EAE mice treated with MOG, a steady increase in proteinuria was observed: day 0: 7.2 ± 0.8 mg/ml; day 30: 13.6 ± 2.5 mg/ml; day 40: 21.8 ± 3.8 mg/ml. The increase after 40 days became significantly different from control animals (**Figure 10C**). CBA mice from 0 to 40 days demonstrated increase in urine protein concentration from 1.6 ± 0.08 to 2.5 ± 0.23 mg/ml (**Figure 10D**). High level of EAE mice proteinuria at three months may be due to the fact that these mice demonstrate spontaneous development of autoimmune processes, which is stimulated by their immunization by MOG. Immunization of non-autoimmune CBA mice also leads to remarkable increase in proteinuria, but after 40 days it is lower 3 mg/ml (**Figure 10D**).

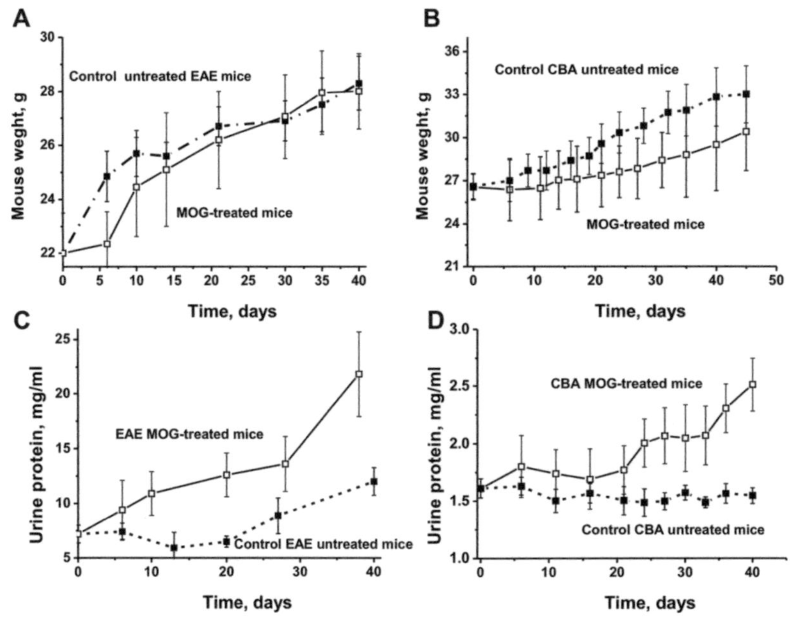

Figure 10. In time changes in weight of C57B2/6 (A) and CBA (B) mice, as well as relative concentration of urine proteins of C57B2/6 (C) and CBA (D) mice in the case of MOG-treated and untreated animals (see Panels) [110, 111].

The sera of healthy humans and mammals usually contain auto-Abs to many various antigens, including DNA [13–21, 59]. For example, the average concentration of anti-DNA Abs for BALB and CBA non-autoimmune mice is approximately 0.03–0.04 A450 units, which is comparable with that for healthy MRL-lpr/lpr mice (0.032 A450 units); then after the spontaneous development of SLE it increases to 0.2 A450 units [24]. Untreated C57BL/6 mice demonstrated an approximately 3.5-fold higher concentration of anti-DNA Abs (0.12 ± 0.04 A450 units) at 3 months of age (day 0) comparing with MRL-lpr/lpr mice. For untreated C57BL/6 mice, the change in anti-DNA Abs during 0–40 days was statistically insignificant (**Figure 11A**). Comparing to healthy control individuals and other neurological diseases of non-AI origin, the sera of MS patients contain anti-DNA Abs at a higher concentration (0.22 A450 units) [19, 21]. Immunization of C57BL/6 mice with MOG during 30 days (0.24 A450 units) led to a near-linear statistically significant twofold increase in anti-DNA Ab concentration, and then to a further additional increase to 0.42 A450 units, which is higher than that for spontaneous disease (0.12 A450 units) (**Figure 11A**), but lower than that for MRL-lpr/lpr mice immunized with DNA (0.6 A450 units) [24].

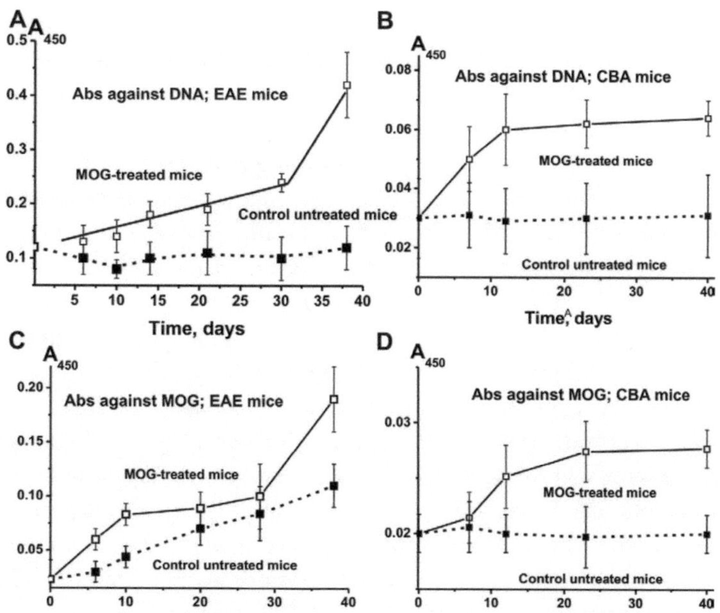

Figure 11. Relative concentrations of Abs to DNA in the case of C57B2/6 (A) and CBA (B) mice as well as to MOG for C57B2/6 (C) and CBA (D) untreated and treated with MOG (see Panels) [110, 111]. Anti-MOG and anti-MBP antibody concentrations in the sera of C57B2/6 and CBA mice were measured by ELISA (sera was diluted 50-fold). The concentration of plasma anti-DNA Abs was determined using standard ELISA plates with immobilized double-stranded DNA (sera was diluted 100-fold).

Untreated CBA mice demonstrated at zero time fourfold lower average concentration of anti-DNA Abs (0.03 A450 units) comparing with EAE mice (0.12 A450 units), and their concentration was not increase remarkably during 40 days (**Figure 11B**). After CBA mice treatment with

MOG, the average concentration of anti-DNA Abs increased ~twofold at 12 days (0.06 A450 units) and then was the same up to 40 days (**Figure 11B**). Finally at 40 days, anti-DNA concentration in treated CBA mice was ~sevenfold lower than for EAE mice immunized with MOG (**Figure 11**). Thus, the immunization of CBA mice with MOG can somehow stimulate their immune response to DNA in these healthy mice, but it is significantly lower than that in the case of autoimmune EAE C57BL/6 mice.

Human healthy donors show a relative average index of anti-MBP Abs – 0.08 ± 0.04 A450, which is ~four- and fivefold lower than that for MS patients (0.32 ± 0.08 A450 units) [44]. The concentration of anti-MOG Abs in the sera of C57BL/6 control (untreated) mice demonstrated a near-linear statistically significant approximately 4.8-fold increase during 40 days (from 0.023 to 0.11 A450 units; **Figure 11C**). After treatment of mice, a significant rise in the titter at 10 days (from 0.023 to 0.083 A450 units) was revealed, followed by a temporary plateau and then an additional increase to 0.18 A450 units. The concentrations of anti-MOG Abs at zero time for C57BL/6 and CBA mice were to some extent comparable (~0.02 A450 units). However, in contrast to EAE mice, CBA mice did not demonstrate remarkable change in anti-MOG Abs over time (**Figure 11D**). The treatment of CBA mice with MOG led to an increase in the average concentration of anti-MOG Abs ~1.4-fold, but this value (0.028 A450 units) is ~6.5- and ~fourfold, respectively lower than those for treated (0.18 A450 units) and untreated (0.11 A450 units) EAE mice (**Figure 11**). Thus, the immunization of CBA mice with MOG stimulates formation of Abs against this antigen, but these healthy mice in contrast to EAE mice do not demonstrate spontaneous development of autoimmune reactions leading to the formation of anti-MOG antibodies. These data indicate that the mice treatment with MOG leads to the formation of Abs against MOG and to DNA. At the same time, the relative concentrations of Abs to different antigens are not always good indicators of the real development of autoimmune diseases, because the relative titters to autoantigens in healthy humans and mammals can be very different [13–21, 59]. The titters of antibodies against autoantigens in sick patients and animals are usually higher than those in healthy individuals only in very late stages of ADs. As we have shown previously, the detection of DNase Abs in human sera may be considered to be a good indicator for the beginning of, or a significant development in, AI reactions associated with several ADs [13–21]. Moreover, like in AI patients, only DNase and ATPase activities of IgGs can be considered as statistically significant indicators of pre-disease conditions of spontaneous SLE in AI prone MRL-lpr/lpr mice [22–24]. Notably, well detectable DNase and ATPase Abs in MRL-lpr/lpr mice can sometimes be revealed 1–2 months earlier than a statistically reliable increase in Abs against DNA, as well as detection of visual and biochemical indexes of mouse SLE [22–24]. We have estimated the relative DNase and proteolytic activities of IgGs from untreated EAE and CBA and MOG-treated mice (**Figure 12**). Surprisingly, detectable levels of IgGs with all activities (in contrast to MRL-lpr/lpr) were revealed the sera of untreated C57BL/6 mice [22–24] even at the beginning of the experiment (at 3 months of age) and then it increased near-linearly. After 40 days, all activities were statistically significantly higher than at day 0: DNase (6.1-fold), MOG-hydrolyzing (1.8-fold), MBP-hydrolyzing (2.8-fold) (**Figure 12**), while there was no statistically significant increase in the concentrations of anti-DNA Abs (**Figure 11**). Furthermore, the detectable increase in abzymes from immunized EAE mice hydrolyzing DNA, MOG, and MBP was observed at a time corresponding to the outset and acute phase of EAE (6–8 days), followed by a statistically significant increase in their activities at 14 days, and maximal increases at 22 days after treatment with MOG (**Figure 12**). Interestingly, a significant decrease in the activities was revealed at the transition from the acute (18–22 days) to the severe chronic phase of EAE (40 days) induced by MOG.

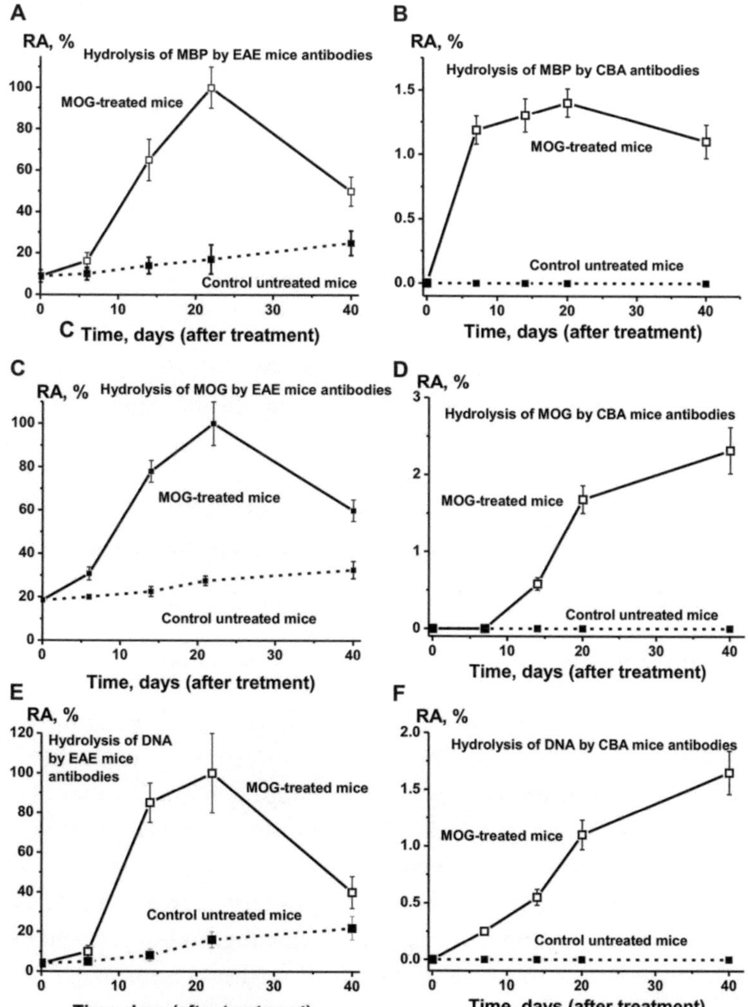

Figure 12. In time changes in the relative average activity of IgGs from sera of untreated and MOG-treated EAE C57B2/6 and CBA mice in the hydrolysis of MBP (A, B), MOG (C, D) and DNA (E, F) [110, 111]. To quantify the MOG-, MBP-, and DNA-hydrolyzing activities of IgGs of different groups, we determined a concentration for each individual IgG preparation (0.03–0.2 mg/ml) and time of incubation (1–24 h) providing hydrolysis (10–40%) of these substrates to their products. Since all measurements (initial rates) were taken within the linear regions of the time courses and Abs concentration curves, the measured RAs for IgGs were normalized to standard conditions and maximal enzymatic activities were taken as 100% of activity analyzed. The average relative activities (RAs) of IgGs corresponding to 7 individual mice for each group are given.

It was shown earlier that Abs from sera of healthy mice and rabbit are completely inactive in the hydrolysis of different substrates including DNA and proteins [13–21]. Immunization of healthy animals with complex DNA and methylated BSA (m-BSA) led to the formation of Abs-hydrolyzing DNA and RNA [116, 117]. The averages relative activities of Abs from sera of immunized animals are usually 100- to 1000-fold lower those from patients with autoimmune diseases [13–21, 115, 116].

IgGs from sera of CBA untreated mice were completely inactive in the hydrolysis of MBP, MOG, and DNA (**Figure 12**). After treatment of CBA mice, IgGs demonstrated detectable activity in the hydrolysis of these substrates, but their maximal relative activities in the hydrolysis of MBP, MOG, and DNA were approximately 40- to 70-fold lower than those for Abs of immunized EAE mice (**Figure 12**). In addition, IgGs from sera of EAE mice at three months of age were significantly more active than maximal activity of Abs of immunized CBA mice in the hydrolysis of all substrates: MBP (6.4-fold), MOG (6.5-fold), and DNA (2.5-fold) (**Figure 12**). It means that spontaneous autoimmune processes and the appearance of the cells producing different Abzs begin to develop in EAE mice before 3 months of their age.

Interestingly, during 40 days, the average relative DNA-hydrolyzing activity increased in EAE mice by a factor of 6.1 (**Figure 12E**), while statistically significant increase in the titters of anti-DNA Abs, there was not observed (**Figure 11A**). Since it was previously shown that the relative content of Abzs to different antigens in the total pools of Abs is usually $\leq 0.01-3\%$, this phenomenon is not surprising, [13–21]. Therefore, the production of a small fraction of specific DNase and protease Abzs may have no detectable effect on the total concentration anti-DNA and anti-MOG Abs.

6.1. Proliferation and apoptosis of lymphocytes in different organs of EAE prone mice

Immunization of healthy and AI-prone mammals usually leads to in an increase in the level of lymphocytes differentiation and proliferation in different organs [19–21]. Different lymphocytes producing Abzs were obtained with a dramatically higher incidence in autoimmune mouse strains than in conventionally used control mouse strains [117, 118]. At the same time, immunization of animals with some antigens usually leads to an increase in apoptosis of some lymphocytes. Apoptotic cells are considered as the primary source of antigens and immunogens in SLE triggering the recognition, perception, processing, and/or presentation of apoptotic autoantigens by antigen-presenting cells and can cause AI processes [60]. DNA-hydrolyzing DNase Abzs from patients with SLE [68] and MS [16], as well as DNase Bence-Jones proteins from multiple myeloma patients [119] are cytotoxic, cause nuclear DNA fragmentation, and induce cell apoptosis. A significant decrease in apoptosis can be an important factor providing the enhancement in the level of specific lymphocytes producing auto-Abs and Abzs, which are normally eliminated in different mammalian organs. Thus, the total number of lymphocytes of various types in different organs after immunization of animals depends on the ratio of possible levels of cell proliferation and apoptosis. The overall level of cytotoxic (harmful) or beneficial to organisms antibodies may depend on this ratio.

We have compared possible lymphocyte proliferation (**Figure 13**) and apoptosis (**Figure 14**) in different organs of EAE and CBA mice. Lymphocyte proliferation in different organs at 3 months of age (zero time) for EAE and CBA mice is to some extent comparable (**Figure 13**).

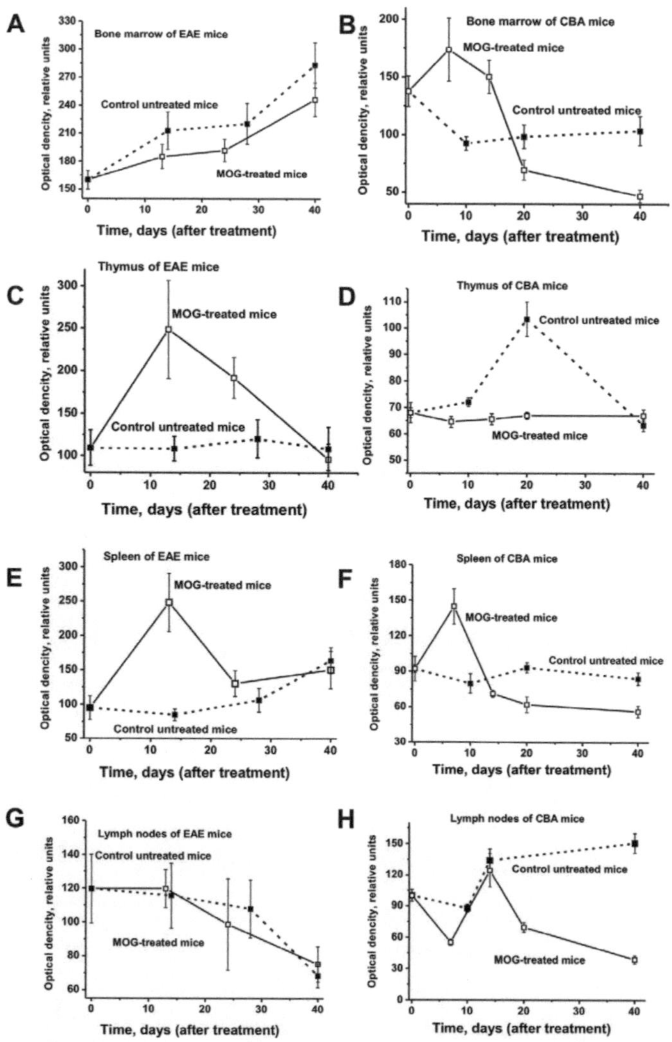

Figure 13. In time changes in lymphocyte proliferation (optical density) in bone marrow, thymus, spleen, and lymph nodes in the case of untreated and MOG-treated EAE and CBA mice; average values corresponding to 7 mice of each group are given [110, 111]. The error in the lymphocyte determination from three independent experiments in the case of every mouse of each group did not exceed 7–10%. Types of mice and their organs are given on panels A–H.

Proliferation of lymphocytes in bone marrow of untreated EAE mice increases constantly over time, and their treatment with MOG slightly decreases the proliferation level (**Figure 13A**). At the same time, untreated CBA mice demonstrate a remarkable decrease in the cell proliferation level over time. However, immunization of these mice with MOG increases their proliferation in the period from 10 to 15 days, but then it is significantly decreased (**Figure 13B**). Maximal observed level of lymphocytes proliferation in bone marrow CBA mice (~26%) is ~threefold lower than that for EAE mice (~77%). The total number of lymphocytes resulting in the brains of EAE mice can be significantly higher than the observed one, since the average level of cell apoptosis in the brains of these mice is about 14.2% and increased up to 22.4% after their treatment with MOG (**Figure 14A**). Interestingly, at three month of age, CBA mice (4.2%) demonstrate ~3.4-fold lower the average level of cell apoptosis comparing with EAE mice, while their immunization with MOG increase it only to 4.6% (**Figure 14B**), 4.9-fold lower than that for EAE mice (**Figure 14A**).

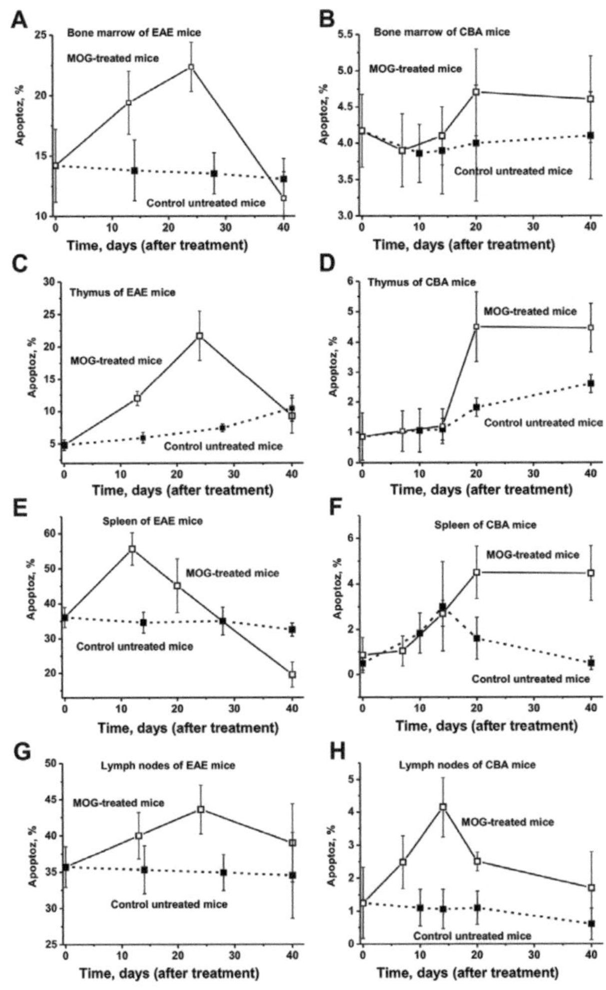

Figure 14. In time changes in cell apoptosis (%) in bone marrow, thymus, spleen, and lymph nodes in the case of untreated and MOG-treated EAE and CBA mice; average values corresponding to 7 mice of each group are given [110, 111]. The error in the cell apoptosis determination from three independent experiments in the case of every mouse of each group did not exceed 7–10%. Types of mice and their organs are given on panels A–H.

The level of lymphocyte proliferation in thymus of untreated EAE mice almost does not change in time (**Figures 13C**), while it increases significantly at 20 days and then return to the level observed at zero time at 40 days (**Figure 13D**). The converse situation is observed for levels of the lymphocytes proliferation of EAE and CBA mice after their immunization with MOG (**Figures 13C** and **D**). Interestingly, the level of the thymus cell apoptosis in healthy CBA (~0.9%) at three month of age is about fivefold lower than that for EAE mice (~4.8%); after mice treatment with MOG, it increases in EAE mice up to 22%, but remains relatively low (~4.8%) in CBA animals. Thus, in contrast to EAE animals, the apoptosis does not affect significantly on the level of lymphocytes proliferation in thymus of CBA mice.

While the level of lymphocytes proliferation in the spleen of untreated EAE mice remarkably increases over time, in CBA mice, it has tendency of only slight decrease (**Figures 13 E** and **F**). At the beginning of autoimmune processes in MOG-immunized EAE mice (7–15 days), there is a strong increase in spleen lymphocytes proliferation for EAE and CBA mice, but the maximum value for autoimmune mice is significantly higher (**Figures 13E** and **F**). Interestingly, the relative level of spleen cell apoptosis in non-immunized EAE mice at three months is very high (~36%) compared to the bone marrow (14.2%) and especially to the thymus (4.8%), but it remains practically unchanged during the spontaneous development of the EAE pathology (**Figure 14E**). At three months of age, CBA mice are characterized by a very low level of spleen cell apoptosis, 0.5%, and its increases at 14 days to 3%, but it returns to 0.5% at 40 days (**Figure 14F**). The treatment of EAE mice leads first (12 days) to an increase in the proliferation from 36% to 55.6%, and then to significant decrease to 19.5% at 40 days. Approximately after 20 days of CBA mice treatment with MOG the cell proliferation increase to ~5%, this is ~11-fold lower than that for EAE mice (**Figure 14F**). Thus, immune processes in the spleen of control healthy CBA mice before and after their treatment with MOG vary relatively weak over time. However, a slow increase in the number of lymphocytes in the spleen of EAE mice during spontaneous develop of the disease and its acceleration after treatment with MOG are associated with strong parallel opposite processes in the lymphocytes proliferation and apoptosis (**Figures 13** and **14E** and **F**). These data are consistent with the fact that immunization of MRL-lpr/lpr mice at three months of age with DNA also leads to a very strong activation of the proliferation and apoptosis in their spleen [22–24].

Lymph nodes of EAE and CBA mice demonstrate different profiles of the cell proliferation over time (**Figures 13 G** and **H**). The level of cell proliferation in lymph nodes of EAE mice before and after animals' treatment with MOG is nearly the same; the cell proliferation is constantly decreased from 3 to 40 days. The level of lymphocytes proliferation in the lymph nodes of CBA mice at 6–10 days before and after their treatment is remarkably decreased (**Figure 13H**). Then, untreated and treated CBA mice show remarkable increase in the proliferation level, but finally control mice at 40 days demonstrate additional increase, while immunized mice—significant decrease in cell proliferation. It should be mentioned that lymph nodes (~36%) similarly to spleen (~36%) of EAE mice are characterized by very high level of cell apoptosis at three months of age, while this level for CBA mice is very low (~1.3%) (**Figure 14H**). Parallel high-level differently directed processes of the cell proliferation and apoptosis in lymph nodes of EAE mice can probably to some extent counterbalance each other. High level of the apoptosis in the lymph nodes of non-treated, but more powerful apoptosis in treated EAE mice can be a reason of a slow decrease in lymphocytes of this organ of autoimmune mice leading to a comparable profiles of the changes over time (**Figures 13** and **14**). The relative changes in the levels of proliferation and apoptosis in lymph nodes of CBA comparing with EAE mice are relatively low (**Figures 13** and **14**).

Overall, the autoimmune EAE and non-autoimmune CBA mice demonstrate very different profiles of differentiation and proliferation of bone marrow stem cells, as well as levels of proliferation and apoptosis of lymphocytes in various organs.

Primary differentiation of lymphocytes begins in the bone morrow of people and animals, and additional differentiation occurs in their various organs. Therefore, possible relative levels of cell differentiation, proliferation, and apoptosis in various organs of mice depends on what type of hematopoietic stem cells was "arrived" to these organs from their bone marrow. As it was mentioned above, autoimmune diseases can originate from defects in hematopoietic stem cells [107]. Therefore, it was very important to understand a possible difference and similarity in differentiation and proliferation of stem cells in the bone marrow of mice, which are prone and unwilling to autoimmune diseases.

6.2. Differentiation of stem cells in the bone marrow of mice

The specific reorganization of the immune system in a profound SLE-like pathology of MRL-lpr/lpr mice during its spontaneous development is associated with changes in the differentiation profile of bone marrow HSCs, leading to the rise of the level of lymphocyte proliferation in combination with the production of different Abzs [22–24]. Since similar to MRL-lpr/lpr, C57BL/6 mice also reveal features of autoimmune-prone mice, it was reasonable to expect similar changes in the HSCs: erythroid burst-forming unit (early erythroid colonies; BFU-E), erythroid burst-forming unit (late erythroid colonies; CFU-E), granulocytic-macrophagic colony-forming unit (CFU-GM), and granulocytic-erythroid-megacaryocytic-macrophagic colony-forming unit (CFU-GEMM) in these mice before and after their immunization with MOG. But it was also very interesting to compare changes in the HSCs for autoimmune C57BL/6 and non-autoimmune CBA mice.

The relative amount of different colonies (BFU-E + CFU-E + CFU-GM + CFU-GEMM) of three monthly autoimmune EAE and normal healthy CBA mice was different. In order to calculate the relative amount of four different types of colonies, we have estimated a relative percent of every type of the colonies with respect to the total number of colonies taken as 100% (**Table 2**). It was shown that the average relative number of BFU-E (57.3 ± 20.1 and 54.5 ± 7.0%), CFU-GM (34.0 ± 3.9 and 28.2 ± 2.0%) colonies, respectively, for C57BL/6 and CBA mice at three months of age was to some extent comparable (**Table 2**). At the same time, the relative average number of CFU-E (3.2 ± 1.7%) for EAE mice was 4.6 lower than that for CBA mice (14.7 ± 10.5%), while in the case of CFU-GEMM, the reverse situation was observed; this average value for EAE mice (5.6 ± 1.7%) was ~2.2-fold higher than that for CBA mice (2.6 ± 0.78%) (**Table 2**). In time changes in the proliferation profiles of the HSCs, during 40 days, it was observed for untreated and MOG-treated autoimmune C57BL/6 and non-autoimmune CBA mice.

Mice	The average relative content, %			
	BFU-E	CFU-E	CFU-GM	CFU-GEMM
EAE, C57BL/6 (1)**	57.3±20.1	3.2±1.7	34.0±3.9	5.6±1.7
Healthy, CBA (2)	54.5±7.0	14.7±10.5	28.2±2.0	2.6±0.78
Ratio of values 1 and 2 or (2 and 1)	1.1 (0.95)	0.22 (4.6)	1.2 (0.83)	2.2 (0.46)

*

Total amount of four types of colonies was taken for 100 %; the average meaning± average deviation are given.

**

Parameters 1 and 2 from [110] and [111], respectively.

Table 2. The average relative content of different colonies of EAE and CBA mice at three month of age (zero time).

It was revealed that there was a constant increase in the relative amount of BFU-E in untreated EAE mice to 28–30 days and then was observe a small decrease (**Figure 15A**). After the treatment of EAE mice with MOG, there was a significant decrease in BFU-E colonies up to 18–20 days and then there was a significant increase (**Figure 15A**). In the case of healthy CBA mice, we revealed quite opposite situation; the relative number of BFU-E in time for untreated mice was decreased, while after treatment with MOG it was significantly increased (**Figure 15B**).

In time changes of CFU-E, before and after treatment of EAE mice was comparable; first there was significant increase from 0 to 10 days and then from 10 to 40 days the number of these colonies slowly, but strongly decreased (**Figure 15C**). CFU-E colonies demonstrated different changes over time in the case of CBA mice. Before and after CBA mice treatment, the relative number of CFU-E cells was remarkably decreased from 0 to approximately 10–12 days (**Figure 15D**). At the same time, later we observed significant increase in CFU-E for MOG-treated CBA mice, but brightly expressed decrease of the cells in the case of the untreated mice (**Figure 15D**).

Quite opposite types in the differentiation were also observed for CFU-GM forming units in the case of the EAE and CBA mice (**Figures 15 E** and **F**). While the relative number of CFU-GM cells in EAE mice over time was dramatically decreased (0–30 days), in the case of CBA mice, it was remarkably increased (0–40 days). The MOG-treatment of EAE mice led to a slight increase in the number of the CFU-GM colonies, while for CBA mice there was observed a constant decrease the number of these colonies (**Figure 15E** and **F**).

Interestingly, a significant decrease in the CFU-GEMM units in treated EAE mice was observed at 10–40 days, while the level of their decrease for untreated mice was observed only after 20 days (**Figure 15G**). In the case of untreated CBA mice, the relative number of CFU-GEMM units was significantly increased from 0 to 25 days, but then it began to decrease, while treatment of CBA mice with MOG stimulated a constant decrease in the number of these colonies (**Figure 15H**). Thus, the autoimmune C57BL/6 and non-autoimmune CBA mice of three-month age demonstrate comparable percent of BFU-E and CFU-GM colonies, but significant difference in the relative number of CFU-E and CFU-GEMM units (**Figure 15**). In addition, these mice show a completely opposite profile of stem cells differentiation before and after their treatment with MOG (**Figure 15**). However, changes in the differentiation profile in the case of untreated CBA mice are not associated with the appearance of cells producing Abzs; Abs from the sera of these mice are completely catalytically inactive. Immunization of CBA mice with MOG stimulates production of Abs-hydrolyzing MBP, MOG, and DNA, but the activities of these Abzs are very low comparing with those for EAE mice. Specific differentiation of bone marrow stem cells of EAE mice even before three months of their age leads to the appearance of cells producing abzyme with relatively high activity. During spontaneous development of EAE in C57BL/6 mice, there is a significant increase in such cells and Abzs, while their immunization stimulates a very strong increase in the Abzs activities.

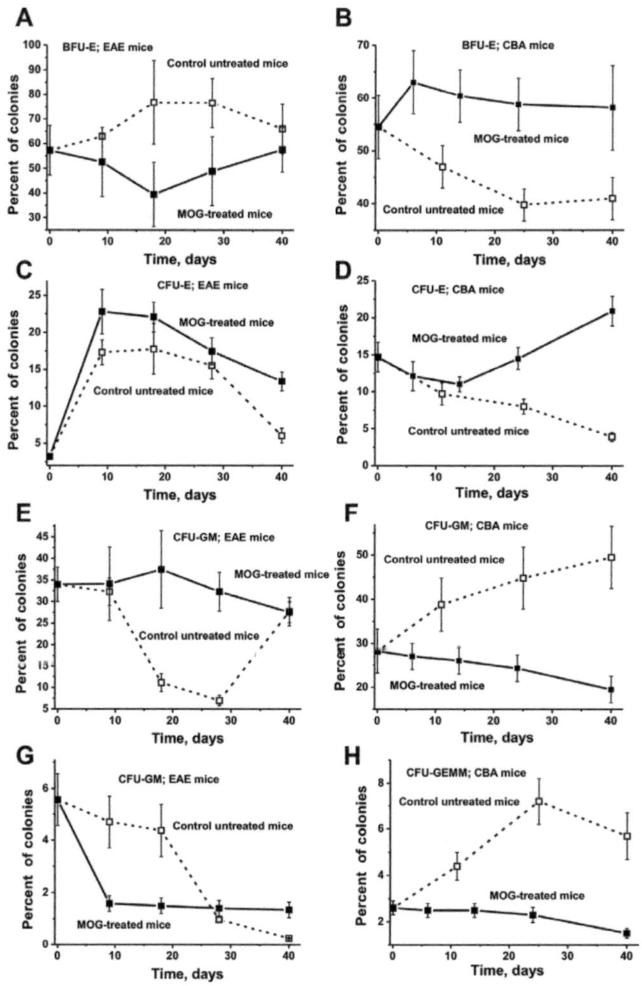

Figure 15. In time changes of an average relative content (%) of colony-forming units of bone marrow progenitor colonies of different type in the case of untreated and MOG-treated mice; average percent of different colonies (BFU-E + CFU-E + CFU-GM + CFU-GEMM) corresponding to 7 mice of each group of autoimmune C57B2/6 and non-autoimmune CBA mice are given; types of progenitor colonies and mice analyzed are shown on panels A–H.

Cuprizone-induced demyelination is a widely used experimental model to study processes of de- and remyelination in the central nervous system [120–123]. We used EAE C57BL/6 mice to assess effects of cuprizone-induced demyelination on different parameters associated with autoimmune inflammation [124]. It was shown that treatment of mice with cuprizone (0–40 days) leads to a significant decrease in the size of the brain corpus callosum when compared with untreated mice. In addition, cuprizone treatment leads to a significant decrease of several indexes, which characterize spontaneous and MOG-induced EAE: increased levels of proteinuria, titters of anti-DNA and anti-MOG antibodies, the generation of Abzshydrolyzing DNA, myelin basic protein (MBP), and MOG. As it mentioned above, spontaneous and MOG-induced EAE is associated with a specific reorganization of the immune system resulting in changes in the profile and level of proliferation of mice HSCs. At day 40 of the experiment, cuprizone decreases the summed proliferation of HSCs (BFU-E, CFU-E, CFU-GM and CFU-GEMM) colony units ~1.2-fold in comparison with untreated mice, but does not significantly change the differentiation profile of BFU-E, CFU-GM, and CFU-GEMM cells. Our data indicate that cuprizone treatment is associated with demyelination, but not with stimulation of autoimmune processes.

It was shown that cuprizone has selective specificity against oligodendrocytes [120, 121]. Acute demyelination following treatment with cuprizone is associated with apoptosis of oligodendrocytes, activation of microglia, and phagocytosis of myelin sheaths [122, 123]. Cuprizone causes demyelination processes all over the brain, with the corpus callosum being the most affected structure. Also distinct foci of demyelination are found in the hippocampus, cerebellum, putamen, and the ventral part of caudal nuclei.

According to our data, cuprizone-induced demyelination is likely not associated with the development of typical autoimmune processes observed after spontaneous or MOG-induced EAE. It looks more like a specific poisoning of mice with cuprizone, leading to the manifestation of some symptoms seen in EAE. The effect of a cuprizone leading to the suppression of cell proliferation and activation of apoptosis [120–123] is consistent with our data on the decrease in the level of lymphocyte proliferation and inhibition of profile differentiation changes of stem cells in the bone marrow. A maximal decrease in the RAs of all Abzs after EAE mice treatment with cuprizone correlates with twofold decrease in the proliferation only CFU-E cells, while its effect on proliferation of other cells was negligible. The relative number of CFU-E colonies over time is significantly decreased in untreated CBA mice (**Figure 15D**), which Abs are completely inactive in the hydrolysis of MBP, MOG, and DNA (**Figure 12**). In addition, maximal activities of Abzs (**Figure 12**) correlate with maximal increase of CFU-E cells in treated CBA mice (**Figure 15**). Moreover, maximal increase in the activities of Abzs in MOG-treated EAE mice at 10–20 days (**Figure 12**) correlates with a sharp increase in the relative amount of these cells at this time (**Figure 15C**). The totality of our data suggests that it is the CFU-E cells may be early progenitors of cells producing catalytic antibodies.

On the one hand, in the debut of various autoimmune diseases usually occurs production of auto-antibodies to different autoantigens and abzyme with different catalytic activities. On the other hand, the repertoires of abzymes with different enzymatic activities and autoantibodies to various autoantigens are constantly expanding. This is indicative of the fact that the basis of all autoimmune diseases may be to some extent similar.

7. Comparison of stem cell differentiation in SLE and EAE mice

C57BL/6 and MRL-lpr–lpr are two various mouse models spontaneously developing two different autoimmune diseases, EAE and SLE, respectively. Stimulation of EAE pathology development usually occurs after immunization of C57BL/6 mice with MOG [112, 113], while SLE after treatment of MRL-lpr–lpr mice with DNA [22–24]. It was interesting to understand a possible difference or similarity in the changing of the differentiation profiles of stem cells of the bone marrow in the case of these models comparing with those for the control CBA mice before and after their treatment with MOG and with DNA. **Figure 16** demonstrates the relative levels BFU-E, CFU-E, CFU-GM, and CFU-GEMM units (%) at the beginning (zero time), spontaneous changes and after mice treatment with MOG (57BL/6) and DNA (MRL-lpr–lpr) at 40 days of the experiments. One can see that the relative content of BFU-E colonies (%) constantly decrease in autoimmune EAE and SLE mice at transition from zero time to spontaneous development of these diseases (40 days) and acceleration of their development by treatment with MOG and DNA at 40 days (**Figure 16A**).

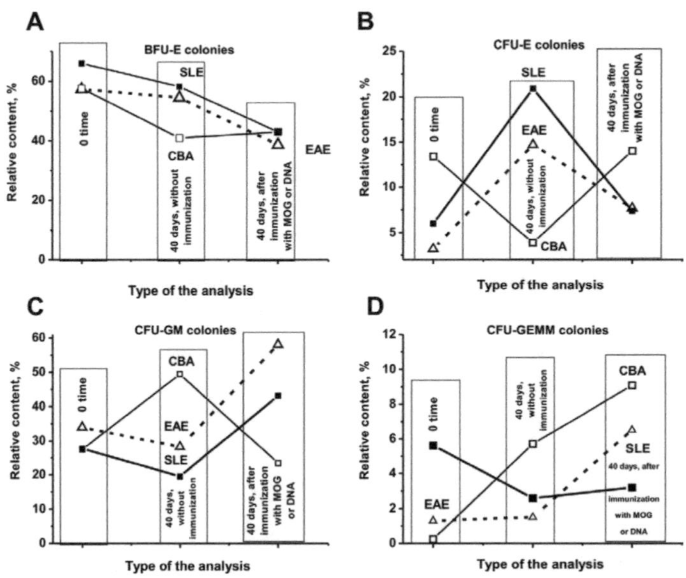

Figure 16. Change in the relative percent (sum of four types of colonies was taken for 100%) of BFU-E (A), CFU-E (B), CFU-GM (C), and BFU-GEMM (D) types of colonies in comparison with zero time of the experiments (first group of values) in the case of spontaneous development of EAE and SLE by respectively C57BL/6 and MRL-lpr–lpr mice after 40 days and changes of differentiation profile of HSCs in CBA mice after 40 days (second group of values); third group of values corresponds to relative amount of the colonies after 40 days in the case C57BL/6 and CBA mice treated with MOG [110, 111] and MRL-lpr–lpr mice immunized with DNA [22–24].

Non-autoimmune CBA mice demonstrate at 40 days a decrease in the percent of BFU-E, when their treatment with MOG leads to remarkable increase in the relative number of these cells. Very similar regularities in the changes of the relative content of CFU-E (**Figure 16B**) and CFU-GM (**Figure 16C**) are observed for EAE and SLE mice, and they are directly opposite than that for the CBA mice. There is a remarkable but not essentially important difference in the curves corresponding relative number of CFU-GEMM colonies for EAE and SLE mice, but they are very different to that for CBA mice (**Figure 16D**). Thus, it is obvious that over time some changes in the profile of stem cell differentiation can occur in the case of non-autoimmune and autoimmune mice. However, these changes are very different or even opposite for non-autoimmune and autoimmune mice during their growth (CBA) or spontaneous development of ADs (SLE and EAE) as well as after immunization of mice with different specific stimulators of autoimmune processes. Thus, one can suppose that SLE and EAE pathologies in two different autoimmune lines of mice on overall demonstrate very similar regularities of change in differentiation profiles of bone marrow stem cells. Interestingly, at 40 days corresponding to spontaneous development of SLE in MRL-lpr/lpr and EAE in 57BL/6 mice demonstrating high activities of different Abzs, there is a strong increase in CFU-E colonies (**Figure 16B**). At the same time, very strong reduction in the relative number of only CFU-E colonies is observed in the case of CBA mice showing catalytically inactive antibodies (**Figure 16B**). This again is indicative of the fact that CFU-E can be precursors of cells producing Abzs in different organs. In this connection, it should be mentioned that IgGs from CSF of patients with MS 30- to 50-fold more active in the hydrolysis of MBP, DNA, and oligosaccharides comparing with Abs from sera of the same patients [110, 111]. It means, that even CSFs of patients with MS contain specific cells producing these catalytically active Abs.

8. Conclusion

It is obvious that in MS patients auto-Abs directed to nucleic acids, proteins, and polysaccharides with different catalytic functions may be induced by primary antigens. During the development of spontaneous and MOG-induced EAE in C57BL/6 mice, a specific reorganization of the immune system of mice takes place. This causes the generation of harmful catalytically active IgGs-hydrolyzing MOG, MBP, and DNA, as well as changes in differentiation of HSCs and to the increase in proliferation of lymphocytes and apoptosis in different organs [110]. Treatment of control non-autoimmune CBA mice with MOG led to different differentiation and proliferation of HSCs comparing with EAE C57BL/6 mice [111].

It was shown that DNA-, RNA-, oligosaccharide-, and MBP-hydrolyzing IgGs and/or IgAs and IgMs from patients with Ms are catalytically very heterogeneous; these Abzs can contain kappa- and lambda-types of light chains, demonstrate different affinity for substrates, different pH optima, may be metal-dependent or independent, and catalyze the hydrolysis of MBP as serine-like or metalloproteases. IgGs of four subclasses (IgG1–IgG4) are catalytically active in the hydrolysis of DNA and MBP, with their different contribution to the total activity of these Abzs in the hydrolysis of these substrates.

MS patients demonstrate some similarity with SLE patients in the development of the same medical, biochemical, immunological indexes including specific plaques in the brain, which appear on late stages of these diseases. Anti-DNA Abs is known as the main important diagnostic index for SLE, but these Abs were also identified as a major component of the intrathecal IgGs in brain and CNS cells of MS patients [40].

It is known that demyelinating plaques appear at relatively late stages in the development of MS, and their presence detected by brain MRI are essential for the diagnosis according to Mc Donald's criteria. At the same time, the detection of Abzs with DNase- and MBP-hydrolyzing activities was shown to be the earliest indicator of development of MS. Catalytic activities of nuclease and protease Abzs are usually very easily detectable at the onset of MS and other autoimmune diseases when the total concentrations of Abs to DNA, MBP, or other auto-antigens are still low and correspond to their ranges in healthy donors. Although Abzs with low activity can sometimes be detected in conventionally healthy people, the RAs of Abzs from MS and SLE patients are usually 1–3 orders of magnitude higher. Therefore, an appearance of some Abzs or a 10- to 100-fold increase in the activity of others over the average Abzs indices for healthy donors may be used as the earliest markers of autoimmune reactions in patients with MS and other autoimmune diseases.

Recognition and degradation of MBP peptides by serum auto-Abs was stated as a novel biomarker for MS [82]. But IgGs from SLE patients also efficiently hydrolyze MBP and oligopeptides corresponding to different AGDs of MBP [84, 85]. Thus, it is clear that early diagnostics of MS requires the use of all known independent methods to exclude SLE and probably other possible diseases leading to a formation of DNA- and MBP-hydrolyzing Abzs. Nevertheless, even revealing of DNase and RNase Abzs on early stages of MS may be very useful. For example, in the case of three patients, we have suggested the possibility of initial stages of MS, but the symptoms did not meet all Poser's and Mc Donald′s criteria. However, Abs found in the sera of these patients demonstrated a high DNase activity speaking in favor of a possibility of an early stage of MS. One and a half years later, these patients met Poser's and Mc Donald′ criteria, and after 2–3 consecutive years, brain plaques were also found in these patients.

The immune systems of individual MS patients generate Abzs, which can attack MBP of myelin-proteolipid shell of axons, while an established MS therapeutic Copaxone inhibits specific MBP-hydrolyzing activity of Abzs [82]. It means that the development of MS and probably SLE or other diseases associated with demyelination can be suppressed by specific inhibitors of MBP-hydrolyzing IgGs, IgAs, and IgMs.

All data indicative of the fact that CFU-E cells can be precursors of cells producing Abzs in different organs. In this connection, it should be mentioned that IgGs from CSF of patients with MS 30- to 50-fold more active in the hydrolysis of MBP, DNA, and oligosaccharides, then Abs from sera of the same patients [110, 111]. It means that even CSFs of patients with MS contain specific cells producing these catalytically active Abs. Moreover, DNase Abzs form SLE and MS patients are cytotoxic and induce apoptotic cell death. SLE and MS Abzs efficiently hydrolyzed polysaccharides. Therefore, it is very possible that abzymes with DNase, amylase, and MBP-hydrolyzing activities may in addition to other different factors cooperatively promote important neuropathological mechanisms in MS and SLE pathogenesis development.

Acknowledgements

This research was made possible by grants mainly from Russian Science Foundation (No. 16-15-10103 to G. A. Nevinsky), purification of IgGs was made grants from the Presidium of the Russian Academy of Sciences (Molecular and Cellular Biology Program, 6.7) and from Russian Foundation for Basic Research (No. 16-04-00603, and 14-04-31281)

Abbreviations

Abs, antibodies; Abzs, abzymes, or catalytically active antibodies; AGDs, antigenic determinants; AI, autoimmune; AD, autoimmune disease; AIDS, human immunodeficiency syndrome; a/u, arbitrary units; BSA, bovine serum albumin; CC, correlation coefficient; HSCs, hematopoietic stem cells; CBA, (CBAxC57BL)F1 mice; MBP, human myelin basic protein; OP-17, OP-19, OP-21, and OP-25—17-25mer oligopeptides corresponding to four known MBP cleavage sites; MS, multiple sclerosis; m-BSA, methylated BSA; nat-DNA and den-DNA, native and denatured DNA, respectively; ODN, oligonucleotide, OP, oligopeptide; SLE- systemic lupus erythematosus, SDS-PAGE, SDS-polyacrylamide gel electrophoresis; RA, relative activity.

Author details

Georgy A. Nevinsky

Address all correspondence to: nevinsky@niboch.nsc.ru

Institute of Chemical Biology and Fundamental Medicine of Siberian Division of Russian Academy of Sciences, Novosibirsk, Russia

References

[1] Pollack SJ, Jacobs JW, Schultz PG. Selective chemical catalysis by an antibody. Science. 1986;234:1570–1573.

[2] Tramontano A, Janda KD, Lerner RA. Catalytic antibodies. Science. 1986;234:1566–1570.

[3] Tramontano A, Janda KD, Lerner RA. Chemical reactivity at an antibody binding site elicited by mechanistic design of a synthetic antigen. Proc Natl Acad Sci U S A. 1986;83:6736–6740.

[4] Lerner RA, Tramontano A. Antibodies as enzymes. Trends in Biochem Sci. 1987;12:427–438.

[5] Stewart JD, Benkovic SJ. Recent developments in catalytic antibodies. Int Rev Immunol. 1993;10:229–240.

[6] Martin AB, Schultz PG. Opportunities at the interface of chemistry and biology. Trends Cell Biol. 1999;9:24–28.

[7] Nevinsky GA, Semenov DV, Buneva VN. Catalytic antibodies (abzymes) induced by stable transition-state analogs. Biochemistry (Moscow). 2000;65:1233–1244.

[8] Keinan EE, editor. Catalytic antibodies. Germany: Wiley-VCH Verlag GmbH and Co. KgaA; 2005. 586 p. doi:10.1002/3527603662

[9] Paul S, Volle DJ, Beach CM, Johnson DR, Powell MJ, Massey RJ. Catalytic hydrolysis of vasoactive intestinal peptide by human autoantibody. Science. 1989;244:1158–1162.

[10] Shuster AM, Gololobov GV, Kvashuk OA, Bogomolova AE, Smirnov IV Gabibov AG. DNA hydrolyzing autoantibodies. Science. 1992;256:665–667.

[11] Buneva VN, Andrievskaia OA, Romannikova IV, Gololobov GV, Iadav RP, Iamkovoi VI, Nevinskii GA. Interaction of catalytically active antibodies with oligoribonucleotides. Mol Biol (Moscow). 1994;28:738–743.

[12] Suzuki H. Recent advances in abzyme studies. J Biochem. 1994;115:138–143.

[13] Nevinsky GA, Kanyshkova TG, Buneva VN. Natural catalytic antibodies (abzymes) in normalcy and pathology. Biochemistry (Moscow). 2000;65:1245–1255.

[14] Nevinsky GA, Buneva VN. Human catalytic RNA- and DNA-hydrolyzing antibodies. J Immunol Meth. 2002;269:235–249.

[15] Nevinsky GA, Favorova OO, Buneva VN. Natural catalytic antibodies—new characters in the protein repertoire. In: Golemis E, editor. Protein-Protein Interactions; A Molecular Cloning Manual. New York, Cold Spring Harbor: Spring Harbor Lab. Press; 2002. p. 532–534.

[16] Nevinsky GA, Buneva VN. Catalytic antibodies in healthy humans and patients with autoimmune and viral pathologies. J Cell Mol Med. 2003;7:265–276.

[17] Nevinsky GA, Buneva VN. Natural catalytic antibodies-abzymes. In: Keinan E, editor. Catalytic Antibodies. Weinheim: Wiley-VCH Verlag GmbH and Co. KgaA; 2005. p. 503–567.

[18] Nevinsky GA, Buneva VN. Natural catalytic antibodies in norm, autoimmune, viral, and bacterial diseases. Sci World J. 2010;10:1203–1233. doi:10.1100/tsw.2010.98

[19] Nevinsky GA. Natural catalytic antibodies in norm and in autoimmune diseases. In: Brenner KJ, editor. Autoimmune Diseases: Symptoms, Diagnosis and Treatment. New York, USA: Nova Science Publishers; 2010. p. 1–107.

[20] Nevinsky GA. Natural catalytic antibodies in norm and in HIV-infected patients. In: Fyson Hanania Kasenga, editor. Understanding HIV/AIDS Management and Care—Pandemic Approaches the 21st Century. Rijeka, Croatia: InTech; 2011. p. 151–192.

[21] Nevinsky GA, Buneva VN. Autoantibodies and natural catalytic antibodies in health, multiple sclerosis, and some other diseases. Adv Neuroimmune Biol. 2012;3:157–182. doi:10.3233/NIB-2012-012042

[22] Andryushkova AA, Kuznetsova IA, Orlovskaya IA, Buneva VN, Nevinsky GA. Antibodies with amylase activity from the sera of autoimmune-prone MRL/MpJ-lpr mice. FEBS Lett. 2006;580:5089–5095. doi:10.1016/j.febslet.2006.08.036

[23] Andryushkova AS, Kuznetsova IA, Orlovskaya IA, Buneva VN, Nevinsky GA. Nucleotide-hydrolyzing antibodies from the sera of autoimmune-prone MRL-lpr/lpr mice. Int Immunol. 2009;21:935–945. doi:10.1093/intimm/dxp060

[24] Andryushkova AS, Kuznetsova IA, Buneva VN, Toporkova LB, Sakhno LV, Tichonova MA, Chernykh ER, Orlovskaya IA, Nevinsky GA. Formation of different abzymes in autoimmune-prone MRL-lpr/lpr mice is associated with changes in colony formation of haematopoetic progenitors. J Cell Mol Med. 2007;11:531–551 doi:10.3233/NIB-2012-012042

[25] Wentworth P, Liu Y, Wentworth AD, Fan P, Foley MJ, Janda KD. A bait and switch hapten strategy generates catalytic antibodies for phosphodiester hydrolysis. Proc Natl Acad Sci U S A. 1998;95:5971–5975.

[26] Tellier C. Exploiting antibodies as catalysts: potential therapeutic applications. Transfus Clin Biol. 2002;9:1–8.

[27] Zhou YX, Karle S, Taguchi P, Planque S, Nishiyama Y, Paul S. Prospects for immunotherapeutic proteolytic antibodies. J Immunol Meth. 2002;269:257–268.

[28] Zouali M. B cell tolerance to self in systemic autoimmunity. Arch Immunol Ther Exp (Warsz). 2001;49:361–365.

[29] Pisetsky D. Immune response to DNA in systemic lupus erythematosus. Isr Med Ass J. 2001;3:850–853.

[30] Earnshaw WC, Rothfield N. Identification of a family of human centromere proteins using autoimmune sera from patients with scleroderma. Chromosoma. 1985;91:313–321.

[31] Raptis L, Menard HA. Quantitation and characterization of plasma DNA in normals and patients with systemic lupus erythematosus. J Clin Invest. 1980;66:1391–1399.

[32] O'Connor KC, Bar-Or A, Hafler DA. Neuroimmunology of multiple sclerosis. J Clin Immunol. 2001;21:81–92.

[33] Barbas CF, Heine A, Zhong G, Hoffmann T, Gramatikova S, Bjornestedt R, List B, Anderson J, Stura EA, Wilson IA, Lerner RA. Immune versus natural selection: antibody aldolases with enzymic rates but broader scope. Science. 1997;278:2085–2092.

[34] Kolesnikov AV, Kozyr AV, Alexandrova ES, Koralewski F, Demin AV, Titov MI, Avalle B, Tramontano A, Paul S, Thomas D, Gabibov AG, Friboulet, A. Enzyme mimicry by the antiidiotypic antibody approach. Proc Natl Acad Sci U S A. 2000;97:13526–13531.

[35] Archelos JJ, Storch MK, Hartung HP. The role of B cells and autoantibodies in multiple sclerosis. Ann Neurol. 2000;47:694–706.

[36] Hemmer B, Archelos JJ, Hartung HP. New concepts in the immunopathogenesis of multiple sclerosis. Nat Rev Neurosci. 2002;3:291–301.

[37] Niehaus A, Shi J, Grzenkowski M, Diers-Fenger M, Archelos J, Hartung HP, Toyka K, Bruck W, Trotter J. Patients with active relapsing-remitting multiple sclerosis synthesize antibodies recognizing oligodendrocyte progenitor cell surface protein: implications for remyelination. Ann Neurol. 2000;48:362–371.

[38] Iglesias A, Bauer J, Litzenburger T, Schubart A, Linington C. T- and B-cell responses to myelin oligodendrocyte glycoprotein in experimental autoimmune encephalomyelitis and multiple sclerosis. Glia. 2001;36:220–234.

[39] Cross AH, Trotter JL, Lyons, J. B cells and antibodies in CNS demyelinating disease. J Neuroimmunol. 2001;112:1–14.

[40] Williamson RA, Burgoon MP, Owens GP, Ghausi O, Leclerc E, Firme L, Carlson S, Corboy J, Parren PW, Sanna PP, Gilden DH, Burton DR. Anti-DNA antibodies are a major component of the intrathecal B cell response in multiple sclerosis. Proc Natl Acad Sci U S A. 2001;98:1793–1798.

[41] Ershova NA, Garmashova NV, Buneva VN, Mogel'nitskii AS, Tyshkevich OB, Doronin B M, Konenkova LP, Boiko AN, Slanova AV, Nesterova VA, Gusev EI, Favorova OO, Nevinskii GA. Association between DNA antibodies levels in the blood of patients with multiple sclerosis and clinical presentation of the disease. Zh Nevrol Psikhiatr Im S. S. Korsakova. 2003;2:25–33.

[42] Ershova NA, Garmashova NV, Mogel'nitskii AS, Tyshkevich OB, Doronin BM, Konenkova LP, Buneva VN, Nevinskii GA. Antibodies to DNA in the blood of patients with multiple sclerosis. Russ J Immunol. 2007;1:229–245.

[43] Bezuglova AM, Konenkova LP, Doronin BM, Buneva VN, Nevinsky GA. Affinity and catalytic heterogeneity and metal-dependence of polyclonal myelin basic protein-hydrolyzing IgGs from sera of patients with systemic lupus erythematosus. J Mol Recognit. 2011;24:960–974.

[44] Polosukhina DI, Garmashova NV, Tyshkevich OB, Doronin BM, Buneva VN, Nevinskii GA. Autoantibodies to myelin basic protein in patients with multiple sclerosis. Int J Immunorehabilatation (Russian). 2009;11:10–18.

[45] Poser CM. The Diagnosis of Multiple Sclerosis. New York: Thieme-Stratton; 1984.

[46] Gusev EI, Demina TL, Boiko AN. Multiple Sclerosis. Moscow: Oil and Gas; 1997.

[47] Steinman L. Multiple sclerosis: a two-stage disease. Nat Immunol. 2001;2:2762–2764.

[48] Polosukhina DI, Kanyshkova T, Doronin BM, Tyshkevich OB, Buneva VN, Boiko AN, Gusev EI, Favorova OO, Nevinsky GA. Hydrolysis of myelin basic protein by polyclonal catalytic IgGs from the sera of patients with multiple sclerosis. J Cell Mol Med. 2004;8:359–368.

[49] Polosukhina DI, Buneva VN, Doronin BM, Tyshkevich OB, Boiko AN, Gusev EI, Favorova OO, Nevinsky GA. Hydrolysis of myelin basic protein by IgM and IgA antibodies from the sera of patients with multiple sclerosis. Med Sci Monit. 2005;11:BR266- BR272.

[50] Polosukhina DI, Buneva VN, Doronin BM, Tyshkevich OB, Boiko AN, Gusev EI, Favorova OO, Nevinsky GA. Metal-dependent hydrolysis of myelin basic protein by IgGs from the sera of patients with multiple sclerosis. Immunol Lett. 2006;103:75–81.

[51] Legostaeva GA, Polosukhina DI, Bezuglova AM, Doronin BM, Buneva VN, Nevinsky, GA. Affinity and catalytic heterogeneity of polyclonal myelin basic protein-hydrolyzing IgGs from sera of patients with multiple sclerosis. J Cell Mol Med. 2010;14:699–709.

[52] Parkhomenko TA, Doronin VB, Castellazzi M, Padroni M, Pastore M, Buneva VN, Granieri E, Nevinsky GA. Comparison of DNA-hydrolyzing antibodies from the cerebrospinal fluid and serum of patients with multiple sclerosis. PLoS One. 2014;9:e93001.

[53] Doronin VB, Parkhomenko TA, Castellazzi M, Padroni M, Pastore M, Buneva VN, Granieri E, Nevinsky GA. Comparison of antibodies hydrolyzing myelin basic protein from the cerebrospinal fluid and serum of patients with multiple sclerosis. PLoS One. 2014;9:e107807.

[54] Baranovskii AG, Kanyshkova TG, Mogelnitskii AS, Naumov VA, Buneva VN, Gusev EI, Boiko AN, Zargarova TA, Favorova OO, Nevinsky GA. Polyclonal antibodies from blood and cerebrospinal fluid of patients with multiple sclerosis effectively hydrolyze DNA and RNA. Biochemistry (Moscow). 1998;63:1239–1248.

[55] Baranovskii AG, Ershova NA, Buneva VN, Kanyshkova TG, Mogelnitskii AS, Doronin BM, Boiko AN, Gusev EI, Favorova OO, Nevinsky GA. Catalytic heterogeneity of polyclonal DNA- hydrolyzing antibodies from the sera of patients with multiple sclerosis. Immunol Lett. 2001;76:163–167.

[56] Baranovskii AG, Buneva VN, Doronin BM, Nevinsky GA. Innunoglobulins from blood of patients with multiple sclerosis like catalytic heterogeneous nucleases. Russian J Immunol. 2008;2:405–419.

[57] Saveliev AN, Ivanen DR, Kulminskaya AA, Ershova NA, Kanyshkova TG, Buneva VN, Mogelnitskii AS, Doronin BM, Favorova OO, Nevinsky GA, Neustroev KN. Amylolytic activity of IgM and IgG antibodies from patients with multiple sclerosis. Immunol Lett. 2003;86:291–297.

[58] Ivanen DR, Kulminskaya AA, Shabalin KA, Isaeva-Ivanova LV, Saveliev AN, Nevinsky GA, Shabalin KA, Neustroev KN. Catalytic properties of IgMs with amylolytic activity isolated from patients with multiple sclerosis. Med Sci Monit. 2004;10:BR273-BR280.

[59] Shoenfeld Y, Ben-Yehuda O, Messinger Y, Bentwitch Z, Rauch J, Isenberg DI, Gadoth N. Autoimmune diseases other than lupus share common anti-DNA idiotypes. Immunol Lett. 1988;17:285–291.

[60] Founel S, Muller S. Antinucleosome antibodies and T-cell response in systemic lupus erythematosus. Ann Med Interne (Paris). 2002;153:513–519.

[61] Semenov DV, Kanyshkova TG, Karotaeva NA, Krasnorutskii MA, Kuznetsova IA, Buneva, VN, Nevinsky GA. Catalytic nucleotide-hydrolyzing antibodies in breast milk and serum of clinically healthy human mothers. Med Sci Monit. 2004;10:BR23-BR33.

[62] Doronin VB, Parkhomenko TA, Castellazzi M, CesnikE, Buneva VN, Granieri E, Nevinsky GA. Comparison of antibodies with amylase activity from cerebrospinal fluid and serum of patients with multiple sclerosis. PLoS One. 2016;11:e0154688.

[63] Savel'ev AN, Eneyskaya EV, Shabalin KA, Filatov MV, Neustroev KN. Antibodies with amylolytic activity. Prot Pept Lett. 1999;6:179–184.

[64] Ivanen DR, Kulminskaya AA, Ershova NA, Eneyskaya EV, Shabalin KA, Savel'ev AN, Kanyshkova TG, Buneva VN, Nevinsky GA, Neustroev KN. Human autoantibodies with amylolytic activity. Biologia. 2002;11:253–260.

[65] Savel'ev AN, Kulminskaya AA, Ivanen DR, Nevinsky GA, Neustroev KN. Human antibodies with amylolytic activity. Trends Glycosci Glycotechnol. 2004;16:17–31.

[66] Neustroev KN, Ivanen DR, Kulminskaya AA, Brumer IH, Saveliev AN, Saveliev AN, Nevinsky GA. Amylolytic activity and catalytic properties of IgM and IgG antibodies from patients with systemic lupus erythematosus. Hum antibodies. 2003;12:31–34.

[67] Savel'ev AN, Kanyshkova TG, Kulminskaya AA, Buneva VN, Eneyskaya EV, Filatov MV, Nevinsky GA, Neustroev KN. Amylolytic activity of IgG and sIgA immunoglobulins from human milk. Clin Chim Acta. 2001;314:141–152.

[68] Kozyr AV, Kolesnikov AV, Aleksandrova ES, Sashchenko LP, Gnuchev NV, Favorov PV, Kotelnikov MA, Iakhnina EI, Astsaturov IA, Prokaeva TB, Alekberova ZS, Suchkov SV, Gabibov AG. Novel functional activities of anti-DNA autoantibodies by proteases

from sera of patients with lymphoproliferative and autoimmune diseases. Appl Biochem Biotechnol. 1998;75:45–61.

[69] Andrievskaya OA, Buneva VN, Naumov VA, Nevinsky GA. Catalytic heterogeneity of polyclonal RNA-hydrolyzing IgM from sera of patients with lupus erythematosus. Med Sci Monit. 2000;6:460–470.

[70] Andrievskaya OA, Buneva VN, Baranovskii AG, Gal'vita AV, Benzo ES, Naumov VA, Nevinsky GA. Catalytic diversity of polyclonal RNA-hydrolyzing IgG antibodies from the sera of patients with systemic lupus erythematosus. Immunol Lett. 2002;81:191–198.

[71] Vlasov AV, Baranovskii AG, Kanyshkova TG, Prints AV, Zabara VG, Naumov VA, Breusov AA, Giege R, Buneva VN, Nevinskii GA. Substrate specificity of serum DNA- and RNA-hydrolyzing antibodies of patients with polyarthritis and autoimmune thyroiditis. Mol Biol (Moscow). 1998;32:559–569.

[72] Vlassov A, Florentz C, Helm M, Naumov V, Buneva V, Nevinsky G, Giege R. Characterization and selectivity of catalytic antibodies from human serum with RNAse activity. Nucl Acid Res. 1998;26:5243–5250.

[73] Vlassov AV, Helm M, Florentz C, Naumov V, Breusov AA, Buneva VN, Giege R, Nevinsky GA. Variability of substrate specificity of serum antibodies obtained from patients with different autoimmune and viral deseases in reaction of tRNA hydrolysis. Russ J Immunol. 1999;4:25–32.

[74] Vlasov AV, Helm M, Naumov VA, Breusov AA, Buneva VN, Florentz C, Giege R, Nevinskii GA. Features of tRNA hydrolysis by autoantibodies from blood serum of patients with certain autoimmune and virus diseases. Mol Biol (Moscow). 1999;33:866–872.

[75] Kuznetsova IA, Orlovskaya IA, Buneva VN, Nevinsky GA. Activation of DNA-hydrolyzing antibodies from the sera of autoimmune-prone MRL-lpr/lpr mice by different metal ions. Biochim Biophys Acta. 2007;1774:884–896.

[76] Breusov AA, Gal'vita AV, Benzo ES, Baranovskii AG, Prints AV, Naumov VA, Buneva VN, Nevinsky GA. Comparison of the level of DNA-hydrolyzing polyclonal IgG antibodies in sera of patients with Hashimoto's thyroiditis and nontoxic nodal goiter. Rus J Immunol. 2001;6:17–28.

[77] Berneman A, Cuilbert B, Enschrich S, Avrames S. IgG auto- and polyreactivities of normal human sera. Mol Immunol. 1993;30:1499–1510.

[78] Coutinho A, Kazatchkine MD, Avrameas S. Natural autoantibodies. Curr Opin Immunol. 1995;7:812–818.

[79] Kostrikina IA, Buneva VN, Nevinsky GA. Systemic lupus erythematosus: molecular cloning of fourteen recombinant DNase monoclonal kappa light chains with different catalytic properties. Biochim Biophys Acta. 2014;1840:1725–1737.

[80] Botvinovskaya AV, Kostrikina IA, Buneva VN, Nevinsky GA. Systemic lupus erythematosus: molecular cloning of several recombinant DNase monoclonal kappa light chains with different catalytic properties. J Mol Recognit. 2013;26:450–460.

[81] Kostrikina IA, Odintsova ES, Buneva VN, Nevinsky GA. Systemic lupus erythematosus: molecular cloning and analysis of recombinant DNase monoclonal light chain NGK-1. Int Immunol. 2014;26:439–450. doi:10.1093/intimm/dxu047

[82] Ponomarenko NA, Durova OM, Vorobiev II, Belogurov AA, Kurkova IN, Petrenko AG, Telegin GB, Suchkov SV, Kiselev SL, Lagarkova MA, Govorun VM, Serebryakova MV, Avalle B, Tornatore P, Karavanov A, Morse HC 3rd, Thomas D, Friboulet A, Gabibov AG. Autoantibodies to myelin basic protein catalyze site-specific degradation of their antigen. Proc Natl Acad Sci U S A. 2006;103:281–286.

[83] Odintsova ES, Baranova SV, Dmitrenok PS, Calmels C, Parissi V, Andreola ML, Buneva VN, Nevinsky GA. Anti-integrase abzymes from the sera of HIV-infected patients specifically hydrolyze integrase but nonspecifically cleave short oligopeptides. J Mol Recognit. 2012;25:193–207. doi:10.1002/jmr.2159

[84] Bezuglova AM, Dmitrenok PS, Konenkova LP, Buneva VN, Nevinsky GA. Multiple sites of the cleavage of 17- and 19-mer encephalytogenic oligopeptides corresponding to human myelin basic protein (MBP) by specific anti-MBP antibodies from patients with systemic lupus erythematosus. Peptides. 2012;37:69–78.

[85] Timofeeva AM, Dmitrenok PS, Konenkova LP, Buneva VN, Nevinsky GA. Multiple sites of the cleavage of 21- and 25-mer encephalytogenic oligopeptides corresponding to human myelin basic protein (MBP) by specific anti-MBP antibodies from patients with systemic lupus erythematosus. PLoS One. 2013;8:e51600. doi:10.1371/journal.pone.0051600

[86] Kalaga R, Li L, O'Dell JR, Paul S. Unexpected presence of polyreactive catalytic antibodies in IgG from unimmunized donors and decreased levels in rheumatoid arthritis. J Immunol. 1995;155:2695–2702.

[87] Odintsova ES, Buneva VN, Nevinsky GA. Casein-hydrolyzing activity of sIgA antibodies from human milk. J Mol Recognit. 2005;18:413–421.

[88] Odintsova ES, Kharitonova MA, Baranovskii AG, Siziakina LP, Buneva VN, Nevinsky GA. Proteolytic activity of IgG antibodies from blood of acquired immunodeficiency syndrome patients. Biochem (Moscow). 2006;71:251–261.

[89] Odintsova ES, Zaksas NP, Buneva VN, Nevinsky GA. Metal dependent hydrolysis of beta-casein by sIgA antibodies from human milk. J Mol Recognit. 2011;24:45–59. doi: 10.1002/jmr.1022

[90] Baranova SV, Buneva VN, Kharitonova MA, Sizyakina LP, Calmels C, Andreola ML, Parissi V, Nevinsky GA. HIV-1 integrase-hydrolyzing antibodies from sera of HIV-infected patients. Biochimie. 2009;91:1081–1086. doi:10.1016/j.biochi.2009.06.018

[91] Baranova SV, Buneva VN, Kharitonova MA, Sizyakina LP, Calmels C, Andreola ML, Parissi V, Zakharova OD, Nevinsky GA. HIV-1 integrase-hydrolyzing IgM antibodies from sera of HIV-infected patients. Int Immunol. 2010;22:671–680. doi:10.1093/intimm/dxq051

[92] Timofeeva AM, Buneva VN, Nevinsky GA. Systemic lupus erythematosus: molecular cloning and analysis of 22 individual recombinant monoclonal kappa light chains specifically hydrolyzing human myelin basic protein. J Mol Recognit. 2015;28:614–627. doi:10.1002/jmr.2476

[93] Timofeeva AM, Ivanisenko NV, Buneva VN, Nevinsky GA. Systemic lupus erythematosus: molecular cloning and analysis of recombinant monoclonal kappa light chain NGTA2-Me-pro-ChTr possessing two different activities-trypsin-like and metalloprotease. Int Immunol. 2015;27:633–645. doi:10.1093/intimm/dxv042

[94] Love JD, Hewitt RR. The relationship between human serum and human pancreatic DNase I. J Biol Chem. 1979;254:12588–12594.

[95] Suck D. DNA recognition by DNase I. J Mol Recognit. 1994;7:65–70.

[96] Baranovskii AG, Buneva VN, Nevinsky GA. Human deoxyribonucleases. Biochem (Moscow). 2004;69:587–601.

[97] Horl WH, Wanner C, Schollmer P. Proteinases in catabolism and malnutrition. JPEN J Parenter Enteral Nutr. 1987;11:98S–103S.

[98] Rao MB, Tanksale AM, Ghatge MS, Deshhange VV. Molecular and biotechnological aspects of microbial proteases. Microbiol Mol Biol Rev. 1998;62:597–635.

[99] Parkhomenko TA, Legostaeva GA, Doronin BM, Buneva VN, Nevinsky GA. IgGs containing light chains of the k and l type and of all subclasses (IgG1-IgG4) from sera of patients with multiple sclerosis hydrolyze DNA. J Mol Recognit. 2010;23:486–494. doi:10.1002/jmr.1016

[100] Galvita AV, Baranovskii AG, Kuznetsova IA, Vinshu NV, Galenok VA, Buneva VN, Nevinsky GA. A peculiarity of DNA hydrolysis by antibodies from patients with diabetes. Russ J Immunol. 2007;1:116–131.

[101] Baranovskii AG, Matushin VG, Vlassov AV, Zabara VG, Naumov VA, Buneva VN, Nevinskii GA. DNA- and RNA-hydrolyzing antibodies from the blood of patients with various forms of viral hepatitis. Biochem (Moscow). 1997;62:1358–1366.

[102] Parkhomenko TA, Buneva VN, Tyshkevich OB, Generalov II, Doronin BM, Nevinsky GA. DNA-hydrolyzing activity of IgG antibodies from the sera of patients with tick-borne encephalitis. Biochimie. 2010;92:545–554. doi:10.1016/j.biochi.2010.01.022

[103] Nevinsky GA, Breusov AA, Baranovskii AG, Prints AV, Kanyshkova TG, Galvita AV, Naumov VA, Buneva VN. Effect of different drugs on the level of DNA-hydrolyzing

polyclonal IgG antibodies in sera of patients with Hashimoto's thyroiditis and nontoxic nodal goiter. Med Sci Monit. 2001;7:201–211.

[104] Ermakov EA, Smirnova LP, Parkhomenko TA, Dmitrenok PS, Krotenko NM, Fattakhov NS, Bokhan NA, Semke AV, Ivanova SA, Buneva VN, Nevinsky GA. DNA-hydrolysing activity of IgG antibodies from the sera of patients with schizophrenia. Open Biol. 2015;5:150064. doi:10.1098/rsob.150064

[105] Odintsova ES, Kharitonova MA, Baranovskii AG, Siziakina LP, Buneva VN, Nevinskii GA. DNA-hydrolyzing IgG antibodies from the blood of patients with acquired immune deficiency syndrome. Mol Biol (Moscow). 2006;40:857–864.

[106] Nevinsky GA. Structural, thermodynamic, and kinetic basis for the activities of some nucleic acid repair enzymes. J Mol Recognit. 2011;24:656–677. doi:10.1002/jmr.1096

[107] Ikehara S, Kawamura M, Takao F. Organ-specific and systemic autoimmune diseases originate from defects in hematopoietic stem cells. Proc Natl Acad Sci U S A. 1990;87:8341–8344.

[108] Dubrovskaya VV, Andryushkova AS, Kuznetsova IA, Toporkova LB, Buneva VN, Orlovskaya IA, Nevinsky GA. DNA-hydrolyzing antibodies from sera of autoimmune-prone MRL/MpJ-lpr mice. Biochem (Moscow). 2003;68:1081–1088.

[109] Ponomarenko NA, Durova OM, Vorobiev II, Telegin GV, Chamborant OG, Sidorik LL, Suchkov SV, Alekbarova ZS, Gnuchev NV, Gabibov AG. Catalytic antibodies in clinical and experimental pathology: human and mouse models. J Immunol Methods. 2002;269:197–211.

[110] Doronin VB, Parkhomenko TA, Korablev A, Toporkova LB, Lopatnikova JA, Alshevskaja AA, Sennikov SV, Buneva VN, Budde T, Meuth SG, Orlovskaya IA, Popova NA, Nevinsky GA. Changes in different parameters, lymphocyte proliferation and hematopoietic progenitor colony formation in EAE mice treated with myelin oligodendrocyte glycoprotein. J Cell Mol Med. 2015: in press. doi:10.1111/jcmm.12704

[111] Doronin VB, Parkhomenko TA, Toporkova LB, Lopatnikova JA, Sennikov SV, Buneva VN, Budde T, Meuth SG, Orlovskaya IA. Popova NA, Nevinsky GA. Comparison of changes in different parameters, lymphocyte proliferation and hematopoietic progenitor colony formation in EAE and CBA mice treated with myelin oligodendrocyte glycoprotein: private communication.

[112] Mouse EAE models. Overview and Model Selection. Lawrence, USA: Hooke Laboratories, Inc; 2011–2013.

[113] Simmons SB, Pierson ER, Lee SY, Goverman JM. Modeling the heterogeneity of multiple sclerosis in animals. Trends Immunol. 2013;34:410–422. doi:10.1016/j.it.2013.04.006

[114] Cheetham SA, Smith AL, Armstrong SD, Beynon RJ, Hurst JL. Limited variation in the major urinary proteins of laboratory mice. Physiol Behav. 2009;96:253–261. doi:10.1016/j.physbeh.2008.10.005

[115] Krasnorutskii MA, Buneva VN, Nevinsky GA. Antibodies against DNA hydrolyze DNA and RNA. Biochem (Moscow). 2008;73:1547–1560.

[116] Krasnorutskii MA, Buneva VN, Nevinsky GA. Antibodies against RNA hydrolyze RNA and DNA. J Mol Recognit. 2008;21:337–346.

[117] Nishi Y. Evolution of catalytic antibody repertoire in autoimmune mice. J Immunol Meth. 2002;269:213–233.

[118] Tawfik DS, Chap R, Green BS, Sela M, Eshhar Z. Unexpectedly high occurrence of catalytic antibodies in MRL/lpr and SJL mice immunized with a transition-state analog: is there a linkage to autoimmunity? Proc Natl Acad Sci U S A. 2002;92:2145–2149.

[119] Sinohara H, Matsuura K. Does catalytic activity of Bens-Jones proteins contribute to the pathogenesis of multiple myeloma. Appl Biochem Biotechnol. 2000;83:85–94.

[120] Blakemore WF, Franklin RJ. Remyelination in experimental models of toxin-induced demyelination. Curr Top Microbiol Immunol. 2008;318:193–212.

[121] Lassmann H. Experimental models of multiple sclerosis. Rev Neurol (Paris). 2007;163:651–655.

[122] Komoly S. Experimental demyelination caused by primary oligodendrocyte dystrophy. Regional distribution of the lesions in the nervous system of mice. Ideggyogy Sz. 2005;58:40–43.

[123] Stidworthy MF, Genoud S, Suter U, Mantei N, Franklin RJ. Quantifying the early stages of remyelination following cuprizone-induced demyelination. Brain Pathol. 2003;13:329–339.

[124] Doronin VB, Korablev A, Toporkova LB, Buneva VN, Budde T, Meuth SG, Orlovskaya IA, Popova NA, Nevinsky GA*. Changes in disease parameters and hematopoietic progenitor colony formation in brain inflammation and demyelinization: private communication. *Institute of Chemical Biology and Fundamental medicine of RAS, Novosibirsk, Russia

Chapter 5

Multiple Sclerosis and Its Relationship with Oxidative Stress, Glutathione Redox System, ATPase System, and Membrane Fluidity

Genaro G. Ortiz, Fermín P. Pacheco-Moisés,
Erandis D. Torres-Sánchez, Tanya E. Sorto-Gómez,
Mario Mireles-Ramírez, Alfredo León-Gil,
Héctor González-Usigli, Luis J. Flores-Alvarado,
Erika D. González-Renovato,
Angelica L. Sánchez-López,
Margarita Cid-Hernández and
Irma E. Velázquez-Brizuela

Additional information is available at the end of the chapter

http://dx.doi.org/10.5772/64737

Abstract

Multiple sclerosis (MS) is an autoimmune disease of the central nervous system (CNS) with a focus on inflammation, demyelination, and damage to axons leading to neurological deficits. MS pathology is associated with excessive reactive oxygen species (ROS) and generation of reactive nitrogen species (RNS), causing oxidative/nitrosative stress. Deregulation of glutathione homeostasis and alterations in glutathione-dependent enzymes are implicated in MS. Reactive oxygen species enhance both monocyte adhesion and migration across brain endothelial cells. In addition, ROS can activate the expression of the nuclear transcription factor-kappa, which upregulates the expression of many genes involved in MS, such as tumor necrosis factor-α and nitric oxide synthase, among others, leading to mitochondrial dysfunction and energy deficits that result in mitochondrial and cellular calcium overload. Loss of mitochondrial membrane potential can increase the release of cytochrome c, one pathway that leads to neuronal apoptosis. Clinical studies suggest that omega-3 long-chain polyunsaturated fatty acids (PUFAs) including eicosapentaenoic acid (EPA) and docosahexaenoic acid (DHA) have anti-inflammatory, antioxidant, and neuroprotective effects in MS and animal models of MS. Here, we review the relationship of oxidative stress, the glutathione redox system, the ATPase system, and membrane fluidity with the development of MS. In addition, we describe the main findings of a clinical trial conducted with relapsing-remitting MS patients who received a diet supplemented with 4 g/day of fish oil or olive oil. The effects of PUFAs supplementation on the parameters indicated above are analyzed in this work.

Keywords: multiple sclerosis, oxidative stress, mitochondria, membrane fluidity, ATPase

1. Introduction

Multiple sclerosis (MS) is a chronic inflammatory demyelinating disease of the central nervous system (CNS) with partially known etiology. It is the most common cause of neurological disability in young adults. Nutrition is commonly accepted as one of the possible environmental factors involved in the pathogenesis of MS. Omega-3 polyunsaturated fatty acids (PUFAs) such as eicosapentaenoic acid (EPA) and docosahexaenoic acid (DHA) are fatty acids that possess several carbon–carbon double bonds. A diet supplemented with PUFAs has clinical and biochemical effects in patients with autoimmune diseases such as MS. Eicosapentaenoic acid and DHA are found in high proportions in fish oil, and these molecules may have anti-inflammatory, antithrombotic, antioxidant, immunomodulatory functions, and neuroprotective effects on the synaptogenesis and biogenesis of the neuronal membrane. Oxidative stress (OS) that is characterized by excessive production of reactive oxygen species and a reduction in antioxidant defense mechanisms have been implicated in the pathogenesis of MS. In consequence, a reduction in this phenomenon could be beneficial for MS patients [1]. In this work, we describe the relationship of several oxidative stress markers (glutathione redox system, mitochondrial ATPase activity, and membrane fluidity) with the development of MS. Furthermore, we describe the main findings of a clinical trial conducted with relapsing–remitting MS patients who received a diet supplemented with 4 g/day of fish oil or olive oil.

Pathologically, MS is characterized by perivenous infiltration of lymphocytes and macrophages in the brain parenchyma. There are four clinical manifestations of MS: relapsing–remitting, primary progressive, secondary progressive, and progressive-relapsing. The MS lesions are typically scattered, and the clinical picture can vary from a benign self-limiting disorder to severe and highly disabling disease. MS is a multifactorial disease involving genetic, immunological, and environmental factors that trigger the autoimmune process leading to the pathological changes of the disease. In this regard, it has been proposed that a viral infection in which self-antigens that generate molecular mimicry with myelin proteins cause a loss of tolerance against it, which results in the destruction of myelin mediated by activated T lymphocytes in white matter of the brain and sometimes extending into the gray matter, resulting in defects in the conduction of nerve impulses that leads to symptoms, depending on the affected site of the brain or spinal cord [1] (**Figure 1**).

According to the areas of myelin destruction, sensory or motor symptoms are affected (balance or vision disorders). The symptoms can change between an "outbreak" or relapse (emergence of new neurological symptoms or worsening of previous ones) and remission. Demyelinating lesions or "plaques" of different sizes and locations are spread throughout the CNS, and the onset of symptoms and response to treatment is unique to each patient [2].

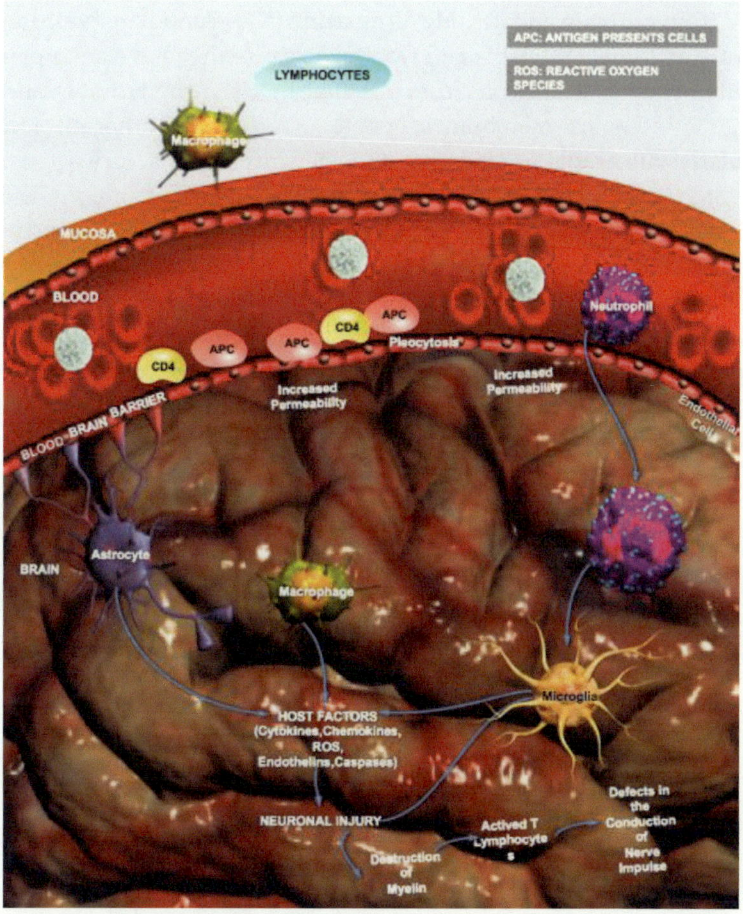

Figure 1. Immune-mediated destruction of myelin components in multiple sclerosis. Pathway Builder Online Tool was used to draw the figure [27].

2. Oxidative stress and multiple sclerosis

OS is a cellular state where the homeostasis of redox reactions is altered when the production of reactive oxygen (ROS) and reactive nitrogen species (RNS) exceed their elimination. These reactive species are generated, among other causes, by oxidative metabolism. Neurons of the CNS are very active in oxidative metabolism, as they are constantly exposed to low-to-moderate levels of ROS, and these species are removed by antioxidants (melatonin, vitamin D, vitamin E, glutathione) and antioxidant enzymes (superoxide dismutase, catalase, glutathione peroxidase, etc.). In chronic inflammatory diseases, such as MS, antioxidant defenses are overcome, which leads to oxidative stress [3].

Collectively, the ROS are reactive species derived from oxygen that include the superoxide anion (O^-), hydrogen peroxide (H_2O_2), and the hydroxyl radical (•OH). The RNS are reactive species derived from nitrogen and include nitric oxide (NO•) and peroxynitrite ($ONOO^-$). The ROS and RNS are extremely unstable and reactive because they have an unpaired electron in their outer orbital. They take electrons from proteins, lipids, carbohydrates, and nucleic acids, causing damage to biological membranes, genetic material, and other macromolecules. The CNS is particularly vulnerable to oxidative damage since it has a very active mitochondrial metabolism, which leads to high levels of intracellular superoxide anions. Moreover, oligodendrocytes have low levels of antioxidant enzymes and a high concentration of iron. Unsaturated fatty acids are the most vulnerable to free radicals, and because myelin has a high lipid-to-protein ratio, it is a preferred target of ROS [4]. The ROS are generated by a number of cellular oxidative and metabolic processes including activity of the enzymes of the mitochondrial respiratory chain, xanthine oxidase, NADPH oxidase, monoamine oxidases, and metabolism of arachidonic acid (AA) mediated by the activity of lipoxygenases (LOX), and ROS are produced primarily by leakage of electrons in the mitochondrial respiratory chain [3].

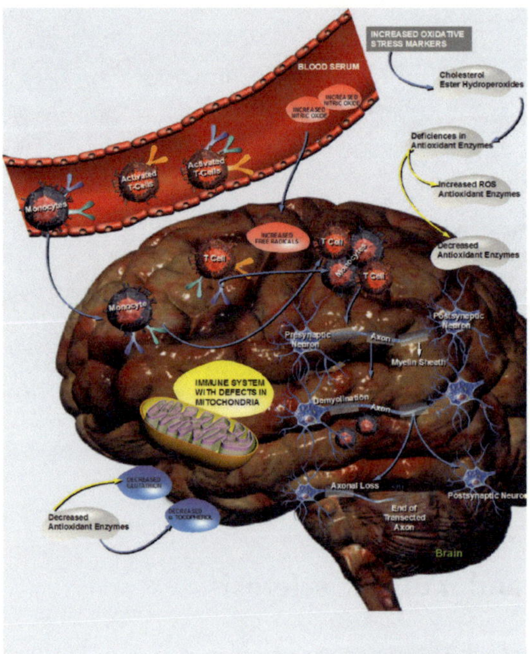

Figure 2. Oxidative stress levels are directly related to the progression of MS. Pathway Builder Online Tool was used to draw the figure [27].

http://dx.doi.org/10.5772/64737

Numerous studies in MS patients have shown an increase in the production of OS markers (such as cholesteryl ester hydroperoxides) and lower levels of uric acid (a $ONOO^-$ scavenger). These changes are accompanied by significant deficiencies in antioxidant enzymes compared to healthy subjects. The increase in ROS coupled with decreased antioxidant capacity is not enough to entirely explain the pathogenesis of MS [4, 5]. Other reports suggest that the loss of myelin nerve sheath is possible because the immune system participates in combination with defects in the mitochondria, and these defects cause the generation of ROS and RNS. Macrophages and monocytes release mediators of OS that degrade the unsaturated fatty acids. The ROS have also been implicated as a mediator of demyelination of axonal damage in MS and experimental autoimmune encephalomyelitis (EAE) [6]. It is important to mention that in assessing platelets in MS patients, increased activity of free radicals with decreased levels of important antioxidants such as glutathione and alpha-tocopherol has been reported [7] (**Figure 2**).

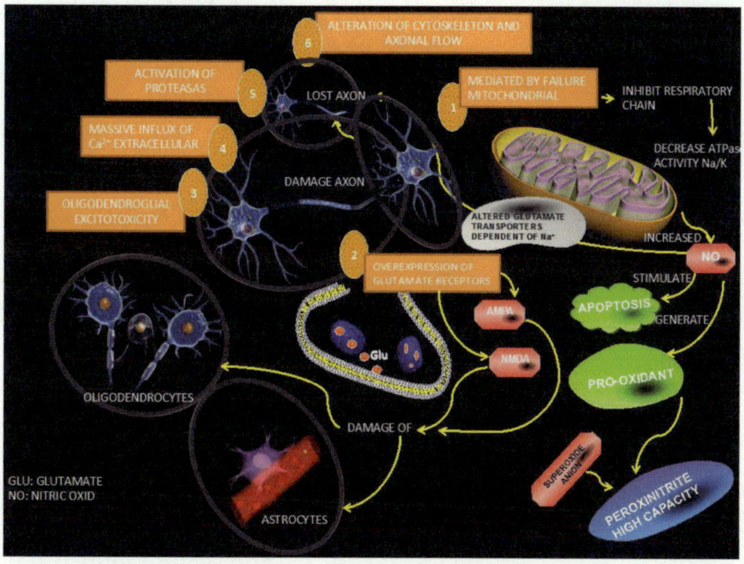

Figure 3. Damage to axons. Pathway Builder Online Tool was used to draw the figure [27].

The molecular mechanisms proposed to explain how ROS could specifically mediate brain damage are the following: (1) The lower levels of antioxidants can promote increased activity of lipoxygenase in CNS stimulating leukotriene production, thereby increasing the immunoinflammatory processes in the cerebral cortex; (2) the damage to myelin can be caused by activation of T cells that may be activated for the presence of free radicals produced by the synthesis route of AA. Then appear the markers of OS associated with reduced activity of superoxide dismutase and the increase in glutamine, followed by increases of •OH and the production of peroxides which ultimately has a negative impact on myelin. After that, the evident changes in mitochondrial activity and finally changes in membrane fluidity (particularly, mitochondrial membranes) appear [8].

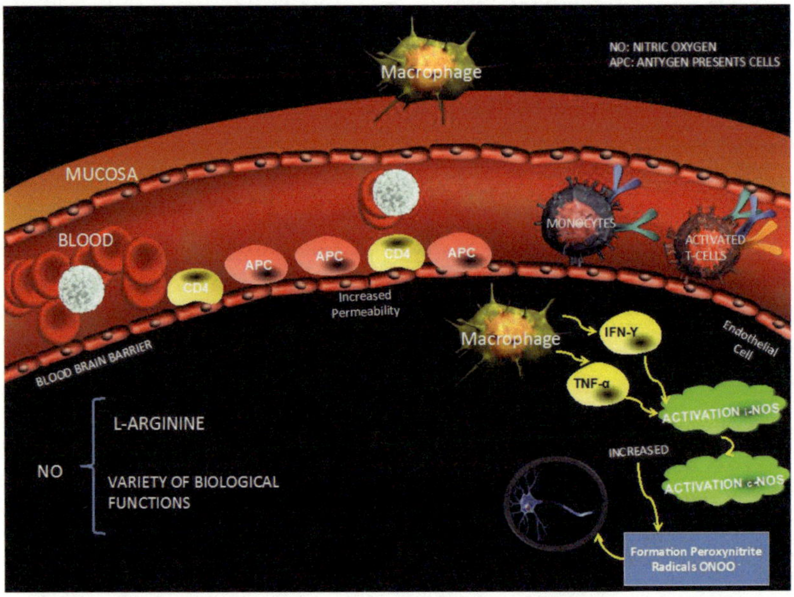

Figure 4. Effect of nitric oxide in inflammation. Pathway Builder Online Tool was used to draw the figure [27].

Paraclinical studies have shown an increased metabolism of the RNS in serum, lymphocytes, and cerebrospinal fluid of MS patients, which correlate to pathology studies. $ONOO^-$ is also closely associated with acute inflammatory lesions [9]. Damage to axons is mediated by the following: (1) failure in mitochondrial energy metabolism due to inhibition of the respiratory chain by nitric oxide, which in turn causes a decrease in Na^+/K^+ ATPase activity and alters Na $^+$-dependent glutamate transporters, (2) over-expression of glutamate receptors, (3) oligodendroglial excitotoxicity, (4) massive influx of extracellular Ca^{++}, (5) activation of proteases, and (6) impaired axonal transport. These mechanisms produce glutamate excitotoxicity and increased generation of nitric oxide leading to nitrosative stress. Nitric oxide is a highly toxic element that by itself blocks nerve conduction, especially in demyelinated axons, and stimulates apoptosis. When nitric oxide is combined with the superoxide anion, it generates a potent free radical, the pro-oxidant peroxynitrite. Glutamate in turn causes neurodegeneration through the AMPA and NMDA receptors in oligodendrocytes and astrocytes (**Figure 3**). It is possible to explain the role of mediators using an experimental model of autoimmune encephalitis: Protection against the experimental disease occurs after administration of a glutamate antagonist [10].

Under physiologic conditions, nitric oxide is produced from L-arginine by constitutive nitric oxide synthase (cNOS) and participates in a variety of important biological functions such as immunoregulation of inflammatory reactions, the downregulation of tumor necrosis factor (TNF)-α production, MHC II expression in macrophages, induction of apoptosis in CD4 cells, physiological regulation of the mitochondrial respiratory chain, inhibition of antigen presentation, and leukocyte adhesion and migration. However, during inflammatory reactions, exposure of macrophages to interferon (IFN)-γ and TNF-α results in the activation of the inducible isoenzyme of NOS (iNOS), which increases up to 10 times the levels of nitric oxide. Nitric oxide facilitates the formation of peroxynitrite radicals. Only cells capable of generating a high flow of NO• have the potential for causing nitrosative stress. The role of nitric oxide in MS is therefore complex, and in fact, peroxynitrite is definitely more toxic than nitric oxide [9] (**Figure 4**).

3. Reactive oxygen species, cytokines, and axonal damage in multiple sclerosis

Mechanisms of axonal damage are the consequence of the presence of TNF-α, matrix metalloproteinases (MMPs), ROS, antibodies, increased glutamate, and aspartate, and these molecules cause excitotoxicity in MS patients. Glutamate is increased in MS patients (active lesions) especially in white matter of normal appearance. Mature oligodendrocytes and astrocytes are highly sensitive to glutamate due to the expression of AMPA and NMDA receptors [9]. The myelin sheath can be damaged by cytokines, autoantibodies, ROS, proteolytic enzymes, and phagocytosis. Increased ROS by activated microglia (specialized macrophages of the CNS) during the immune response gives a state of increased lipid peroxidation, and the oligodendrocyte cell is the cell most susceptible to damage by ROS. Myelin degradation may be the result of lipid peroxidation mediated by peroxides, but the role of these specific toxic factors in the pathogenesis of MS remains partially elusive [9].

4. Glutathione system and multiple sclerosis

In a recent study, the oxidation of DNA in the nucleus of oligodendrocytes and oxidation of lipids in the myelin of oligodendrocytes and axons were observed. This oxidation was associated with the active process of demyelination and neurodegeneration. Active lesions in relapsing-remitting MS (RRMS) and progressive course patients were associated with inflammation, lipid peroxidation, and DNA oxidation [11]. Similarly, Ortiz et al. [12] observed an increase in serum lipid peroxides and nitrite/nitrate levels and the activity of glutathione peroxidase in patients with RRMS compared to healthy individuals.

Reduced ubiquinone and vitamin E levels, and reduced activity of the enzyme glutathione peroxidase in lymphocytes and granulocytes were reported (with a decrease in 51 and 78%, respectively), as well as a decrease in glutathione reductase activity in granulocytes (27%) and lymphocytes (8%) [13]. In contrast, in 2012, Tasset et al. [14] found an increase in activity of the glutathione reductase in patients with RRMS when compared to control subjects (1.3 ± 0.9 vs 0.3 ± 0.19, $P < 0.01$), and an increased ratio of reduced glutathione to oxidized glutathione (GSH/GSSG) in these patients (28.2 ± 39.6 vs 4.0 ± 2.9, $P < 0.01$). Similarly, an increase was found in the levels of oxidized glutathione and also increased concentrations of isoprostanes and malondialdehyde (MDA) in patients with MS [15, 16].

4.1. Glutathione deficiency and multiple sclerosis

There are several reports in the literature that relate the decrease or alteration of glutathione (GSH) metabolism with several neurodegenerative diseases. Biochemical analysis of postmortem brains has provided evidence for the generation of oxidative stress during the course of the disease since the total GSH content is reduced by 40–50% compared to controls. Also in several brain regions, we have found increased levels of lipid peroxidation [17]. The ratio GSH/GSSG (usually 10:1) is considered consistent with the concept of oxidative stress as an important part in the pathogenesis of MS. Moreover, low concentrations of GSH appear to be an important indicator of oxidative stress during the progression of MS. Although the decrease in GSH alone is not responsible for the degeneration of glial cells and neurons, reduced GSH could increase the susceptibility to other stressful factors and contribute to neuronal damage at glia and neuron cells. Glutathione has been reported to protect mitochondrial complex I activity against nitrosative stress, as S-nitrosoglutathione is formed. When this complex increases its content of nitrotyrosine and nitrosothiol groups in response to nitrosative stress, its activity is inhibited and therefore ATP production is diminished, which causes neuronal degeneration [10]. The role of glial cells in generating ROS in MS and the selective vulnerability of neurons is due to activated glial cells surrounding these neurons, as these glial cells are also directly involved in GSH levels. The engagement of the glutathione system in astroglial cells contributes to the reduction in its antioxidant defenses and so poor glial defense could contribute to existing neuronal damage (**Figure 5**) [10]. Furthermore, the specific activities of some enzymes that metabolize GSH are high, as in the case of glutathione peroxidase, glutathione reductase, and glutathione S-transferase. Other products of OS are also elevated, as in the case of 4-hydroxynonenal (4-HNE, a product of lipid peroxidation of polyunsaturated omega-6 fatty acids) [17].

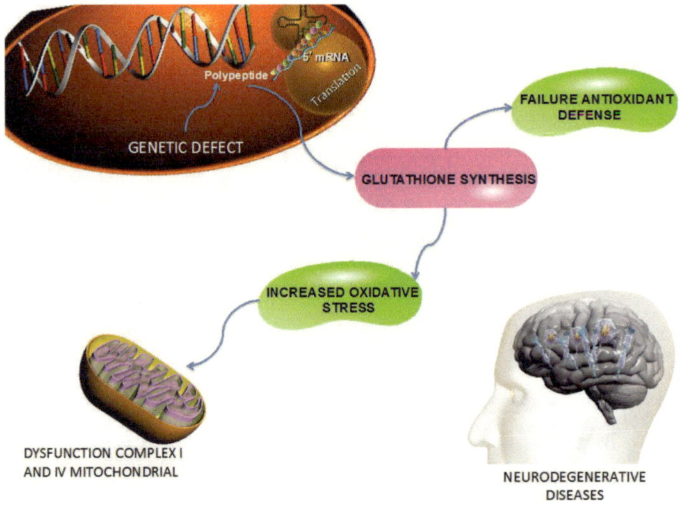

Figure 5. Genetic defect in glutathione synthesis and neurodegenerative diseases. Pathway Builder Online Tool was used to draw the figure [27].

A new proposal is that a genetic defect of glutathione synthesis may be the initial event in the failure of the antioxidant defenses. In neurodegenerative diseases, a decreased GSH level is accompanied by dysfunction of the mitochondrial complex I and complex IV and promotes oxidative stress [18]. We found a significant decrease in GSH levels in the cerebrospinal fluid of patients with this disease, and, in addition, proton magnetic resonance studies have shown a 50% decrease in GSH levels in the frontal cortex of patients with MS (**Figure 5**).

5. Mitochondria

Mitochondria are granular and filamentous organelles found in the cytoplasm of all eukaryotic cells and are the main site of adenosine triphosphate (ATP) synthesis by the processes of oxidative phosphorylation. These organelles vary in size and shape depending on the source and metabolic status, but are often ellipsoids of about 5 microns in diameter and 1 micron long. A typical eukaryotic cell contains more than 2,000 mitochondria, which takes up about one-fifth of the cell volume, an amount that is needed to meet the energy demands of the cell. Its main function is the mitochondrial respiration process in which the reducing power produced in the oxidation reactions enters the electron transport chain and energy is captured in the form of adenosine triphosphate (ATP). Mammalian tissues containing more mitochondria are the heart and brain [19]. The mitochondrion is formed by two membranes: the outer membrane and the inner membrane, which is highly folded, and the inner matrix is gel (approximately 50% water) [20].

The outer mitochondrial membrane contains porin, a pore-forming protein that allows diffusion of up to 10 kD molecules). The inner membrane contains approximately 75% protein and 25% lipids by weight, and it is much richer in outer membrane proteins. The inner membrane is permeable only to carbon dioxide (CO_2), oxygen (O_2), and water (H_2O). The passage of metabolites such as ATP, adenosine diphosphate (ADP), pyruvate, calcium ions (Ca^{2+}), and phosphate (PO_4) is regulated by controlling the transport proteins. This controlled permeability allows the generation of ionic gradients and results in the compartmentalization of metabolic functions between the cytoplasm and mitochondria. The inner membrane components of the respiratory chain are responsible for the synthesis of ATP (ATP synthase F_oF_1) [22], where the enzyme complex is housed. The inner membrane is arranged in ridges, giving it a large surface area: A single mitochondrion may have more than 10,000 sets of electron transfer systems (respiratory chain) and ATP synthase molecules distributed throughout the membrane's internal surface [21]. The inner membrane is, from the functional point of view, the most important because it contains the components of the respiratory chain and proteins necessary for the synthesis of ATP [21]. The mitochondrial matrix is the space delimited by the inner membrane and contains the pyruvate dehydrogenase complex and the enzymes of the tricarboxylic acid cycle (TCA), the fatty acid oxidation, and the oxidation of amino acids [21] (**Figure 6**).

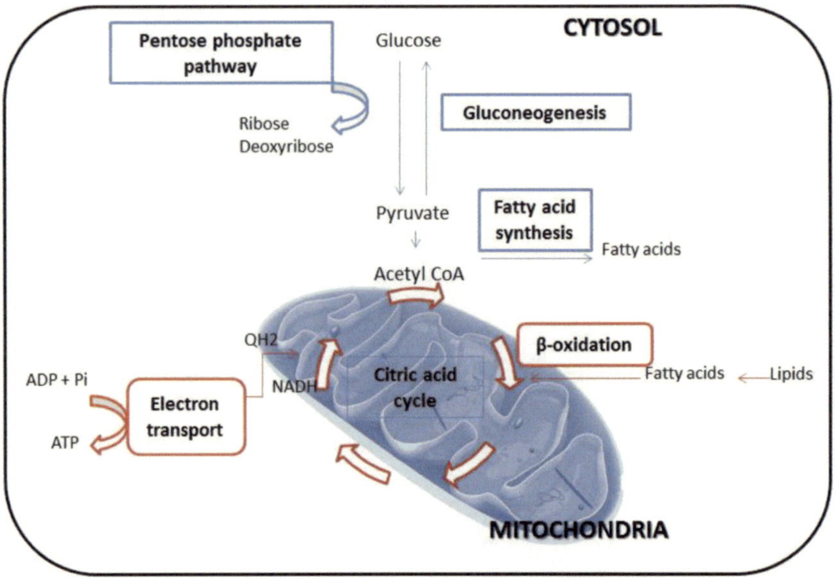

Figure 6. Main mitochondrial metabolic pathways. An important component of metabolic regulation is specialization. Mitochondria have a role in biosynthesis, catabolism, and energy metabolism, including citric acid cycle, oxidative phosphorylation, and fatty acid breakdown pathways.

The chemical energy required for cellular activities such as biosynthesis, transportation of ions and molecules, and mechanical work comes from ATP. Mitochondria generate more than 90% of the energy needed for the proper functioning of tissues that are highly dependent on aerobic metabolism, such as the brain and heart. This subcellular organelle provides the energy necessary for the production of ATP [22]. Depending on cell type and metabolic state, mitochondria consume approximately 90–95% of the oxygen consumed by the cell. The energy of this process, in which electrons are transferred from the substrates of the TCA to oxygen, is coupled to vectorial transport of H^+ from the mitochondrial matrix space [22].

The electron carriers, reduced nicotinamide dinucleotide adenine (NADH) and reduced flavin dinucleotide adenine ($FADH_2$), originating mainly in the TCA cycle, confer the energy that electrons carry. This energy is released gradually along the respiratory chain in the mitochondrial inner membrane. In this membrane, an exchange of electrons between the enzymatic complexes is given by NADH or $FADH_2$ [20].

The complexes are as follows: I (NADH-ubiquinone reductase), II (succinate-ubiquinone reductase), III (ubiquinol-cytochrome c reductase), IV (cytochrome oxidase), and V (ATP synthase complex F_0F_1) [20]. Electron transport is carried out by complexes I, III, and IV that produce a flow of electrons accompanied by a movement of protons from the mitochondrial matrix to the intermembrane space (space between the inner and outer mitochondrial membrane). This produces a difference in proton concentration and a difference in charge across the membrane [20]. The proton-motive force generated thereby drives protons through the F_0F_1-ATP synthase, allowing condensation of a phosphate group to ADP, with the formation of ATP [23]. Meanwhile, the complex F_0F_1-ATP synthase is an enzyme located in the inner membrane of the mitochondria, responsible for ATP synthesis from ADP and a phosphate group (Pi), and the energy is supplied by a flow of protons (H^+). The difference between the terms ATPase and ATP synthase is that the enzyme has a dual function: It breaks down ATP to ADP and Pi (activated ATPase), and it also allows for catalyzing Pi binding of ADP using the proton gradient for ATP synthesis (ATP synthase activity). As complex V has both functions, we can name it indiscriminately when speaking in general terms of the enzyme [23]. This enzyme is constituted by two components: a soluble portion (F_1), located in aqueous medium, and another portion (F_o), which is lipid soluble. The F_o part is inserted into the lipid bilayer and is sensitive to the antibiotic oligomycin (**Figure 7**).

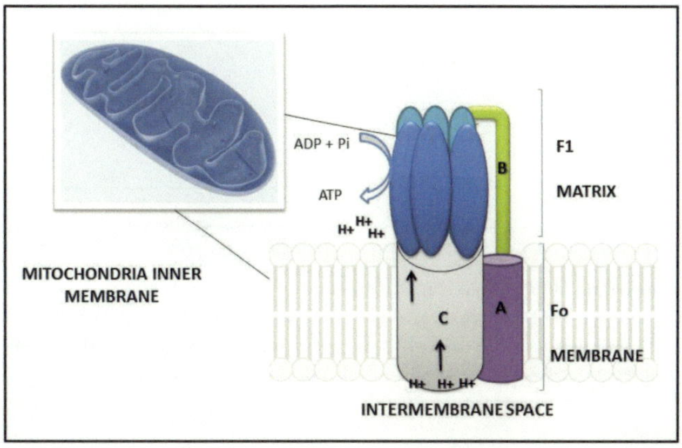

Figure 7. ATP synthase complex structure. The ATP synthase complex plays a central role in energy transduction in living cells that uses energy released by the movement of protons down a transmembrane electrochemical gradient to drive the synthesis of ATP. This enzyme is located in the inner membrane of mitochondria and is constituted by two parts: a soluble portion (F1) in aqueous medium and another portion (Fo) lipid soluble. The Fo part is inserted into the lipid bilayer.

On the other hand, pathophysiological features exhibited the association between mitochondrial dysfunction, decreased activity of complex I and complex IV of the electron transport chain, and the glutathione system in MS [23].

6. Mitochondria and multiple sclerosis

In acute phases of the disease, axonal degeneration correlates with the severity of inflammation. This type of injury has been used in an experimental model of autoimmune encephalomyelitis (EAE), where acute mitochondrial damage within axons is detected and later suffers from focal damage as a preliminary pathological step of axonal damage [15].

Complex IV of the mitochondrial electron transport chain has a binding site for O_2 (The final acceptor in the respiratory chain) and catalyzes the reduction in O_2 to H_2O. Interestingly, nitric oxide inhibits mitochondrial respiration by reacting with either the reduced or the oxidized binuclear site of cytochrome c oxidase, leading to ATP depletion. In cases of excessive nitric oxide production, complete inhibition of cytochrome c oxidase has been shown to contribute to pathology.

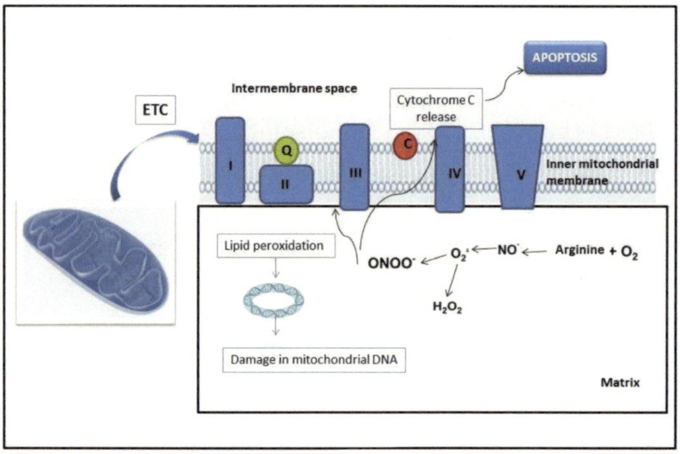

Figure 8. Association of mitochondrial electron transport chain with oxidative stress. The mitochondrial electron transport chain (ETC), which is composed of four multiprotein complexes named complex I–IV, has been recognized as one of the major cellular generators of free radicals. Leakage of electrons directly from the intermediate electron carriers generates reactive oxygen species that leads to membrane lipid peroxidation, mitochondrial DNA damage, and the release of cytochrome C to the cytosol triggering apoptosis.

At the same time, interrupting the electron transport chain by binding of NO to complex IV increases electron release, thus facilitating the formation of reactive oxygen species, firstly superoxide anion and subsequently H_2O_2 and OH.·Peroxynitrite has a direct effect on mitochondria leading to lipid peroxidation of membrane lipids and thus damaging the complexes of the respiratory chain and mitochondrial DNA. Opening of permeability transition pores and release of cytochrome C from mitochondria initiate apoptosis (**Figure 8**).

At the stage of acute inflammation, a set of mechanisms that alter mitochondrial function is produced. The energy deficit causes structural and functional damage to macromolecules by increased ROS that ultimately leads to severe axonal damage. In these events, the mitochondria has an important role; therefore, if we know what the mechanisms involved in glial and neuronal alterations are, we must be able to identify the elements that can be used as effector elements and design drugs to control and reduced harm during the stage of relapse [14].

Many demyelinated axons survive during a relapse, and these can become chronically demyelinated axons, in which case axonal mitochondria develop compensatory mechanisms to cope with the lack of myelin. There are reports in which inactive lesions from chronic demyelinated axons of patients with MS are observed. In such reports, they have found an increase in the activity of mitochondrial complex IV and increased synphilin anchoring protein [19]. However, axons progressively degenerate in chronic lesions of MS patients. In the absence of myelin, redistribution of Na^+ occurs to maintain the transmission of nerve impulses that increases energy demand, and this produces a situation of "virtual hypoxia." At the end, the demand exceeds the capacity of axonal mitochondria to produce enough ATP, which causes an increase in the concentration of Ca^{2+} in the axon. Ca^{2+} pumping and extended levels of intramitochondrial calcium leads to opening pores, rupture of the outer mitochondrial membrane, and release of cytochrome C, finally leading to apoptosis (**Figure 8**).

One of the questions we have not answered is: Why are mitochondria helpless and overwhelmed by the energy demand and how does this happen? Are the axons unable to maintain stable mitochondrial activity in demyelination?. This reflects the inability of the cell to carry and generate mitochondria. Dutta et al. [23] have shown decreased gene expression of 26 nuclear-encoded subunits of the oxidative phosphorylation chain in non-demyelinated motor cortex from MS patients, which coincided with a significant reduction in activity of NADH dehydrogenase and ubiquinol-cytochrome c reductase . In the progressive phase of MS, it is postulated that chronically demyelinated axons are unable to maintain mitochondrial function, and thus, a deficit of ATP synthesis coupled with oxidative stress results in irreversible axonal damage.

7. Effect of fish oil (Omega3) and olive oil on membrane fluidity, ATPase activity in relapsing-remitting multiple sclerosis.

The mechanism of action for omega-3 PUFAs is suggested to be attributed to immunomodulation and antioxidant action [24]. For instance, omega-3 PUFAs decrease the production of inflammatory mediators (eicosanoids, cytokines, and ROS) and the expression of adhesion molecules. They both act directly by replacing AA as an eicosanoid substrate and inhibiting AA metabolism and indirectly by altering the expression of inflammatory genes through effects on transcription factor activation. Omega-3 PUFAs also give rise to anti-inflammatory mediators (resolvins and protectins) [25]. Effects of resolvins and protectins include reducing neutrophil trafficking, cytokine, and ROS regulation and lowering the magnitude of the inflammatory response [26].

Previously, we developed a twelve-month randomized double-blind controlled clinical trial in 50 patients with relapsing-remitting MS. Patients received an oral dose of 4 g/day of fish oil (containing a total of 800 mg of EPA and 1600 mg of DHA) or olive oil. Fasting blood samples were collected at baseline and after 6 and 12 months of the trial, in order to evaluate the effect of consumption of omega-3 PUFAs on some markers of oxidative stress at the peripheral level. The initial findings of this work were the decrease in serum levels of TNFα, IL-1β, IL-6, and nitric oxide metabolites compared with the placebo group [27].

On the other hand, after 12 months of intervention, supplementation with omega-3 PUFAs significantly enhanced the quantities of serum omega-3 highly unsaturated fatty acids compared with baseline values. Additionally, the levels of medium-chain monounsaturated fatty acids were significantly decreased. The olive oil supplementation induced minor decreases in EPA and DHA levels after 12 months of intervention. There were significant increases in both EPA and DHA in the group given fish oil supplementation compared to the control group receiving olive oil. These increases were associated with a concomitant decrease in AA. Consequently, the omega-3 fatty acid index in the fish oil group increased significantly, and the ratios of n-6/n-3 and AA/EPA were decreased [28].

No differences in glutathione reductase activity and content of reduced glutathione, oxidized glutathione, and oxidized/reduced glutathione ratio were seen after 12 months of supplementation with omega-3 PUFAs. However, a trend in favor of omega-3 PUFAs supplementation was observed in GSSG levels and glutathione reductase activity at 12 months of intervention between the study groups [28].

A steady decrease in mitochondrial ATPase activity in platelets was observed in the groups given omega-3 fatty acid and the control group receiving olive oil. Membrane fluidity of platelets was significantly reduced in MS patients. Interestingly, a significant increase in platelet membrane fluidity was observed in the groups receiving omega-3 fatty acid and the control group receiving olive oil. As well, the fluidity of erythrocyte membranes was unchanged for both treatments (Unpublished results).

Epidemiological and experimental studies suggest an increased incidence of MS in populations with a high intake of saturated fats mainly from animal sources. Therefore, by consuming a diet high in fatty acids, without an appropriate number of unsaturates, a shift is produced in the integrity and functionality of the membrane [29]. An optimal balance in the consumption of fatty acids includes 35% polyunsaturated fatty acids and 65% saturated fatty acids, and the appropriate proportion of PUFA to maintain membrane balance is 50% omega-3 with 50% omega-6. The above ratio was a factor that inactivated the CD4 autoreactive cells in the CNS, a phenomenon that prevents the production of proinflammatory cytokines and free radicals [30].

Membrane fluidity depends on the temperature, the ratio of saturated/PUFA fatty acids, the presence of "lipid rafts," and the proportion of cholesterol present at the membrane [31]. Previous studies in patients with rheumatoid arthritis had increased cell membrane rigidity compared to membranes from those receiving immunomodulatory treatment. Our results showed diminished platelet membrane fluidity in MS patients and that proper membrane fluidity is restored with treatment of omega3 PUFAs. The increase in platelet membrane fluidity is directly related to the incorporation of PUFA's. Furthermore, the increase in membrane fluidity is accompanied with a significant decrease in mitochondrial ATPase activity. This ensures that the activity of ATP synthesis in mitochondria remains elevated.

8. Conclusions

The inflammatory process seen in MS is due to an excess production of pro-inflammatory cytokines, which leads to increased secretion of ROS. Oxidative stress plays a preponderant, key role in the pathogenesis of MS. Reactive oxygen species generated by macrophages have been implicated as mediators of demyelination and axonal damage in EAE and MS. The main findings of a clinical trial conducted with relapsing-remitting MS patients who received a diet supplemented with 4 g/day of fish oil or olive oil are the following:

1. Fish oil supplementation resulted in a high increase in proportions of EPA and DHA, leading to a decrease in AA concentrations as well as the AA/EPA ratio. These changes in fatty acids are indicative of a reduction in the production of inflammatory eicosanoids from AA and an increase in anti-inflammatory mediators such as resolvins and protectins.
2. No differences in glutathione reductase activity, content of reduced and oxidized glutathione, and GSH/GSSG ratio were seen after 12 months of supplementation. However, fish oil supplementation resulted in a smaller increase in GR compared with the control group. In addition, there was a significant change in glutathione reductase activity within subjects in the fish oil group after 6 months of treatment, while no significant differences within subjects were observed in the control group, suggesting a possible effect of fish oil on antioxidant defense mechanisms of the cell. Although glutathione reductase activity was not significantly different between the groups, fish oil supplementation resulted in a smaller increase in GR compared with the control group, suggesting a possible antioxidant effect of fish oil supplementation.
3. Membrane fluidity of platelets was significantly reduced in MS patients. That membrane property steadily increased in the groups given omega-3 fatty acid and the control group receiving olive oil. The increases in membrane fluidity of platelets were associated with a decrease in mitochondrial ATPase. As well, the fluidity of erythrocyte membranes was unchanged for both treatments (unpublished results).

Author details

Genaro G. Ortiz[1*], Fermín P. Pacheco-Moisés[2], Erandis D. Torres-Sánchez[1], Tanya E. Sorto-Gómez[1], Mario Mireles-Ramírez[3], Alfredo León-Gil[3], Héctor González-Usigli[3], Luis J. Flores-Alvarado[4], Erika D. González-Renovato[1], Angelica L. Sánchez-López[1], Margarita Cid-Hernández[2] and Irma E. Velázquez-Brizuela[5]

*Address all correspondence to: genarogabriel@yahoo.com

1 Laboratory of Mitochondria-Oxidative Stress and Pathology, Neurosciences Division, Occidental Biomedical Research Center, The Mexican Social Security Institute, Guadalajara, Jalisco, México

2 Department of Chemistry, Centre of Exact Sciences and Engineering, University of Guadalajara, Guadalajara, Jalisco, México

3 Department of Neurology, Sub-specialty Medical Unit, National Occidental Medical Center, The Mexican Social Security Institute, Guadalajara, Jalisco, México

4 Department of Biochemistry, Health Sciences Center, University of Guadalajara, Guadalajara, Jalisco, México

5 Health Sciences Center, University of Guadalajara, Guadalajara, Jalisco, México

References

[1] Mejía BL, Agudelo RC, Gómez HJC, Cabrera HD. Genética de la EM: An epidemiological and molecular perspective. Archivos de medicina 2009;5(1:5).

[2] Lassmann H. The pathology of MS and its evolution. Phil Trans R. Soc. Lond B 1999;354:1635–40.

[3] Coronado HM, Vega y León S, Gutiérrez TR, García FB, Díaz G. omega-3 and omega-6 fatty acids Nutrición, Bioquímica y Salud 2009;REB 25(3):72–79.

[4] Reinhart GA. (1996), Review of w-3 Fatty acids and dietary influences on tissue concentration en recent advances en canine and feline nutritional research. Edit Carey D. P., Ohio 235–242.

[5] Villegas P, Vidal S, Bray GM, Aguayo T. (2005), Axonal regeneration and synapse formation in the superior colliculus by retinal ganglion cells in the adult rat. Journal of Neuroscience 2005;7:2894–2909.

[6] Valenzuela A, Nieto S. Ácido docosahexanoico (DHA) en el desarrollo fetal y en la nutrición materno infantil. Revista Médica de Chile 2001;129:1203–1211.

[7] Bazan G, Bodker M, Serhan N, Marcheselli V, Lukiw W. A role for docosahexaenoic acid-derived neuroprotectin D1 in neural cells survival and Alzheimer disease. Journal Clinic Investigation 2005;115:2774–2780.

[8] White P. (1995) Essential fatty acids in medicine veterinary, Bayer AG. S Business group animal health supplement, Germany.

[9] Li S, Vana AC, Ribeiro R, Zhang Y. Distinct role of nitric oxide and peroxynitrite in mediating oligodendrocyte toxicity in culture and in experimental autoimmune encephalomyelitis. Neuroscience 2011;184:107–119.

[10] Ferreira B, Mendes F, Osório N, et al. Glutathione in multiple sclerosis. Br J Biomed Sci 2013;70(2):75–79.

[11] Fischer MT, Sharma R, Lim JL et al. NADPH oxidase expression in active multiple sclerosis lesions in relation to oxidative tissue damage and mitochondrial injury. Brain: A Journal of Neurology 2012;135:886–899.

[12] Ortiz GG, Macias-Islas MA, Pacheco-Moises FP, et al. Oxidative stress is increased in serum from Mexican patients with relapsing-remitting multiple sclerosis. Dis Markers 2009;26:35–39.

[13] Jensen GE, Clausen J. Glutathione peroxidase and reductase, glucose-6-phosphate dehydrogenase and catalase activities in multiple sclerosis. Journal of the Neurological Sciences, 1984;63:45–53.

[14] Tasset I, Agüera E, Sánchez-López F, et al. Peripheral oxidative stress in relapsing–remitting multiple sclerosis. Clinical Biochemistry 2012;45:440–444.

[15] Greco A, Minghetti L, Sette G, et al. Cerebrospinal fluid isoprostane shows oxidative stress in patients with multiple sclerosis. Neurology 1999 Nov 10;53(8):1876–1879.

[16] Karg E, Klivényi P, Németh I, et al. Nonenzymatic antioxidants of blood in multiple sclerosis. J Neurol. 1999;246(7):533–539.

[17] Hauser S, Oksenberg J. The neurobiology of multiple sclerosis: genes, inflammation, and neurodegeneration. Neuron 2006;52:61–76.

[18] Correale J, Tenembaum S. Myelin basic protein and myelin oligodendrocyte glycoprotein T-cell repertoire in childhood and juvenile multiple sclerosis. Multiple sclerosis 2006;12:1–9.

[19] Westermann B. (2002), Merging mitochondria matters: Cellular role and molecular machinery of mitochondrial fusion. European Molecular Biology Organization, 2002;3(6):527–531.

[20] Frey Terrence G, Mannella Carmen A. The internal structure of mitochondria, Review. TIBS 2000;Jul;25(7) 319–24

[21] Lehninger (2000) Principles of Biochemistry 3rd, Ed. Worth Publishers, pp. 389, 391, Capitulo 5, Capitulo 8, Capitulo 1, Capitulo 14, Capitulo 19.

[22] Lee CL, Hanay J, Hrachovy R. (2001) Spatial learning deficits without hippocampal loss in a model of early-onset epilepsy. Neuroscience 2001;107:71–84.

[23] Dutta R, McDonough J, Yin X, Peterson J, Chang A, et al. Mitochondrial dysfunction as a cause of axonal degeneration in multiple sclerosis patients. Ann Neurol 2006;59:478–489.

[24] Mehta LR, Dworkin RH, Schwid SR. Polyunsaturated fatty acids and their potential therapeutic role in multiple sclerosis. Nat Clin Pract Neurol 2009;5:82–92.

[25] Calder PC. n-3 Polyunsaturated fatty acids, inflammation, and inflammatory diseases. Am J Clin Nutr 2006;83(6 suppl):1505S–19S.

[26] Serhan CN, Ariel A. Resolvins and protectins in the termination program of acute inflammation. Trends Immunol 2007;28:176–183.

[27] Ramirez-Ramirez V, Macias-Islas MA, Ortiz GG, Pacheco-Moises F, Torres-Sanchez ED, et al. Efficacy of fish oil on serum of TNF-α, IL-1 β, and IL-6 oxidative stress markers in multiple sclerosis treated with interferon beta-1b. Oxid Med Cell Longev. 2013;2013:709493.

[28] Effect of Fish Oil on glutathion redox system in multiple sclerosis. Am J Neurodegenertive Dis 2016; 5(2): 145–151.

[29] Shinitzky M. Membrane fluidity and cellular functions. Physiology of membrane fluidity. Boca Raton: CRC Press 1984;1–151.

[30] Kantarci OH, Weinshenker BG. Natural history of multiple sclerosis. Neurol Clin 2005;23(1):17–38.

[31] Comparán A, Interés de los brotes en la EM, Fisiopatología y tratamiento. Rev Neurol 2003;36:1058–64.

Section 2

Environmental Risk Factors and Clinical Issues in MS

Chapter 6

Pediatric Multiple Sclerosis

Ozgul Ekmekci

Additional information is available at the end of the chapter

http://dx.doi.org/10.5772/63919

Abstract

Multiple sclerosis (MS) is an autoimmune inflammatory demyelinating disorder of the central nervous system. Although pediatric and adult-onset MS have similar neurologic symptoms, there are some differences from adults in radiologic findings, cognitive features, clinical course, and diagnostic criteria of pediatric MS. Diagnostic criteria and radiologic features of pediatric MS have been defined in recent years. There are no large, randomized, controlled therapeutic trials in pediatric MS. In this chapter, clinical characteristics, diagnostic criteria, laboratory findings, differential diagnosis, and treatment of pediatric MS are summarized.

Keywords: multiple sclerosis, pediatric multiple sclerosis, childhood multiple sclerosis, demyelinating disorders, demyelination

1. Introduction

Multiple sclerosis (MS) is an autoimmune chronic inflammatory disease of the central nervous system; it is characterized by demyelination and axonal loss. MS primarily affects young adults. Recently, it has been increasingly recognized in children and adolescents. Approximately 2–5% of all MS patients have onset before age 18 [1, 2]. Onset before 10 years of age occurs in less than 1% of all patients. There are some differences, including clinical presentation, magnetic resonance imaging (MRI) findings, and neuroimmunologic features, between pediatric and adult MS patients. The first attack can be acute disseminated encephalomyelitis, particularly in young children. Relapses are more frequent in pediatric MS patients than in adults, though improvement is better. Cognitive impairment including linguistic dysfunction and reduction in IQ scores also differs from adults. T2 lesion burden is higher in pediatric patients in MRI as compared to adult MS patients. These differences are more marked in prepuberal children [3]. The still developing central nervous and immune systems may be responsible for these differences. However, studies on pathogenesis and pathology of pediatric MS are limited.

2. Epidemiology

The incidence of pediatric MS is unknown, but its estimated prevalence has been reported to be 1.35–2.5 per 100,000 children [4]. The gender ratio varies with the age of onset: in patients older than 10 years, the female-to-male ratio is similar to adults; there is female dominance. In children younger than 10 years old, the female-to-male ratio decreases. This difference may be due to hormonal influence or gender-specific genetic influence on immunological reactivity [5].

3. Etiology and risk factors

Pediatric MS has a complex etiology related to both genetic and environmental factors. Vitamin D deficiency has been implicated as a risk factor for MS in children, as it is in adults. Mowry et al. have demonstrated an association between relapse rate and vitamin D level in pediatric MS patients [6]. Smoking has been considered as a risk factor in adults, whereas passive smoke exposure has been recognized as a risk factor in children [7]. One of the most studied environmental risk factors is viral exposure and studies have found that viral exposure in childhood may predispose some individuals to the development of MS. Epstein-Barr seropositivity and serum anti-EBV antibody titers tend to be higher in MS patients than they are in normal individuals. The relationship between the Epstein-Barr virus and MS has also been shown in pediatric MS [8]. Another risk factor is obesity. Childhood and adolescent obesity has been suggested as a risk factor for the development of MS in both adults and children [9]. Genetic susceptibility is also a risk factor for MS. HLA-DRB1 locus has been associated with multiple sclerosis in children. Twin studies have demonstrated a concordance rate of 27% in monozygotic twins. The incidence for first-degree relatives of patients with MS is 2–5%, whereas the incidence for the general population is under 0.1% [10].

4. Pathogenesis

Multiple sclerosis is a neuroimmunologic disorder characterized pathologically by inflammation, demyelination, and axonal loss. Neuropathological findings and animal models such as experimental allergic encephalomyelitis support the immunopathogenesis in multiple sclerosis. HLA Class II genes which are associated with MS risk are also related to the immune system.

The first step in the immunopathogenesis of MS is peripheral activation of CD4+ T lymphocytes in response to an antigen. This antigen is unknown. It has been suggested that molecular mimicry between this antigen and central nervous system antigens causes cross reactivity. Subsequently, activated T lymphocytes migrate through the blood-brain barrier into the central nervous system [10, 11]. Lymphocyte migration represents an important step in MS pathogenesis. This multistep process includes adhesion, chemoattraction, and active infiltration into the central nervous system. Adhesion molecules, chemokines, and cytokines play an important role in these steps [10]. $\alpha 4\beta 1$ integrin (VLA-4, very late activating antigen) is an adhesion molecule which is expressed on the lymphocyte surface and binds to the vascular cell adhesion molecule-1 (VICAM-1) located on the endothelium. As a result of this interaction, lymphocytes adhere to the endothelium and transmigrate across the endothelial cell layer into the central nervous system [12]. Chemokines regulate migration of immune cells into the brain; they also manipulate the lymphocyte transendothelial migration and locomotion within the tissue along chemoattractant gradients. Reactivation of infiltrating immune cells within the central nervous system leads to perivascular inflammation and injury. This injury results in the release of additional central nervous system antigens such as myelin proteins and leads to immune responses to these self-antigens (antigen spreading/epitope spreading). T cells reactive to myelin proteins including myelin basic protein (MBP), myelin oligodendrocyte glycoprotein (MOG), and myelin proteolipid protein (PLP) are involved in the central nervous system inflammatory response of MS patients [10]. Myelin-reactive T cells have differences in MS patients as compared with healthy controls. In MS patients myelin-reactive T cells differ by having memory phenotype. Memory T cells play an important role in MS pathogenesis. Other immune cells including proinflammatory and anti-inflammatory/regulatory CD4+ T cells (helper T lymphocytes), CD8+ T cells (cytotoxic T lymphocytes), myeloid cell subsets, B cells, and natural killer cells contribute to the pathogenesis of MS in adults. After activation by antigen-presenting cells such as dendritic cells, naïve T cells differentiate into one of the several subsets with different effector functions. Th1 lymphocytes secrete proinflammatory cytokines such as interferon gamma, while Th2 lymphocytes produce anti-inflammatory cytokines such as interleukin 4, interleukin 10. The imbalance between proinflammatory and anti-inflammatory cytokines has been invoked in MS pathogenesis. Proinflammatory cytokines play crucial roles in MS pathogenesis including peripheral immune activation, enhancement of trafficking of activated immune cells into the CNS, and direct damage to oligodendrocytes, myelin, and axons [10, 12]. Th17 lymphocytes are also a subgroup of CD4+ T cells that produce the proinflammatory cytokines interleukin 17A and interleukin 17F. Th17 lymphocytes are developmentally distinct from Th1 and Th2 lineages. Interleukin 23 produced by macrophages and dendritic cells contributes to development of Th17. High Th17 to Th1 ratios are associated with T cell infiltration and inflammation in the brain parenchyma [13]. The presence of interleukin 17 in MS lesions and increased interleukin 17 expression in both blood and CSF of MS patients have been demonstrated [14, 15]. Other subgroups of T cells also have been implicated in the immunopathogenesis of MS. Regulatory T (Treg) cells control potentially pathogenic autoreactive T cells. Studies demonstrated that regulatory T cell functions are altered in MS. In a study, similar T cell responses to myelin basic protein and myelin oligodendrocyte glycoprotein epitopes have been found in both adult and pediatric MS patients [16]. Vargas Lowy demonstrated increased CD4+ T cell proliferation to myelin peptides in children with MS and also found an increased proportion of dividing CD4+ T cell to myelin peptides with a memory phenotype which produced interleukin 17 [10].

Humoral immunity has also been implicated in MS pathogenesis. B lymphocytes, plasma cells, immunoglobulins, and complement deposition have been shown in MS lesions. Anti-myelin oligodendrocyte glycoprotein antibodies (anti-MOG) have been reported in pediatric cases with inflammatory demyelinating diseases, predominantly in children with ADEM-like first episodes and in pediatric MS patients younger than 10 years of age at disease onset. Anti-MOG antibodies have also been observed in pediatric patients with recurrent optic neuritis and seronegative NMO [10, 17]. The presence of anti-MOG antibodies has been reported in a subgroup of adults with seronegative NMO but only rarely in adults with MS [18]. Moreover, antibody-independent functions of B lymphocytes such as cytokine production play a role in MS immunopathogenesis.

Neurodegeneration and axonal damage are other processes in the pathogenesis of MS. Mechanisms of axonal damage in multiple sclerosis include a specific immunologic attack on axons; the presence of soluble mediators such as proteases, cytokines, and free radicals released during the inflammatory process and lack of neurotrophic factors provided to the axon by oligodendrocytes as a result of chronic demyelination [10, 19].

5. Pathology

The cellular content of MS lesions includes primarily T lymphocytes (CD4+ and CD8+) and macrophages. Lucchinetti et al. have described four distinct pathological patterns of demyelination in autopsy and biopsy samples from adult MS patients. Patterns I and II showed T cell/macrophage inflammation and there was also T cell plus antibody-mediated autoimmune damage in pattern II. Patterns III and IV were suggestive of a primary oligodendrocyte dystrophy. Oligodendrocyte apoptosis or death and lesser macrophage-T cell inflammation were observed in patterns III and IV [20]. In another study, Trapp et al. demonstrated axonal damage in normal appearing white matter [21]. Additionally, subpial cortical, intracortical, and leukocortical lesions were found in adult-onset multiple sclerosis patients' biopsy specimens. Immune cells were also identified within the pia-arachnoid in adult-onset multiple sclerosis and ectopic B-cell follicles with germinal centers were detected in the meninges of patients with secondary progressive multiple sclerosis. All these pathological findings were identified in adult patients [10, 22, 23]. Neuropathological studies are limited in pediatric multiple sclerosis [10]. Tumefactive demyelinating lesions have been investigated in pediatric patients with MS [24]. The pathological characteristics of tumefactive demyelinating lesions include relative axonal preservation, perivascular and parenchymal lymphocyte and macrophage inflammation [25].

http://dx.doi.org/10.5772/63919

6. Diagnostic criteria

In 2007, the International Pediatric Multiple Sclerosis Study Group (IPMSSG) proposed a consensus on definitions for pediatric acquired demyelinating disorders of the central nervous system and pediatric MS. Pediatric MS referred to "children" (under the age of 10) and "adolescents" (aged 10 and above but younger than 18) in this definition. In 2012, the study group revised the criteria in consideration of studies that had applied 2007 pediatric MS criteria and the 2010 revised McDonald's criteria for adults [26–28].

According to the 2012 revised criteria, pediatric MS can be satisfied by any of the following:

- Two or more non-encephalopathic (e.g. not ADEM-like) clinical central nervous system (CNS) events with a presumed inflammatory cause, separated by more than 30 days and involving more than one area of the CNS.
- One non-encephalopathic episode typical of MS which is associated with MRI findings consistent with the 2010 revised McDonald criteria for DIS (dissemination in space) and in which a follow-up MRI shows at least one new enhancing or non-enhancing lesion consistent with DIT (dissemination in time) MS criteria.
- One ADEM attack followed by a non-encephalopathic clinical event, three or more months after the onset of symptoms, which is associated with new MRI lesions that fulfill the 2010 revised McDonald DIS criteria.
- A first single, acute event that does not meet ADEM criteria and whose MRI findings are consistent with the 2010 revised McDonald criteria for DIS and DIT (applies only to children ≥ 12 years old).

7. Clinical features

Most of the patients with pediatric MS have a relapsing remitting course. A primary progressive course is extremely rare in pediatric MS. The definition of an attack (relapse/exacerbation) in pediatric MS is similar to that in adults. An attack is defined as "the appearance of new symptoms and neurologic signs, or worsening of old symptoms and signs due to an acute inflammatory demyelinating event in the CNS, with duration of at least 24 hours in the absence of fever or infection," and the onset of the attack should be separated from the onset of a previous attack by at least 30 days [27].

Visual, sensory, motor, brainstem, cerebellar symptoms, sphincter, and cognitive dysfunctions may also occur in pediatric MS, as they do in adults. Polysymptomatic and ADEM-like onset are more common in prepuberal patients, particularly in very young children. Visual and sensory symptoms may go unnoticed in very young children. In adolescents, the presentation of monosymptomatic and sensorimotor symptoms is frequent, and optic neuritis is the most common initial presentation. The interval between the initial demyelinating event and the second attack varies, and this interval may be longer in very young children. Relapses are more frequent and may be more severe in pediatric patients but recovery is often better than it is in adults. The accumulation of disability takes a long time in pediatric MS; however, over the long term, patients can become disabled at a younger age. The transition to secondary progressive MS occurs at a younger age in pediatric-onset MS than in adult-onset MS. The risk of transition to secondary progressive MS in pediatric patients is associated with a higher frequency of relapses and shorter intervals between attacks in the first few years of the disease [2, 29–31].

Cognitive disturbance is an important feature in pediatric MS. Cognitive impairment can occur even in the first few years of the disease and does not correlate with physical disability, number of relapses, and disease duration. The onset of multiple sclerosis in very young children increases the risk of cognitive impairment [3]. In adult MS patients, the most commonly affected cognitive functions include processing speed, visual-spatial function, memory, and executive functions. The most commonly affected cognitive areas in pediatric MS are attention span, processing speed, and visual-motor skills as adults. Receptive language, verbal fluency, and intelligence also are affected in pediatric MS, and they are affected differently than they are in adult MS. Linguistic involvement (verbal fluency, naming, and comprehension) is an important neuropsychological difference between pediatric and adult-onset MS [32, 33]. Pediatric MS patients are also at risk for a lower IQ [3]. Differences in cognitive dysfunctions between pediatric MS and adult MS may be due to the effect of inflammatory demyelination on the developing central nervous system and neuronal networks. All patients with pediatric MS should be checked for cognitive dysfunction because it occurs in the early stages of the disease and is unrelated to physical disability [29, 30, 33].

Psychiatric disorders such as depression or anxiety are common in pediatric MS, as they are in adults. Fatigue is also reported in patients with pediatric MS. Cognitive impairment, depression, and fatigue disrupt the child's academic performance and quality of life [3].

8. Diagnostic evaluation

8.1. Magnetic resonance imaging features

MRI is the most important paraclinical tool for the diagnosis of MS, and it also provides information for differential diagnosis.

Demyelinating plaques are demonstrated as an increased signal on T2 and FLAIR sequences and are typically located in deep white matter, corpus callosum, periventricular zone, juxtacortical, and posterior fossa. Hypointense lesions occur on T1 sequences. These hypointense lesions are named "black holes." Black holes are a result of tissue loss due to previous inflammatory events. Acute MS plaques may appear to be T1 hypointense as a result of transient edema, but these are not true T1-black holes. T1 hypointensity may remain for months after an acute event with such lesions evolving to isointensity (loss of edema or repair) or persisting as chronic, permanent hypointensity [34]. Active demyelinating plaques may show gadolinium enhancement due to a blood-brain barrier breakdown and enhancement is often incomplete around the periphery (open ring sign) (**Figures 1** and **2**).

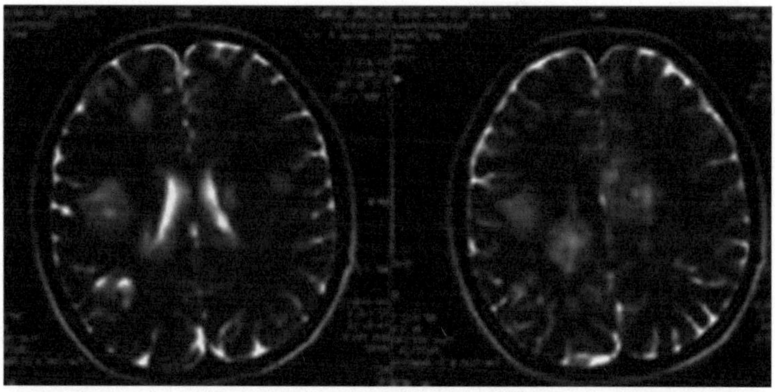

Figure 1. Large, hyperintense lesions on T2-weighted sequences.

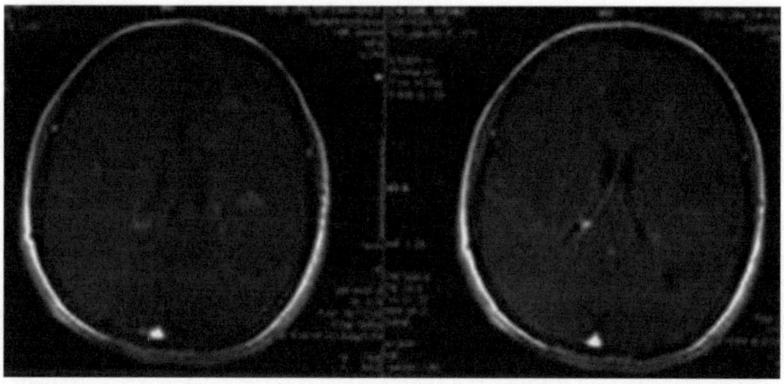

Figure 2. Gadolonium enhanced demyelinating plaques and black holes on T1-weighted sequences.

MRI findings in McDonald's diagnostic criteria are important and provide a diagnosis of MS at the first demyelinating event. According to McDonald's diagnostic criteria, dissemination in space (DIS) can be demonstrated by one or more T2 lesions in at least two of four areas of the CNS (periventricular, juxtacortical, infratentorial, spinal cord) and dissemination in time (DIT) can be demonstrated by a new T2 and/or gadolinium-enhancing lesion(s) on a follow-up MRI, with reference to a baseline scan, irrespective of the timing of the baseline MRI or the simultaneous presence of asymptomatic gadolinium-enhancing and non-enhancing lesions at any time [10]. These criteria have been found to be highly sensitive (100%) and highly specific (86%) for children older than 12 years with non-ADEM presentation, but they may not be appropriate for young children [35].

There are some differences in MRI findings between children and adults, particularly in prepuberal cases: T2-hyperintense lesion volume and lesion load in the infratentorial area are higher in children than they are in adults; first presentation may be as ADEM; there is an increased incidence of larger, tumefactive lesions in young children; spinal cord lesions may be longer than three vertebral segments in children with MS as in neuromyelitis optica [29, 36].

8.2. Cerebrospinal fluid (CSF) features

Analysis of CSF provides information about both the inflammatory process and differential diagnosis such as infection and malignancy. Cell count, presence of oligoclonal bands, and IgG index are examined in CSF analysis. A mild lymphocytic pleocystosis may be seen in children, but it has been shown that children younger than 11 years have more neutrophils in the CSF than older children. Oligoclonal band positivity has been found in 92% of patients with pediatric MS [37, 38]. An increased IgG index is more common in adolescents than in young children.

8.3. Evoked potentials

Evoked potentials help to demonstrate subclinical demyelination and to evaluate prior demyelination [39]. Visual evoked potentials are more informative than brainstem auditory and somatosensory evoked potentials.

9. Differential diagnosis

Other immune-mediated central nervous system demyelinating disorders (clinically isolated syndrome, acute disseminated encephalomyelitis, neuromyelitis optica) must be excluded in pediatric patients presenting a first demyelinating attack.

Clinically isolated syndrome (CIS) is a monofocal (optic neuritis, brainstem syndrome, transverse myelitis, cerebellar syndrome, or hemispheric syndrome) or polyfocal clinical CNS event with a presumed inflammatory demyelinating cause without a prior clinical history of a CNS demyelinating disease and encephalopathy. MRI features do not meet McDonald's criteria. Therefore, a follow-up check for the possibility of developing MS is necessary; however, the likelihood of developing MS is low in patients with a normal brain MRI [28].

Acute disseminated encephalomyelitis (ADEM) is an inflammatory demyelinating disease which is characterized by acute encephalopathy and polyfocal neurologic deficits. Encephalopathy is an important feature and diagnostic criterion. Encephalopathy is defined as an alteration in consciousness or behavioral change unexplained by fever, systemic illness, or postictal symptoms in IPMSSG criteria 2012. Encephalopathy is an unexpected finding in MS. MRI features are also defined for pediatric ADEM in the 2012 IPMSSG criteria [28]. Diffuse, large (>1–2 cm), poorly demarcated hyperintense lesions are detected in cerebral white matter on T2-weighted and fluid-attenuated inversion recovery (FLAIR) sequences; T1 hypointense lesions are rare and deep gray matter lesions can be present in the thalamus or basal ganglia. White matter lesions are multiple, bilateral, and asymmetrical in the cerebral hemispheres, cerebellum, brainstem, and spinal cord. Deep gray matter lesions are usually symmetrical and more characteristic of ADEM than of MS. The presence of T1 hypointense lesions in white matter leads to a diagnosis of MS. Periventricular lesions are less common. Cerebrospinal fluid (CSF) oligoclonal bands are rarely observed and usually transient in ADEM. Anti-MOG antibodies may be transiently present in the serum. ADEM is usually a monophasic disorder.

Clinical and radiologic findings may fluctuate in the first 3 months after the onset of disease. A second attack of ADEM may occur rarely, and it is named "multiphasic ADEM" [28]. This second ADEM event can involve either new neurologic symptoms and MRI findings or the re-emergence of prior neurologic symptoms and MRI findings. In the 2012 IPMSSG criteria, multiphasic ADEM is defined as two episodes consistent with ADEM separated by 3 months but not followed by any further events [28]. Sometimes pediatric ADEM may be the first manifestation of pediatric MS. Mikaeloff et al. showed that 18% of patients with pediatric ADEM had a second attack suggesting MS [40]. The second attack usually occurs within 2 years of the initial event.

Neuromyelitis optica (NMO) is an inflammatory disorder characterized by severe acute transverse myelitis and optic neuritis. Pediatric NMO can be monophasic or relapsing. Optic neuritis and myelitis are more severe in NMO and the prognosis is worse than it is for MS. Atypical presentations such as encephalopathy, persistent hiccups, nausea, and vomiting may occur. A brain MRI does not meet the criteria for MS and can show lesions in the supratentorial area, periaquaductal gray matter, hypothalamus, medial thalamus, dorsal pons, and medulla. The presence of longitudinally extensive spinal cord lesions (more than three vertebral segments) in a spinal MRI is an important finding and a supportive criterion. Anti-aquaporin-4 IgG seropositivity is another supportive criterion and it is 99% specific and 60–70% sensitive in children [41]. CSF oligoclonal bands are generally absent.

Other causes such as vasculitis, vascular, infectious, or neoplastic diseases must be excluded in pediatric patients with acute neurologic deficits. The presence of encephalopathy, persistent headaches, fever, polyneuropathy, and hearing loss, the involvement of other organs such as arthritis, skin rashes, oral/genital ulcers, lymphadenopathy, nephropathy, or hepatopathy with a progressive course should be suggestive of other causes. A progressive course and the involvement of the peripheral nervous system usually occur in mitochondrial diseases or neurometabolic disorders such as leukodystrophies. The diseases that should be kept in mind in the differential diagnosis are shown in **Table 1**. Markedly elevated pleocytosis, low glucose, and increased protein in CSF analysis should rouse suspicions. Persistent gadolinium enhancement and continued enlargement of lesions, leptomeningeal enhancement, T2 hyperintensities in the basal ganglia, thalamus, and hypothalamus, and calcifications in an MRI should also eliminate the diagnosis of MS.

Other demyelinating disorders	
	Clinically isolated syndrome
	ADEM
	Neuromyelitis optica
Vasculitis/inflammatory diseases	
	Primary CNS angiitis
	Systemic lupus erythematosus
	Sjögren syndrome
	Behcet disease

	Neurosarcoidosis
Cerebrovascular disorders	
İnfection	
	Neurborreliosis
	Tuberculosis
	Viral encephalitis
	HIV
	Progressive multifocal leukoencephalopathy (PML)
Neurometabolic/genetic disorders	
	Mitochondrial diseases
	Leukodystrophies
Neoplasm	
	CNS lymphoma
	Other CNS tumors

Table 1. Differential diagnosis of pediatric MS.

10. Treatment

10.1. Treatment of the acute demyelinating attack

A mildly acute demyelinating attack that does not impair the patient's functions may not require treatment. The first option in the treatment of an acute demyelinating attack is a high-dose intravenous corticosteroid. Corticosteroids increase the speed of recovery and reduce the number of gadolinium-enhancing lesions on an MRI. The presumed mechanisms of action are modification of cytokine responses, reduction in T cell activation, and reduction in blood-brain barrier permeability. Intravenous corticosteroid is administered as 20–30 mg/kg (up to 1 g/day) methyl prednisolone over 3–5 days in children. There is no consensus on tapering oral corticosteroid. Oral prednisone may be administered to patients with incomplete recovery after intravenous treatment. Plasma exchange can be considered for patients with severe, life-threatening attacks or patients who were unresponsive to intravenous steroid treatment. The typical course is 5–7 exchanges over the course of 10–14 days. Plasma exchange therapy is an invasive treatment; its side effects include infection, blood clotting issues, and electrolyte disturbances. Another option is intravenous immunoglobulin (IVIG) if the steroids are contraindicated or the response is inadequate. There have been no controlled studies for the efficiency of this treatment in pediatric MS. IVIG influences cytokine production, T cell proliferation, and autoantibodies against myelin. It is given at a dose of 2 g/kg over 2–5 days. Side effects include fever, headache, aseptic meningitis, thromboembolism, and allergic reactions. Severe allergic reactions may develop in people with IgA deficiency; therefore, serum IgA levels should be examined before treatment [42, 43].

10.2. Disease-modifying therapy

The aims of treatment are to reduce disease activity, prevent disability, and preserve cognitive functions. Therefore, it is recommended to start treatment at an early stage.

First-line disease-modifying therapy includes interferon beta and glatiramer acetate. These drugs are used in adults for 15–20 years. Their efficacy, side effects, and safety are well known in adults. Both interferon beta and glatiramer acetate reduce relapse rates by approximately 30% and the accrual of new lesions on the MRI. There have been no randomized controlled trials in pediatric patients.

Glatiramer acetate is a synthetic amino acid polymer that resembles myelin basic protein. Its mechanism is not clear. It modulates T cells, shifts the population of T cells from proinflammatory Th1 cells to regulatory Th2 cells, and reduces antigen presentation. Standard dosage is 20 mg daily by subcutaneous injection. Its side effects include injection reactions, lipoatrophy at injection sites, chest pain, and a post-injection reaction (anxiety, flushing, palpitations, dyspnea, and chest pain) [42–44].

Interferon beta inhibits autoreactive T cells, increases production of anti-inflammatory cytokines, reduces proinflammatory cytokines, and decreases the migration of inflammatory cells into CNS. There are two subgroups: interferon beta 1a and 1b. Interferon beta 1a is given three times a week at a dose 22 or 44 μg via subcutaneous injection or intramuscularly at a dose of 30 μg a week. A pegylated form of interferon beta 1a is used in adults, but the safety and efficacy of this form in children and adolescents have not been established. The standard dose of interferon beta-1b is 0.25 mg (8 MIU), injected subcutaneously every other day. Dose titration is recommended at the start of treatment for interferons. Most pediatric patients tolerate the adult dose. The most frequent side effects are flu-like symptoms, injection site reaction, transient transaminase elevation, bone marrow suppression, thyroid dysfunction, and depression. Paracetamol and ibuprofen are effective in managing the flu-like symptoms. Liver transaminases, blood counts, and a thyroid function test should be carried out following the treatment.

The aim of disease-modifying therapy is to reduce clinical and radiological disease activity. Disease activity is defined as clinical relapses, new or enlarging lesions on an MRI, or gadolinium-enhancing lesions on an MRI. When the first-line disease-modifying therapy remains insufficient to reduce disease activity, second-line therapies can be used. The second-line therapies that have been used in pediatric MS include natalizumab, rituximab, and cyclophosphamide [42–44].

Natalizumab is a humanized monoclonal antibody. Natalizumab selectively binds to the 4-integrin component of adhesion molecules found in lymphocytes, monocytes, eosinophils and inhibits the $\alpha 4$-mediated adhesion of leukocytes to their counter-receptors. It decreases clinical relapse rate by about 70% and reduces the accumulation of new or enlarging T2 hyperintense lesions. Natalizumab is given at a dose of 300 mg intravenously every 4 weeks. Its side effects include hypersensitivity and headaches. The most serious risk is progressive multifocal leukoencephalopathy (PML) in adults. This fatal risk is higher in patients who have been exposed to the JC virus and have been treated with immunosuppressive drugs previously.

There is also a relationship between the duration of natalizumab therapy and an increased risk. There have been no controlled, randomized trials in pediatric MS to date.

Rituximab is a monoclonal antibody. It selectively depletes CD20+ B lymphocytes. There have been no controlled, randomized trials. Salzer et al. suggested that rituximab treatment is safe, effective, and well tolerated in their case series with pediatric MS [45].

Trials on the safety and efficacy of new oral therapies including fingolimod, dimethyl fumarate, and teriflunamide in pediatric MS patients have not been finalized.

10.3. Symptomatic treatment

Spasticity, fatigue, tremor, neuropathic pain, paroxysmal symptoms, epileptic seizures, bladder dysfunctions, and depression can be persistent symptoms in MS and affect patient's quality of life. Medical drugs can be effective in the treatment of these symptoms as in adult patients.

Baclofen, tizanidine, and benzodiazepines are effective for spasticity. Amantadine, modafinil, methylphenidate can be used for fatigue. Antiepileptic drugs such as carbamazepine, gabapentine are effective for both paroxysmal symptoms and neuropathic pain [42]. Anticholinergic agents (oxybutynin, tolterodine) can be used for detrusor hyperreflexia, and desmopressin may be beneficial for nocturia.

10.4. Rehabilitation

The aim of MS rehabilitation is to reduce symptoms including spasticity, gait disturbances, imbalance, bladder-bowel dysfunction, speech and swallowing disorders, fatigue, pain and improve quality of life. Rehabilitation interventions for MS symptoms include methods such as exercise (stretching/strengthening), gait training, endurance training, aerobic training, hydrotherapy, physiotherapy, exercise-pelvic floor training, occupational therapy, psychological training [46]. Rehabilitation interventions should be selected according to patient's characteristics such as age and functional deficits.

Cognitive rehabilitation is an important part of MS rehabilitation, but there is no specific cognitive rehabilitation intervention for pediatric MS. Rehabilitative strategies include rehabilitation of attention and language based on other disease such as trauma, stroke, and tumor [47].

11. Conclusion

Two to 5% of all MS patients have their first attack during childhood or adolescence. Pediatric MS has different clinical features from adult-onset MS, particularly in very young children. ADEM can occur as first attack in children, especially those under 10 years of age. The relapse rate in pediatric MS is higher than in adult MS, but recovery from relapse is better than in adults. However, the onset of secondary progression occurs at a younger age as compared

http://dx.doi.org/10.5772/63919

with adult-onset MS. The primary progressive form of MS is extremely rare in pediatric patients. Primary progressive course should suggest other diagnoses in children. Cognitive impairment is one of the most important causes of disability and has different characteristics from adults. Linguistic dysfunction and decrease in IQ scores can occur during the first year of disease. Despite all these differences from adult MS, the therapeutic approach is based on information in adult MS. There are no randomized controlled trials on efficacy and safety of immunomodulatory and immunosuppressive drugs. Studies on pathogenesis are also limited in pediatric MS. One of the most important differences in the pathogenesis of pediatric-onset and adult-onset MS is the presence of anti-MOG antibodies in children. More studies on pathogenesis will provide insight into clinical differences and the development of more safe and effective treatment.

Author details

Ozgul Ekmekci

Address all correspondence to: ozgul.ekmekci@ege.edu.tr

Ege University, Faculty of Medicine, Department of Neurology, Izmir, Turkey

References

[1] Duquette P, Murray TJ, Pleines J, et al.: Multiple sclerosis in childhood: clinical profile in 125 patients. J Pediatr. 1987;111:359–363. DOI: 10.1016/S0022-3476(87)80454-7.

[2] Ghezzi A, Deplano V, Faroni J, et al.: Multiple sclerosis in childhood: clinical features of 149 cases. Mult Scler. 1997;3:43–46. DOI: 10.1177/135245859700300105.

[3] Bigi S, Banwell B: Pediatric multiple sclerosis. J Child Neurol. 2012;27(11):1378–1383. DOI: 10.1177/0883073812452784

[4] Gadoth N: Multiple sclerosis in children. Brain Dev. 2003;25:229. DOI: 10.1016/S0387-7604(03)00035-4.

[5] Banwell B, Ghezzi A, Bar-Or A, Mikaeloff Y, Tardieu M: Multiple sclerosis in children: clinical diagnosis, therapeutic strategies, and future directions. Lancet Neurol. 2007;6:887–902. DOI: 10.1016/S1474-4422(07)70242-9.

[6] Mowry EM, Krupp LB, Milazzo M, et al.: Vitamin D status is associated with relapse rate in pediatric onset multiple sclerosis. Ann Neurol. 2010;67(5):618–624. DOI: 10.1002/ana.21972.

[7] Mikaeloff Y, Cardidade C, Tardieu M, Suissa S: Parental smoking at home and risk of childhood onset multiple sclerosis in children. Brain. 2007;130:2589–2595. DOI: 10.1093/brain/awm198.

[8] Ascherio A, Munger KI: Environmental risk factors for multiple sclerosis: part 1: the role of infection. Ann Neurol. 2007;61(4):288–289. DOI: 10.1002/ana.21117.

[9] Langer-Loud A, Brara SM, Beaber BE, et al.: Childhood obesity and risk of pediatric multiple sclerosis and clinically isolated syndrome. Neurology. 2013;80(6):548–552. DOI: 10.1212/WNL.0b013e31828154f3.

[10] Vargas-Lowy D, Chitnis T: Pathogenesis of pediatric multiple sclerosis. J Child Neurol. 2012;27(11):1394–1407. DOI: 10.1177/0883073812456084.

[11] Chitnis T: The role of CD4 T cells in the pathogenesis of multiple sclerosis. Int Rev Neurobiol. 2007;79:43–72. DOI: 10.1016/S0074-7742(07)79003-7.

[12] Ciccarelli O, Barkhof F, Bodini B, et al.: Pathogenesis of multiple sclerosis: insights from molecular and metabolic imaging. Lancet Neurol. 2014;13:807–822. DOI: 10.1016/S1474-4422(14)70101-2.

[13] Stromnes IM, Cerretti LM, Liggitt D, et al.: Differential regulation of central nervous system autoimmunity by TH1 and TH17 cells. Nat Med. 2008;14:337–342. DOI: 10.1038/nm1715.

[14] Lock C, Hermans G, Pedotti R, et al.: Gene-microarray analysis of multiple sclerosis lesions yields new targets validated in autoimmune encephalomyelitis. Nat Med. 2002;8:500–508. DOI: 10.1038/nm0502-500.

[15] Graber JJ, Allie SR, Mullen KM, et al.: Interleukin-17 in transverse myelitis and multiple sclerosis. J Neuroimmunol. 2008;196:124–132. DOI: 10.1016/j.jneuroim.2008.02.008.

[16] Correale J, Tenembaum SN: Myelin basic protein and myelin oligodendrocyte glycoprotein T-cell repertoire in childhood and juvenile multiple sclerosis. Mult Scler. 2006;12:412–420. DOI: 10.1191/135248506ms1282oa.

[17] Fernandez-Carbonell C, Vargas-Lowy D, Musallam A, et al.: Clinical and MRI phenotype of children with MOG antibodies. Mult Scler J. 2016;22(2):174–184. DOI: 10.1177/1352458515587751.

[18] Kitley J, Woodhall M, Waters P, et al.: Myelinoligodendrocyte glycoprotein antibodies in adults with a neuromyelitis optica phenotype. Neurology. 2012;79:1273–1277. DOI: 10.1212/WNL.0b013e31826aac4e.

[19] Chitnis T, Imitola J, Khoury SJ.: Therapeutic strategies to prevent neurodegeneration and promote regeneration in multiple sclerosis. Curr Drug Targets Immune Endocr Metabol Disord. 2005;5:11–26.

[20] Lucchinetti C, Bruck W, Parisi J, et al.: Heterogeneity of multiple sclerosis lesions: implications for the pathogenesis of demyelination. Ann Neurol. 2000;47:707–717.

[21] Trapp BD, Peterson J, Ransohoff RM, et al.: Axonal transection in the lesions of multiple sclerosis. N Engl J Med. 1998;338:278–285. DOI: 10.1056/NEJM199801293380502.

[22] Kutzelnigg A, Lucchinetti CF, Stadelmann C, et al.: Cortical demyelination and diffuse white matter injury in multiple sclerosis. Brain. 2005;128(pt 11):2705–2712. DOI: 10.1093/brain/awh641.

[23] Kutzelnigg A, Faber-Rod JC, Bauer J, et al.: Widespread demyelination in the cerebellar cortex in multiple sclerosis. Brain Pathol. 2007;17:38–44. DOI: 10.1111/j.1750-3639.2006.00041.x.

[24] McAdam LC, Blaser SI, Banwell BL.: Pediatric tumefactive demyelination: case series and review of the literature. Pediatr Neurol. 2002;26:18–25. DOI: 10.1016/S0887-8994(01)00322-8.

[25] Lucchinetti CF, Gavrilova RH, Metz I.: Clinical and radiographic spectrum of pathologically confirmed tumefactive multiple sclerosis. Brain. 2008;131(7):1759–1775. DOI: 10.1093/brain/awn098.

[26] Krupp LB, Banwell B, Tenenbaum S: Consensus definitions proposed for pediatric multiple sclerosis and related disorders. Neurology. 2007;68:S7–S12. DOI: 10.1212/01.wnl.0000259422.44235.a8.

[27] Polman CH, Reingold SC, Banwell B, et al.: Diagnostic criteria for multiple sclerosis: 2010 revisions to the McDonald criteria. Ann Neurol. 2011;69:292–302. DOI: 10.1002/ana.22366.

[28] Krupp LB, Tardieu M, Amato MP et al.: International Pediatric Multiple Sclerosis Study Group criteria for pediatric multiple sclerosis and immune-mediated central nervous system demyelinating disorders: revisions to the 2007 definitions. Mult Scler. 2013;19(10):1261–1267. DOI: 10.1177/1352458513484547.

[29] Narula S: New perspectives in pediatric neurology-multiple sclerosis. Curr Probl Pediatr Adolesc Health Care. 2016:46(2):62–69. DOI: 10.1016/j.cppeds.2015.11.002.

[30] Pena JA, Lotze TE: Pediatric multiple sclerosis: current concepts and consensus definitions. Autoimmune Dis. 2013:2013, Article ID 673947:12 p. DOI: 10.1155/2013/673947.

[31] Huppke B, Ellenberger D, Rosewich H, Friede T, Gartner J, Huppke P: Clinical presentation of pediatric multiple sclerosis before puberty. Eur J Neurol. 2014;21(3): 441–446. DOI: 10.1111/ene.12327.

[32] Cardoso M, Olmo NR, Fragoso YD: Systematic review of cognitive dysfunction in pediatric and juvenile multiple sclerosis. Pediatr Neurol. 2015;53:287–292. DOI: 10.1016/j.pediatrneurol.2015.06.007.

[33] Suppiej A, Cainelli E: Cognitive dysfunction in pediatric multiple sclerosis. Neuropsychiatr Dis Treat. 2014;10:1385–1392. DOI: 10.2147/NDT.S48495.

[34] Simon JH, Li D, Traboulsee A, et al.: Standardized MR imaging protocol for multiple sclerosis: consortium of MS centers consensus guidelines. Am J Neuroradiol. 2006;27:455–461.

[35] Sadaka Y, Verhey LH, Shroff MM, et al.: 2010 McDonald criteria for diagnosing pediatric multiple sclerosis. Ann Neurol. 2012;72(2):211–223. DOI: 10.1002/ana.23575.

[36] Waubant E, Chabas D, Okuda T, et al.: Difference in disease burden and activity in pediatric patients on brain magnetic resonance imaging at time of multiple sclerosis onset vs adults. Arch Neurol. 2009;66(8):967–971. DOI: 10.1001/archneurol.2009.135.

[37] Ghezzi A, Pozzilli C, Liguori M, et al.: Prospective study of multiple sclerosis with early onset. Mult Scler. 2002;8(2):115–118. DOI: 10.1191/1352458502ms786oa.

[38] Pohl D, Rostasy K, Reiber H, Hanefeld F: CSF characteristics in early-onset multiple sclerosis. Neurology. 2004;63(10):1966–1967. DOI: 10.1212/01.WNL.0000144352.67102.BC.

[39] Pohl D, Rostasy K, Treiber H et al.: Pediatric multiple sclerosis: detection of clinically silent lesions by multimodal evoked potentials. J Pediatr. 2006;149:125–127. DOI: 10.1016/j.jpeds.2006.01.003.

[40] Mikaeloff Y, Suissa S, Vallée L, Lubetzki C, et al.: First episode of acute CNS inflammatory demyelination in childhood: prognostic factors for multiple sclerosis and disability. J Pediatr. 2004;144(2):246–252. DOI:10.1016/j.jpeds.2003.10.056.

[41] Banwell B, Tenenbaum S, Lennon VA, et al.: Neuromyelitis optica-IgG in childhood inflammatory demyelinating CNS disorders. Neurology. 2008;70(5):344–352. DOI: 10.1212/01.wnl.0000284600.80782.d5.

[42] Narula S, Hopkins SE, Banwell B: Treatment of pediatric multiple sclerosis. Curr Treat Options Neurol. 2015;17:10. DOI: 10.1007/s11940-014-0336-z.

[43] Bernton JN, Banwell BL. Therapeutic approach to the management of pediatric demyelinating disease: multiple sclerosis and acute disseminated encephalomyelitis. Neurotherapeutics. 2016;13:84–95. DOI: 10.1007/s13311-015-0396-0.

[44] Kornek B. Treatment of pediatric multiple sclerosis. Neuropediatrics. 2013;44(06):309–313. DOI: 10.1055/s-0033-1359308.

[45] Salzer J, Lycke J, Wickstrom R, Naver H: Rituximab in paediatric onset multiple sclerosis: a case series. J Neurol. 2016;263(2):322–326. DOI: 10.1007/s00415-015-7979-x.

[46] Beer S, Khan F, Kesselring J. Rehabilitation interventions in multiple sclerosis: an overview. J Neurol. 2012;259(9):1994–2008. DOI: 10.1007/s00415-012-6577-4.

[47] Portaccio E, Goretti B, Zipoli V, et al.Cognitive rehabilitation in children and adolescents with multiple sclerosis. Neurol Sci. 2010;31(Suppl 2):S275–S278. DOI: 10.1007/s10072-010-0377-3.

Chapter 7

Association Between Multiple Sclerosis Risk and Human Immunodeficiency Virus Infection: Insights and Challenges

Ehtishamul Haq, Insha Zahoor and
Mushfiquddin Khan

Additional information is available at the end of the chapter

http://dx.doi.org/10.5772/63828

Abstract

Multiple sclerosis (MS) is a convoluted autoimmune and inflammatory disease of the central nervous system (CNS) in which the protective myelin sheath is eroded and the underlying nerve fibers are damaged. There is no conclusive knowledge on the role played by different etiological factors in its development, and studies have shown that it primarily results due to complex interactions between the genetic, geographic and infectious components. Among the risk factors reported to have a possible role in MS development, retroviruses also appear to influence it. Studies suggest human immunodeficiency virus (HIV) infection to be inversely related to MS risk, but to date, the association between the two remains enigmatic. This protective inverse association has become an area of active research and the most plausible explanations for this may be immune suppression and/or antiretroviral medications. The purpose of writing this chapter is to provide background information on the unfathomable relationship between HIV infection and the risk of developing MS while at the same time providing description of the insights garnered from recent studies. While highlighting the application of ART (antiretroviral therapy) as budding future alternative for MS management, this chapter provides momentum for further studies.

Keywords: multiple sclerosis, etiology, human immunodeficiency virus, epidemiology, ART

1. Introduction

Multiple sclerosis (MS) is a complex, debilitating neurologic disease characterized by demyelination of axons in the brain and spinal cord and caused by an immune attack against the myelin sheath. The disease is highly prevalent in North America and Europe (>100/100,000 inhabitants). According to the recently revised 2013 Atlas of MS published by the World Health Organization (WHO) and Multiple Sclerosis International Federation (MSIF) (http://www.atlasofms.org), the prevalence rate of 5–20 per 100,000 has been reported for India. Clinically, MS is characterized by a broad spectrum of symptoms [1]. It has autoimmune and inflammatory components, with intense effects on the communication between nerve cells within the brain and spinal cord [1]. The different types of MS vary in terms of severity, prevalence, and degree of progression [2, 3]. The most common phenotype is relapsing remitting (RR) MS, followed by secondary progressive (SP) and then primary progressive (PP). Less prevalent phenotypes have also been reported [2]. MS pathology is characterized by inflammatory plaques caused by demyelination of axons in the central nervous system (CNS). Due to the presence of immune-inflammatory characteristics in MS, treatments targeting T lymphocyte and natural killer (NK) cell activation seem to play a significant role [4].

With intangible and enigmatic etiology having both genetic and environmental backgrounds, MS offers a profound conundrum. Yet, despite incomplete understanding of the basic mechanisms behind its pathogenesis, a growing body of evidence suggests heterogeneous etiology of MS with multiple environmental factors contributing to its development [5–7]. Various studies suggest that intricate interactions between genetic factors and environmental factors elicit it; thus, genetically susceptible individuals who encounter a number of environmental and epigenetic factors are at higher risk (**Figure 1**) [8, 9].

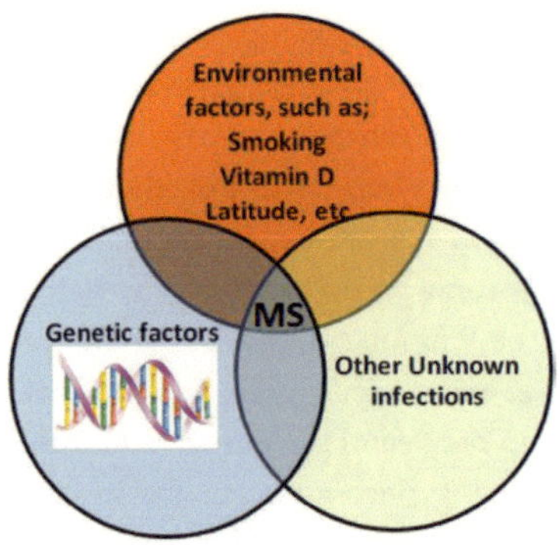

Figure 1. Multiple sclerosis as a complex neurological condition affecting CNS: The etiology of MS is unknown and enigmatic; however, it has a profound role of numerous environmental and genetic components, and multiplex interactions between them lead to its development, thus making it a multifactorial and polygenic heterogeneous disease.

Some risk factors, which have been studied in various populations, include geographic location [10, 11], wheat consumption [11, 12], dairy product consumption [13, 14], fish intake [15], animal fat intake [15], high ultraviolet radiation [16–18], vitamin D deficiency [19], and viral infection [20–22]. The likely association between genetic and infectious components in MS development is shown by the human endogenous retroviruses (HERVs) [23, 24]. Although many viruses have raised suspicions as responsible for MS, not all studies confirm their etiologic role. Thus, each virus has chalked up another obstruction in the MS conundrum. There is escalating evidence suggesting a retroviral connection to MS risk, and the most noteworthy among them is human immunodeficiency virus (HIV). Studies suggest HIV infection to be inversely related to MS risk [25–27] but, to date, the association between the two remains enigmatic [28]. The purpose of this chapter is to provide an overview of the insights garnered from recent studies on the association between HIV and MS risk. While highlighting this association, the main objective of this chapter is to provide an impetus for future studies aimed at precisely establishing the mechanism behind the impact of HIV on MS.

2. Link between HIV and MS risk

The epidemiology of MS shows a latitudinal gradient, and its risk is governed by genetic predisposition as well as local environmental conditions (**Figure 1**). Even though its etiology remains uncertain, quite a few studies have suggested involvement of a virus in its pathogenesis. For example, the association between genetic and infectious components in MS development is suggested by the HERV, which constitutes about 8–30% of the human genome with approximately 98,000 elements [29]. Until 2005, however, no HERVs capable of replication had been identified, only traces of original viruses were identified [30]. were identified. Only one family of HERV viruses has been active, the HERV-K family, comprising <1% of total HERV elements [29, 30]. This family is a candidate for playing a fundamental role in MS pathophysiology. Evidence for this role includes studies that have shown activation of T-cell response against HERV in individuals infected with HIV [31]. This has formed the much needed ground for alternative drug therapy targeted against HERV for elimination of HIV, and it might therefore aid in using HERV proteins as markers for drug designing instead of frequently mutating HIV antigens. One of the HERV proteins reported to be expressed in the active lesions of MS is the MS-associated retrovirus envelope protein (MSRV-Env) [32–34]. There is accumulating evidence suggesting an inverse association between HIV and MS, and large-scale epidemiological studies have supported this notion. Studies have found significantly lower prevalence of MS in people with HIV infection [26]; moreover, there has been only a single case report of MS treatment with antiretroviral drugs in an HIV patient.

With the help of population-based databases, a recent study demonstrated reduced incidence of MS in HIV patients; however, due to a smaller sample size, it proved statistically insignificant [26]. Gold et al. [25] investigated a much larger sample and revealed a statistically significant negative relationship between HIV and MS, reflecting a protective effect of HIV on MS. Still unclear is the exact mechanism behind this association. The protection HIV provides against MS may be mediated by suppression of the immune system due to chronic HIV infection and antiretroviral medications, thus preventing MS progression or treating it completely (**Figure 2**). To date, it is not known whether HIV *per se*, application of antiretroviral therapy (ART), or a combination of the two diminishes MS symptoms. The most plausible explanation for this protective effect may be HIV-induced immunodeficiency targeting a wide continuum of immune cells and signal transduction pathways involved in MS pathogenesis. Alternatively, antiretroviral medications used against HIV may target other viruses involved in MS pathogenesis such as, HERV and herpes.

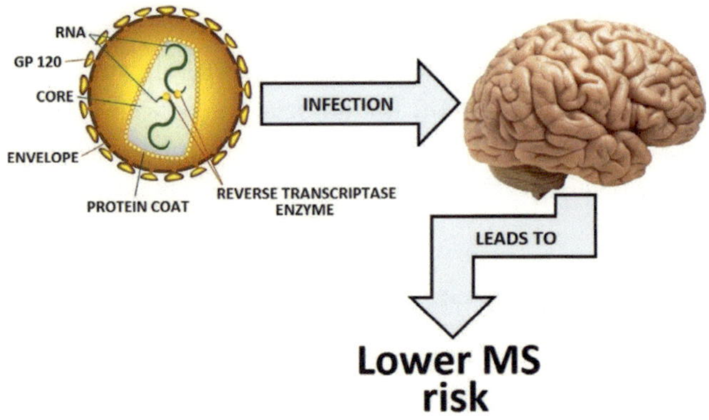

Figure 2. Protective inverse relationship between MS and HIV: HIV infection leads to reduced MS risk, which may be attributed to constant suppression of the immune system by HIV-induced immunodeficiency targeting diverse spectrum of immune cells and signal transduction pathways involved in MS pathogenesis, and/or antiretroviral drugs used to treat the infection, thus preventing MS progression or treating it completely.

The big puzzle of whether and when to start HIV therapy in MS patients remains blurred. Previous studies based on case report and data linkage studies presumed that protective infection was conferred against MS development due to ART treatment rather than HIV infection *per se*. However, in neither case has systematic description been offered about the individuals who were treated with ART and those who were not [27]. There are still different opinions on early [35] and late treatment options due to different aspects such as side effects and drug resistance [36]. Therefore, no clear-cut approach exists on starting ART. In these studies, nothing has been mentioned about exposure to antiretroviral medications and its duration [27]. Moreover, HIV and MS are often misdiagnosed due to the presence of MS-like symptoms in HIV; therefore, focus should be on targeted treatments of MS patients with HIV and vice versa. To fully understand the mechanism behind the apparently MS-protective phenotype of HIV infection, the most plausible research approach would be analysis of data on HIV patients with MS or vice versa and the details on influence of cotreatment with antiretroviral medications and disease-modifying treatments (DMTs).

Due to the presence of immune-inflammatory characteristics in MS, treatments targeting T lymphocyte activation may play a significant role. There is growing evidence that favors suppression of MS pathology by employing anti-HIV therapy, and it has prompted one trial in MS patients for the drug Raltegravir (Isentress) [37] used in HIV treatment and also an immunoglobulin G4 monoclonal antibody called GNbAC1 [4, 38–40] against HERV proteins. The association between HIV and MS can be exploited to replace conventional treatment options for MS by formulating new safe, effective, and long-term therapeutic alternatives. Further investigations are mandatory to provide a deeper insight into the mechanism of action

http://dx.doi.org/10.5772/63828

for HIV/ART on MS risk, and this can be fulfilled by carrying out large-scale clinical, molecular, as well as epidemiological studies.

3. Conclusion

Despite the extensive research on MS, its exact etiology remains hard to pin down. Nevertheless, epidemiological findings across the globe suggest its association with specific retroviruses endogenous to humans. Regardless of the paucity of reports on HIV and MS association, this finding appears to be crucial in the etiology of MS. A comprehensive understanding of this link is needed to elucidate the complex interactions between HIV and MS and also to exploit HIV's protective role in order to develop treatments for MS. Research that unscrambles the relation between the two would, at the same time, provide new insights into the etiopathogenesis of MS and provide therapeutic targets and strategies.

Nevertheless, additional studies on mechanisms of interaction between HIV and MS are required to determine the underlying mediators of this protective association and eventually endow insight into the disease pathogenesis as well as its management. To date, the studies in this milieu hitherto are insufficient, and there is extreme need for an extensive upsurge in large-scale conclusive molecular and epidemiological studies. It is noteworthy that this chapter further enlightens the acuity of an association between HIV (or its treatment) and a reduced risk of developing MS; however, it is flagrant that this association needs to be examined skeptically in order to gain deeper insight into this enigmatic relationship. The need of hour is to establish precisely whether having HIV, being treated for HIV with antiretroviral drugs, or a combination of the two reduces the risk of developing MS, which will certainly open the door for developing better and more promising treatment options for MS.

Acknowledgements

We express our heartfelt gratitude to the Department of Science and Technology (DST), Govt. of India, New Delhi, for providing grants to Insha Zahoor (Principal Investigator), under Women Scientist Scheme-A (WOS-A) project on Multiple Sclerosis.

Author details

Ehtishamul Haq[1*], Insha Zahoor[1] and Mushfiquddin Khan[2]

*Address all correspondence to: haq@kashmiruniversity.ac.in

1 Department of Biotechnology, University of Kashmir, Srinagar, India

2 Department of Pediatrics, Medical University of South Carolina, Charleston, SC, USA

References

[1] Compston A, Coles A. Multiple sclerosis. Lancet 2008;372:1502–17.

[2] Confavreux C, Vukusic S, Adeleine P. Early clinical predictors and progression of irreversible disability in multiple sclerosis: an amnesic process. Brain: A Journal of Neurology 2003;126:770–82.

[3] Pugliatti M, Rosati G, Carton H, Riise T, Drulovic J, Vecsei L, et al. The epidemiology of multiple sclerosis in Europe. European Journal of Neurology 2006;13:700–22.

[4] Curtin F, Perron H, Faucard R, Porchet H, Lang AB. Treatment against human endogenous retrovirus: a possible personalized medicine approach for multiple sclerosis. Molecular Diagnosis & Therapy 2015;19:255–65.

[5] Ascherio A, Munger KL. Environmental risk factors for multiple sclerosis. Part I: the role of infection. Annals of Neurology 2007;61:288–99.

[6] Handunnetthi L, Ramagopalan SV, Ebers GC. Multiple sclerosis, vitamin D, and HLA-DRB1*15. Neurology 2010;74:1905–10.

[7] Ramagopalan SV, Dobson R, Meier UC, Giovannoni G. Multiple sclerosis: risk factors, prodromes, and potential causal pathways. The Lancet Neurology 2010;9:727–39.

[8] Ebers GC. Genetics and multiple sclerosis: an overview. Annals of Neurology 1994;36(Suppl):S12–4.

[9] Ebers GC, Sadovnick AD, Risch NJ. A genetic basis for familial aggregation in multiple sclerosis. Canadian Collaborative Study Group. Nature 1995;377:150–1.

[10] Poser CM. The epidemiology of multiple sclerosis: a general overview. Annals of Neurology 1994;36(Suppl 2):S180–93.

[11] Shatin R. Multiple sclerosis and geography. New interpretation of epidemiological observations. Neurology 1964;14:338–44.

[12] Alter M, Yamoor M, Harshe M. Multiple sclerosis and nutrition. Archives of Neurology 1974;31:267–72.

[13] Agranoff BW, Goldberg D. Diet and the geographical distribution of multiple sclerosis. Lancet 1974;2:1061–6.

[14] Malosse D, Perron H, Sasco A, Seigneurin JM. Correlation between milk and dairy product consumption and multiple sclerosis prevalence: a worldwide study. Neuroepidemiology 1992;11:304–12.

[15] Hutter C. On the causes of multiple sclerosis. Medical Hypotheses 1993;41:93–6.

[16] Islam T, Gauderman WJ, Cozen W, Mack TM. Childhood sun exposure influences risk of multiple sclerosis in monozygotic twins. Neurology 2007;69:381–8.

[17] van der Mei IA, Ponsonby AL, Blizzard L, Dwyer T. Regional variation in multiple sclerosis prevalence in Australia and its association with ambient ultraviolet radiation. Neuroepidemiology 2001;20:168–74.

[18] van der Mei IA, Ponsonby AL, Dwyer T, Blizzard L, Simmons R, Taylor BV, et al. Past exposure to sun, skin phenotype, and risk of multiple sclerosis: case-control study. BMJ 2003;327:316.

[19] Hayes CE. Vitamin D: a natural inhibitor of multiple sclerosis. The Proceedings of the Nutrition Society 2000;59:531–5.

[20] Cook SD, Dowling PC. Multiple sclerosis and viruses: an overview. Neurology 1980;30:80–91.

[21] Handel AE, Williamson AJ, Disanto G, Handunnetthi L, Giovannoni G, Ramagopalan SV. An Updated Meta-Analysis of Risk of Multiple Sclerosis following Infectious Mononucleosis. PLoS ONE 2010; 5(9): e12496.

[22] Alter M, Zhang ZX, Davanipour Z, Sobel E, Zibulewski J, Schwartz G, et al. Multiple sclerosis and childhood infections. Neurology 1986;36:1386–9.

[23] Blond JL, Beseme F, Duret L, Bouton O, Bedin F, Perron H, et al. Molecular characterization and placental expression of HERV-W, a new human endogenous retrovirus family. Journal of Virology 1999;73:1175–85.

[24] Perron H, Geny C, Laurent A, Mouriquand C, Pellat J, Perret J, et al. Leptomeningeal cell line from multiple sclerosis with reverse transcriptase activity and viral particles. Research in Virology 1989;140:551–61.

[25] Gold J, Goldacre R, Maruszak H, Giovannoni G, Yeates D, Goldacre M. HIV and lower risk of multiple sclerosis: beginning to unravel a mystery using a record-linked database study. Journal of Neurology, Neurosurgery, and Psychiatry 2015;86:9–12.

[26] Nexo BA, Pedersen L, Sorensen HT, Koch-Henriksen N. Treatment of HIV and risk of multiple sclerosis. Epidemiology 2013;24:331–2.

[27] van der Kop ML. Does antiretroviral therapy for HIV reduce the risk of developing multiple sclerosis? Journal of Neurology, Neurosurgery, and Psychiatry 2015;86:3.

[28] Khan M, Zahoor I, Haq E. Human immunodeficiency virus and multiple sclerosis risk: probing for a connection. Journal of Multiple Sclerosis 2015;2:100141.

[29] Belshaw R, Pereira V, Katzourakis A, Talbot G, Paces J, Burt A, et al. Long-term reinfection of the human genome by endogenous retroviruses. Proceedings of the National Academy of Sciences of the United States of America 2004;101:4894–9.

[30] Nelson PN, Hooley P, Roden D, Davari Ejtehadi H, Rylance P, Warren P, et al. Human endogenous retroviruses: transposable elements with potential? Clinical and Experimental Immunology 2004;138:1–9.

[31] Garrison KE, Jones RB, Meiklejohn DA, Anwar N, Ndhlovu LC, Chapman JM, et al. T cell responses to human endogenous retroviruses in HIV-1 infection. Plos Pathogens 2007;3:e165.

[32] Antony JM, van Marle G, Opii W, Butterfield DA, Mallet F, Yong VW, et al. Human endogenous retrovirus glycoprotein-mediated induction of redox reactants causes oligodendrocyte death and demyelination. Nature Neuroscience 2004;7:1088–95.

[33] Perron H, Germi R, Bernard C, Garcia-Montojo M, Deluen C, Farinelli L, et al. Human endogenous retrovirus type W envelope expression in blood and brain cells provides new insights into multiple sclerosis disease. Multiple Sclerosis 2012;18:1721–36.

[34] Perron H, Lazarini F, Ruprecht K, Pechoux-Longin C, Seilhean D, Sazdovitch V, et al. Human endogenous retrovirus (HERV)-W ENV and GAG proteins: physiological expression in human brain and pathophysiological modulation in multiple sclerosis lesions. Journal of Neurovirology 2005;11:23–33.

[35] Ho DD. Time to hit HIV, early and hard. The New England Journal of Medicine 1995;333:450–1.

[36] Harrington M, Carpenter CC. Hit HIV-1 hard, but only when necessary. Lancet 2000;355:2147–52.

[37] G G RI. Pilot Study in Relapsing Multiple Sclerosis (INSPIRE). ClinicalTrialsGov registration number: NCT0176770.

[38] Curtin F, Perron H, Kromminga A, Porchet H, Lang AB. Preclinical and early clinical development of GNbAC1, a humanized IgG4 monoclonal antibody targeting endogenous retroviral MSRV-Env protein. MAbs 2015;7:265–75.

[39] Kremer D, Forster M, Schichel T, Gottle P, Hartung HP, Perron H, et al. The neutralizing antibody GNbAC1 abrogates HERV-W envelope protein-mediated oligodendroglial maturation blockade. Multiple Sclerosis 2015;21:1200–3.

[40] Derfuss T, Curtin F, Guebelin C, Bridel C, Rasenack M, Matthey A, et al. A phase IIa randomised clinical study of GNbAC1, a humanised monoclonal antibody against the envelope protein of multiple sclerosis-associated endogenous retrovirus in multiple sclerosis patients. Multiple Sclerosis 2015;21:885–93.

Chapter 8

The Role of Over-Nutrition and Obesity in Multiple Sclerosis

Ema Kantorová, Egon Kurča, Daniel Čierny,
Dušan Dobrota and Štefan Sivák

Additional information is available at the end of the chapter

http://dx.doi.org/10.5772/63992

Abstract

In countries with high standard of living, lowered risk of infectious diseases is parallel to increased incidence of autoimmune diseases. One of the autoimmune disorders, multiple sclerosis, affects genetically susceptible individuals. Genetic susceptibility is supposed to interact with lifestyle and environmental factors in developing autoimmunity in MS. From this point of view, epigenetics provides the bridge between the external environment and the internal genetic system. In MS, environmental burden can modulate gene expression by epigenetic modification of chromatin components, microRNAs or by subtle changes in DNA methylation. Our paper focuses on describing the epigenetic mechanisms linking environmental factors with pathogenesis of multiple sclerosis. We summarise current knowledge about the role of over-nutrition and obesity as epigenetic factors in multiple sclerosis.

Keywords: multiple sclerosis, epigenetics, early life environmental factors, obesity, microRNA, DNA methylation, histone acetylation

1. Introduction

The genomewide association study (GWAS) conducted by International Multiple Sclerosis Genetics Consortium has identified genes conferring susceptibility to multiple sclerosis (MS) [1]. Many of these genes play a role in the immune system with a prominent role for major histocompatibility complex (MHC) class II molecules in particularly defined HLA-DRB1 alleles. GWAS found complete concordance between the rs 3135388A SNP and the HLA-DRB1*1501 genotype [1].

In most cohorts, especially in Caucasian population, genetic burden for MS has been found to be associated with gene clusters in chromosome 6p21.3 [2]. Evident genetic heterogeneity of MS makes identification of single candidate gene impossible. This highlights the role of molecular markers rather than MS-susceptibility genes in indicating the disease status [3]. As the genetic background determines only about 26–30% of the risk of developing MS [4, 5], other factors have been considered to determine heterogeneity of clinical course and MS symptoms [6].

Epigenetics is defined as heritable changes in gene expression that are not due to any alteration in the primary DNA sequence. The changes are responsible for organisation and reading of genetic information [7]. The term epigenetics has evolved to define mechanisms underlying phenotype plasticity due to environmental influences, parent-of-origin effects, gene-dosage control, imprinting, and X-chromosome inactivation. At the molecular level, epigenetics includes modification of DNA base pairs, post-translational modification of histones, and the effects of non-coding RNAs [8]. Moreover, it was found that epigenetic alterations accumulate in time; consequently they can exert their effect on expressed genes longitudinally [9].

Our paper focuses on describing the epigenetic mechanisms linking environmental factors with pathogenesis of multiple sclerosis. We summarise current knowledge about roles of over-nutrition and obesity as epigenetic factors in multiple sclerosis.

1.1. Molecular epigenetic mechanisms

In human DNA, cytosines in the CpG dinucleotide are commonly methylated, and methylation is well-balanced. DNA methylation is involved in normal development and sustaining of cellular homeostasis and functions in adult organisms (particularly for X-chromosome inactivation in females, genomic imprinting, silencing of repetitive DNA elements, regulation of chromatin structure, and control of gene expression). CpG sites are concentrated in short regions of the genome [7, 10, 13]. Another common mechanism that regulates chromatin structure inside a cell involves histone modification. In general, histone acetylation and phosphorylation act as activators of gene expression, whereas histone deacetylation, biotinylation and sumoylation inhibit gene expression [10, 12]. Other described mechanisms of epigenetic regulation of gene function are mediated by miRNAs. They are small non-coding RNAs, 16–29 nucleotides-long, that function primarily as negative gene regulators at the post-transcriptional level. Recently, novel microRNAs (miR) have been identified to be human-specific as well as tissue-specific [7, 11].

Different authors have suggested that epigenetic mechanisms could be directly controlled by metabolic and dietary constituents, metabolic state, or endocrine unbalances [10, 40].

1.2. Early life period and potential epigenetic risks

Recently, studies on humans have indicated that adaptive changes made by foetus in response to intrauterine environment result in permanent changes in early life programming [14–16].

Currently, there are no prospective systematic studies conducted in humans that would evaluate the association of selective environmental factors and risk of MS in humans. However, many environmental factors have been described to be potential epigenetic regulators of MS development [16, 17, 18]. Some of the metabolic and toxic epigenetic factors are listed and included in **Table 1**.

- lower levels of maternal vitamin D and lower exposure to UV light in childhood

- nutritional factors + obesity

- exposure to glucocorticoids, metabolic trigger

- smoking

- epigenetics of endocannabinoid system

- maternal psychosocial stress

Potential epigenetic factor	Mechanism of action	Clinical and immunological consequences	References number
Lower maternal vitamin D Decreased vitamin D in MS patients	blocking of NF for activated T-cells, sequestration of Runt-related TF-1 FokI gene polymorphism (rs10735810) Vitamin-D-mediated trans-repression of the CYP27B1 p450 27B1 gene methylation of CpG sites IL-17 gene expression by blocking of NF, necessary for activating Th-1 cells TF and by HDAC Vitamin-D mediated suppression of IL-12 via HDAC	1,25(OH)2D3 inhibits the production of IFNγ, IL2 and IL12, expansion of dependent Th-1 cells, modification of dendritic cells 58% reduced risk of MS for each 400 IU/day evolution of MS, sex-differences	[19–25]
Lower UV exposure	Similar to vitamin D deficiency	Increase of TNFα and IL-10-impaired antigen-presenting cell function, and antigen -specific Th-cell tolerance, decreased Th-regulatory cells region of birth and low maternal exposure to UV radiation	[26, 27]

Potential epigenetic factor	Mechanism of action	Clinical and immunological consequences	References number
		in the first trimester are independently associated with subsequent risk of MS in offspring	
Higher maternal pre-pregnancy BMI	Oxidative stress, lower vitamin D exposure, over-expression of miR-145,146,155, cluster 17-92 on immune cells Over-expression of Notch1 signalling pathways on oligodendrocytes, impaired neural stem differentiation	No significant relation of weight gain during pregnancy and MS risk when increased pre-pregnancy BMI (OR: 0.39; 0.18–0.85)	[18, 28–31]
Glucocorticoids hyperglycaemia/ diabetes	Reduction of GLUT, dysfunction of cell membrane, impaired DNA methylation of central myelin and genes important in regulating cortisol levels	Blockage of the HPA axis increased risk to MS in offspring	[32–34]
Parental smoking, passive inhalation	Methyl group deficiency, loss of histone H3K9 and H4K20 methylation	24–50% increased risk of MS in women exposed to parental or passive smoking	[18, 30, 31, 35]
Cannabis consumption	Endocannabionoids influence gametogenesis, DNA modulation of reproductive cells, dysregulation of glutamatergic gene expression, findings that would be predictive of impaired synaptic plasticity	Trans-generational effect to next generation, potential modulatory effect to mesolimbic reward-related subregion of the striatum, risk of MS and neurodegenerative disorders	[34, 36]
Lower choline in diet	Impaired DNA methylation of PAD2 promotor, encoding oligodendrocyte activity, developmental type of myelin	Increased inflammatory cytokines: IL-6 and TNFα Increased risk of MS	[37, 38]

http://dx.doi.org/10.5772/63992

Potential epigenetic factor	Mechanism of action	Clinical and immunological consequences	References number
Psychosocial stress in pregnancy, inappropriate maternal immune activation due to stress, maternal separation and obesity	Increased DNA methylation of endocannabionoid receptor-1	Increased IL-6, IL-1, IL-10, increased CD4 and B lymphocytes, decreased Th-regulatory cells, increased permeability of BBB, altered the HPA axis in infants, risk of immune deregulations	[32, 38, 39]

Abbreviations: NF = nuclear factor, TF = transcriptional factor, 1.25(OH)2D3 = 1.25-dihydroxycholecalciferol, FokI = polymorphism of vitamin D receptor, IFNγ = interferon gamma, TNFα = tumour necrosis factor alfa, IL-1,-2,-6,-10,-12,-17 = interleukine 1,-2,-6,-10,-12,-17, Th-1 = autoaggresive T lymphocytes, CYP27B1 p450 27B1 = cytochrome P450 family 27 subfamily B polypeptide 1, CpG = cytosine guanine islands - regions of DNA, HDAC = histone deacetylase, UV = ultraviolet, MS = multiple sclerosis, BMI = body mass index, HPA = hypothalamo-pituitary-adrenal, miR = microRNA, GLUT = glucocorticoid transporters, PAD2 = peptidylarginine deiminase 2, CD4 = Th lymphocytes - helpers, BBB = blood-brain barrier.

Table 1. The list of potential epigenetic risk factors.

1.3. Obesity, nutritional factors and multiple sclerosis

Over the last decade, obesity appears to be a new component of the complex mosaic of autoimmunity [41], suggesting that starvation leads to immunosuppression [42] and that over-nutrition or obesity promotes autoimmunity [8, 41, 43].

Maternal obesity in pre-pregnancy period [measured by body mass index (BMI)], correlated with higher risk of developing MS in children [18], suggests that obesity is a prenatal risk factor. Maternal obesogenic environment is considered to be an epigenetic modulator [40, 43, 44].

Trans-generational epigenetic effects have been supported by nutritional studies that identified a link between food supply during childhood and MS mortality in grandchildren [45, 46]. Although not clearly defined in MS, intergenerational epigenetic effects could explain why the HLA DRB 1*15 frequency is significantly lower in the first-generation affected females, whereas it remains unchanged across the two generations in affected males [46].

Although in one of the retrospective studies, maternal obesity in pre-pregnancy period was associated with risk of MS in children [18], other studies analysed the association of body configuration in adolescence with risk of MS. They found a correlation between higher BMI in adolescence and subsequent development of MS [28, 29, 47], whereas the interaction of obesity and carriage of HLA DRB 1*15 genotype was identified [48]. Munger et al. [28] found that a higher BMI at ages 7–13 years was associated with a significant 1.61–1.95-fold increased risk of MS only among girls. Similarly, another study [49] identified a higher risk of paediatric MS and clinically isolated syndrome (encompassing optic neuritis and transverse myelitis) in extremely obese adolescent girls (BMI ≥ 35 kg/m^2) with an OR = 2.57. In age-adjusted analyses, women with a BMI ≥ 30 kg/m^2 at an age of 18 had a greater than twofold risk of developing MS as compared to women with a BMI between 18.5 and 20.9 kg/m^2. A higher percentage of women who were obese (BMI ≥ 30 kg/m^2) at an age of 18 were smokers at baseline as compared to women with lower BMI [29]. However, body weight at age ≥ 30 was not associated with risk of MS [28], indicating that postnatal life period and adolescence are most important for future development of MS. Other authors did not prove the relationship between obesity and MS in adult patients with ongoing MS symptoms [50, 51]. Moreover, Emamgholipour and colleagues presented a study demonstrating a decreased adipose tissue mass in patients with definite MS compared with healthy individuals (18% MS versus 22.6% in controls) [52]. The negative correlation of MS severity and adipose tissue mass was supposed to result from increased lipolysis and loss of metabolic plasticity.

During over-nutrition, immune cells are increasingly activated and accumulated in adipose tissue, but pro-inflammatory cytokines and chemokines, released from immune cells can also affect other organs [53]. Obesity is associated with accumulation of macrophages, changed from anti-inflammatory M2 to pro-inflammatory M1 phenotype [53]. Obesity selectively promotes an expansion of the Th17 T-cell sub-lineage, producing progressively more IL-17 than lean subjects. IL-6-dependent Th17 expansion is a clinically prominent element in obesity [53]. The results of a small clinical study concurred with the previous investigations. These authors demonstrated stimulation of pro-inflammatory pathways through elevated IL-17 in serum of obese women [54].

Moreover, inflammatory peptides, originated from enlarged adipocytes, have a tendency to change the activity of the HPA axis via hypothalamic receptors [34, 71] and consequently modulate immune responses [58]. Obesity induced by high-fat diet increases blood-brain barrier (BBB) permeability [56] and leads to accumulation of lipids in brain tissue [60, 61], stimulating innate immunity responses. Over-nutrition was correlated with increased number of activated brain microglial cells and oligodendrocytes [61].

MS is one of the autoimmune disorders of the central nervous system (CNS) with not fully known aetiology [6]. Immunological assessments of MS patients have supported the concept of MS as the disorder driven by myelin-specific Th1 helper cells [6], and/or Th17 cells [52]. They were found to migrate into CNS, where they cause demyelination and axonal loss and subsequent neurological disability in MS [6]. Currently, it is known that both innate and adaptive immune processes contribute to MS pathogenesis [42]. Additionally, there is evidence indicating that MS has a neurodegenerative component since neuronal and axonal loss occurs even in the absence of overt inflammation [56]. However, interactions between infiltrating immune cells and resident cells of the CNS require co-stimulatory and additive factors that determine both disease evolution and clinical outcome of MS patients [57]. However, neuro-inflammation cross-talk can have either beneficial or destructive consequences [57], depending on the environmental influences interacting with genetic risks. In MS, environmental exposures might occur long before the disease becomes clinically evident. In addition, the onset of the disease is unknown. Changes in gene expression driven by epigenetic mechanisms play an important role in the predisposition to future disease development [17, 61].

http://dx.doi.org/10.5772/63992

1.4. Epigenetic links between over-nutrition or obesity and multiple sclerosis

1.4.1. Micro RNA

Until today many studies have demonstrated that miR have multiple functions in negative gene 4 regulation and play important roles in neurological disorders, and it seems possible that 5 several epigenetic mechanisms have multiple targets [62].

Interestingly, while obesity increases the expression of the miR-143–145 cluster in adipose tissue/adipocytes via increasing over-expression of tumour necrosis factor alpha (TNFα) secretion and lipolysis [62], recent research has shown miR-145 to be expressed dramatically in peripheral blood mononuclear cells (PBMCs) from patients with MS [63]. Other miR-142-3p, miR-146a, miR-155 and miR-326 were also aberrantly expressed in the PBMCs of MS patients [64].

Obesity-induced over-expression of miR-155, miR-107, and miR-146-5p led to release of pro-inflammatory cytokines, adaptive and innate immune activation [65, 66], while miR-155 and miR-326 were up-regulated in both PBMCs and brain white matter lesions [67].

It has also been found that miR-146a increases IL-17 expression and miR-155 promotes Th1 and Th17 cells [65], determining severity of the disease course [64]. Th17 cell–associated miR-326 expression was highly correlated with disease severity in patients with MS. In vivo silencing of miR-326 resulted in fewer Th17 cells [65]. Moreover, a recent research has revealed that miR-155 over-expression could be implemented into acute BBB dysfunction, as miR-155 was increased at the neurovascular unit in MS lesions when compared to levels in MS normal-appearing white matter [68]. Pro-inflammatory cytokines, such as interferon gamma (IFNγ) and TNFα were able to up-regulate miR-155 in human cells. The findings indicate contribution of miR-155 to cytokine-induced disruption of the brain endothelium via cell-to-cell and cell-to-matrix interactions, leading to an increased permeability of BBB which is typical for MS [68]. Similarly, another study confirmed increased expression of miR-155 on astrocytes in acute MS demyelinated lesions [69], while miR-155-deficient macrophages had a decreased inflammatory potential, and miR-155 inhibited adipogenesis in adipocytes [62].

Pro-inflammatory cytokines, namely IFNγ, secreted from auto-reactive Th-1 lymphocytes in not only MS patients [67] but also in obese individuals [53, 71] could be responsible for up-regulation of miR-155 and dysfunction of BBB.

Another possible cross-link between obesity and MS might be the expression of the miR-17-92 cluster, which was found down-regulated in B lymphocytes of MS patients [72] and also in blood and adipocytes in obese individuals [62]. The immunogenetic study by Steiner and colleagues proposed that miR-17-92 family members potentiate T helper cell proliferation, whereas miR-29 family members specifically inhibited IFNγ [73].

Further studies are needed to investigate whether obesity-induced over-expression of specific miR and release of pro-inflammatory cytokines in periphery could trigger autoimmune reaction against brain structures in sensitive life periods. We hypothesise that maternal over-nutrition or high-fat diet in childhood might stimulate over-expression of miR-145, -146, -155 in several sites including adipocytes and peripheral blood cells. This allows inflammatory cells to release cytokines and cross the BBB and attack myelin in brain white matter.

Reported down-regulation of the cluster miR-17-92 in Th cells both in obese subjects and MS patients [62, 72] supports the theory of common immune pathways, and indirectly supports the role of over-nutrition in autoimmunity and development of MS.

1.4.2. DNA methylation

One of the epigenetic mechanisms, methylation of myelin basic protein (MBP), is important for maintaining protein stability. In MS patients, methylation of MBP was reported to be higher than in healthy controls [74, 75], and some isoforms of MBP (such as the early developmental ones) are implicated in de- and re-myelination attempts during MS [74]. Since the myelin sheath has been described to be developmentally immature due to impaired myelin synthesis via oligodendrocyte failure [76], a post-translational pathogenetic mechanism has been proposed. A recent research confirmed the previous hypothesis, whereas re-expression of the developmental pathway was found to restrict oligodendrocyte maturation [77]. The authors showed that over-expression of Notch1 within and around active MS plaques lacking re-myelination was associated with immature oligodendrocyte phenotype and up-regulation of transforming growth factor beta1 in perivascular extracelullar matrix [77]. It is of interest that animal studies proved maternal high-fat diet to be a potent epigenetic regulator of the Notch signalling pathway that impairs hippocampal development in the offspring. Notch signalling was involved in molecular mechanisms of neurogenesis, whereas over-expression of Notch1 in neural stem cells caused inhibition of the proliferation of neural progenitors [78]. Although in humans the relationship between high-fat diet and inhibition of neural progenitors has not been confirmed yet, we hypothesised that nutritional factors could exert the effect via the same mechanism.

Myelin structure can be altered when an alternative pathway for the reversal of arginine methylation involves the conversion of an arginine in either histone H3 or H4 to a citrulline. This is termed deimination because the methyl group is removed along with the imine group of arginine and is accelerated by peptidylarginine deiminase 4 (PAD4). Converting citrulline back to arginine has not yet been described [7, 10]. It was found that deimination of MBP-bound arginyl residues makes them more susceptible to myelin-associated proteases [75]. The accompanying loss of positive charge compromises the ability of MBP to interact with the lipid bilayer. The conversion of arginine to citrulline in brain is carried out by an enzyme peptidylarginine deiminase 2 (PAD2). The amount of PAD2 in brain was increased in MS normal-appearing white matter. The mechanism responsible for this increase involved hypomethylation of the promoter region in the PAD2 gene in MS [79]. The triggering factor is not fully known. However, the methylation process requires Vitamin B12, which transfers its methyl group to homocysteine via synthesis of methionine, which is then converted to S-adenosylmethionine, the methyl donor in all biological methylation reactions [79]. Cholin, methionine and 5-methyl tetrahydrofolate are major sources of methyl groups in humans [10, 38]. Moreover, they have an importance in suppression of inflammatory processes. Individuals whose diet was rich in choline and betaine had the lowest levels of several inflammatory markers, including C-reactive protein, homocysteine, IL-6 and TNFα [37]. Among the most concentrated sources of dietary choline are fish and fish-caviar, liver, eggs and wheat germ [37]. On the other hand, vulnerability of myelin sheath is caused by disturbed lipid metabolism, while the uptake of external lipids may also play a role in the formation and disturbances of myelin membranes. The pathogenic mechanisms are known from research of neurodegenerative brain disorders [81, 82].

1.4.3. *Histone acetylation*

Histone acetylation is another epigenetic mechanism involved in the pathogenesis of MS. Histone deacetylases (HDACs) are responsible for the removal of the acetyl group from histones, with resulting ability to influence expression of genes encoded by DNA linked to the histone molecule. HDACs are also able to modify a large variety of non-histone proteins whose activity depends on their acetylation status, such as transcription factors, chaperone proteins, signal transduction mediators, structural proteins, and inflammation mediators [83].

Sirtuin-1 (SIRT1), a member of the HDAC class III family of proteins, can induce chromatin silencing through the deacetylation of histones and can modulate cell survival by regulating the transcriptional activities [84]. It was recently reported that SIRT1 was expressed by a significant number of cells in both acute and chronic active lesions in brains of MS patients. Authors found SIRT1 to co-locate with CD4, CD68, oligodendrocytes and glial fibrillar acidic protein (GFAP) cells in MS plaques, when statistically significant decrease in SIRT1 expression correlated with that of histone H3 lysine 9 acetylation (H3K9ac) and methylation (H3K9me2) [84].

HDAC9 has a key role in the development and differentiation of many types of cells, including regulatory Th cells. Dysfunction of Th cells in MS suggests that HDAC9 may act as an epigenetic switch in effector Th cell-mediated systemic autoimmunity [85]. Genetic variability in HDAC9, along with variants in HDAC11, SIRT4 and SIRT5, has also been shown to influence brain volume in MS patients, as assessed using neuroimaging methods [86].

A growing number of the dietary HDAC reported in the literature are generated as metabolites during the course of digestion [83]. Dietary constituents are formed by the metabolism of some vegetables and fruits, olive oil and nuts. Broccoli, cabbage, Brussel sprouts, cauliflower, kale, Savoy cabbage, citruses, grapes, berries and apples contain many HDAC regulators [83]. For example, resveratrol, naturally occurring compound found in grapes, wine and eucalyptus, is a potent activator of sirtuins (class III HDACs) and in particular, SIRT1 [83]. Thus, regular consumption of foods rich in this compound can have protective effect.

2. Conclusion

Until now, a lot of potential epigenetic mechanisms in MS have not been discovered, and also the hypotheses linking nutritional factors and obesity or nutritional compounds have not been proved by prospective epidemiological studies. The relationship among diet, obesity and genetic risk of MS has been studied only occasionally. The included studies were usually focused on a role of vitamin D. Further studies based on both genetic-epigenetic factors and environmental triggers could bring new information about how to determine the MS risk factors more precisely and much earlier in life. Although at present, there is no particular preventive strategy in MS, new findings could help us to work out dietary interventions and other alternative non-conventional therapies.

Acknowledgements

This work was supported by Project APVV 14-0088.2014.

Author details

Ema Kantorová[1*], Egon Kurča[1], Daniel Čierny[2], Dušan Dobrota[2] and Štefan Sivák[1]

*Address all correspondence to: kantorova@jfmed.uniba.sk

1 Neurology Clinic, Jessenius Faculty of Medicine, Comenius University, Martin, Slovakia

2 Department of Clinical Biochemistry, Jessenius Faculty of Medicine, Comenius University, Martin, Slovakia

References

[1] Risk Alleles for Multiple sclerosis identified by a genomewide study. The International Multiple Sclerosis Genetics Consortium. N Engl J Med 2007; 357: 851-862.

[2] Olerup O, Hillert J. HLA class II-associated genetic susceptibility in multiple sclerosis: a critical evaluation. Tissue Antigens 1991; 38(1): 1-15.

[3] Bomprezzi R, Ringnér M, Kim S, et al. Gene expression profile in multiple sclerosis patients and healthy controls: identifying pathways relevant to disease. Hum Mol Gen 2003; 12(17): 2191-2199.

[4] Ebers GC, Bulman DE, Sadovnick AD, et al. A population-based study of multiple sclerosis in twins. N Engl J Med 1986; 315(26): 1638-1642.

[5] Ebers GC, Sadovnick AD, Dyment DA, et al. Parent-of-origin effect in multiple sclerosis: observations in half-siblings. Lancet 2004; 363: 1773-1774.

[6] Weiner HC. Multiple sclerosis is an inflammatory T-cell- mediated autoimmune disease. Arch Neurol 2004; 61(10): 1613-1615.

[7] Chango A, Pogribny IP. Considering maternal dietary modulators for epigenetic regulation and programming of the fetal epigenome. Nutrients 2015; 7: 2748-2770.

[8] Hyunh JL, Casaccia P. Epigenetic mechanisms in multiple sclerosis: implications for pathogenesis and treatment. Lancet Neurol 2013;12(2): 195-206.

[9] van den Elsen PJ, van Eggermond MC, Puentes F, van der Valk P, Baker D, Amor S. The epigenetics of multiple sclerosis and other related disorders. Mult Scler Relat Disord. 2014 Mar;3(2): 163-75. doi: 10.1016/j.msard. 2013.08.007.

[10] Millagro FI, Campión J, Martinez JA. Dietary and metabolic compounds affecting chromatin dynamics/remodelling. In: Handbook of Epigenetics: The New Molecular and Medical Genetics. Trygve Tollefsbol 1st ed. Elsevier Inc; 2011. p. 302-307.

[11] Londin E, Loher P, Telonis AG, et al. Analysis of 13 cell types reveals evidence for the expression of numerous novel primate- and tissue-specific microRNAs. Proc Natl Acad Sci U S A 2015; 112: E1106-E1115.

[12] Kouzarides T. Chromatin modifications and their function. Cell 2007; 128: 693-705.

[13] Butler JS, Koutelou E, Schibler AC, Dent SY. Histone-modifying enzymes: regulators of developmental decisions and drivers of human disease. Epigenomics 2012; 4: 163-177.

[14] Tarantal A, Berglund L. Obesity and lifespan health-importance of the fetal environment. Nutrients 2014; 6(4): 1725-1736.

[15] Martínez JA, Cordero P, Campión J, Milagro FI. Interplay of early-life nutritional programming on obesity, inflammation, and epigenetic outcomes. Proc Nutr Soc 2012; 6: 1-8.

[16] Laker RC, Wlodek ME, Connelly JJ, Yan ZE. Epigenetic origins of metabolic disease: the impact of the maternal condition to the offspring epigenome and later health consequences. Food Sci Hum Wellness 2013; 2: 1-11.

[17] Gardener H, Munger KL, Chitnis T, et al. Prenatal and perinatal factors and risk of multiple sclerosis. Epidemiology 2009; 20(4): 611-618.

[18] Munger KL, Chitnis T, Ascherio A. Body size and risk of MS in two cohorts of US women. Neurology 2009; 73(19): 1543-1550.

[19] Munger KL, Bentzen J, Laursen B, et al. Childhood body mass index and multiple sclerosis risk: a long-term cohort study. Mult Scler J 2013; 19(10):1323-1329.

[20] Ascherio A, Munger KL. Environmental risk factors for multiple sclerosis Part II: noninfectious factors. Ann Neurol 2007; 61(6):504-513.

[21] Ascherio A, Munger KL, Lunemann JD. The initiation and prevention of multiple sclerosis. Nat Rev Neurol 2012; 8: 602-612.

[22] Reynolds RM. Glucocorticoid excess and the developmental origins of disease: two decades of testing the hypothesis-2012 Curt Richter Award Winner. Psychoneuroendocrinology 2013; 38(1): 1-11.

[23] Mirzaei F, Michels KB, Munger K, et al. Gestational vitamin D and the risk of multiple sclerosis in the offspring. Ann Neurol 2011; 70(1): 30-40.

[24] Staples J, Ponsonby AL, Lim L. Low maternal exposure to ultraviolet radiation in pregnancy, month of birth, and risk of multiple sclerosis in offspring: longitudinal analysis. BMJ 2010; 340: 1640.

[25] Coussons-Read ME, Okumn ML, Nettles CD. Psychosocial stress increases inflammatory markers and alters cytokine production across pregnancy. Brain Behav Immun 2007; 21(3): 343-350.

[26] Marquez AH, O'Connor TG, Roth Ch, et al. The influence of maternal prenatal and early childhood nutrition and maternal prenatal stress on offspring immune system development and neurodevelopmental disorders. Front Neurosci 2013; 7: 120.

[27] Ponsonby AL, McMichael A, van der Mei I. Ultraviolet radiation and autoimmune disease: insights from epidemiological research. Toxicology 2002; 181-182: 71-78.

[28] Karatsoreos IN, Thaler JP, Borgland S, et al. Food for thought: hormonal, experiential, and neural influences on feeding and obesity. J Neurosci 2013; 33(45): 17610-17616.

[29] Zeisel SH, da Costa K-A. Choline: an essential nutrient for public health. Nutr Rev 2009; 11: 615-623.

[30] Nijland PG, Moolenar RJ, van der Pol SMA, et al. Differential expression of glucose-metabolizing enzymes in multiple sclerosis lesions. Acta Neuropathol Commun 2015; 3:79.

[31] Hewagama A, Richardson B. The genetics and epigenetics of autoimmune diseases. J Autoimmun 2009; 33: 3-11.

[32] Ramagopalan SV, Maugeri NJ, Handunnetthi L, et al. Expression of the multiple sclerosis-associated MHC class II allele *HLA-DRB1*1501* is regulated by vitamin D. PLoS Genet 2009; 5(2): e1000369. doi:10.1371/journal.pgen.1000369

[33] Čierny D, Michalik J, Kurča E, et al. FokI vitamin D receptor gene polymorphism in association with multiple sclerosis risk and disability progression in Slovaks. Neurol Res 2015; 37(4): 301-308.

[34] Kim MS, Kondo T, Takada I, et al. DNA demethylation in hormone-induced transcriptional derepression. Nature 2009; 461(7266): 1007-1012.

[35] Saccone D, Asani F, Bronman L. Regulation of the vitamin D receptor gene by environment, genetics and epigenetics. Gene 2015; 561(2): 271-280.

[36] Niculescu MD, Zeisel SH. Diet, methyl donors and DNA methylation: interactions between dietary folate, methionine and choline. J Nutr 2002; 132: 2333S-2335S.

[37] Versini M, Jeandel P-Y, Rosenthal E, Shoenfeld Y. Obesity in autoimmune diseases: not a passive bystander. Autoimmun Rev 2014; 13(9): 981-1000. Doi: http://dx.doi.org/10.1016/j.autrev.2014.07.001

[38] Bhat R, Steinman L. Innate and adaptive autoimmunity directed to the central nervous system. Neuron 2009; 64(1): 123-132.

[39] Riccio P. The molecular basis of nutritional intervention in multiple sclerosis: a narrative review. Complement Ther Med 2011; 19: 228-237.

[40] Sookoian S, Gianotii TF, Burgueňo AL. Fetal metabolic programming and epigenetic modifications: a systemic biology approach. Pediatr Res 2013; 73: 531-542.

[41] Pembrey ME, Bygren LO, Kaati G, et al. Sex-specific, male-line transgenerational responses in humans. Eur J Hum Genet 2006; 14(2): 159-166.

[42] Chao MJ, Ramagopolan SV, Herrera BM, et al. Epigenetics in multiple sclerosis susceptibility: difference in transgenerational risk localizes to the major histocompatibility complex. Hum Mol Gen 2009; 18 (2): 261-266.

[43] Hedström AK, Baarnhielm M, Olsson T, Alfredsson L. Exposure to environmental tobacco smoke is associated with increased risk for multiple sclerosis. Mult Scler 2011; 17:788-793.

[44] Hedström AK, Olsson T, Alfredsson L. High body mass index before age 20 is associated with increased risk for multiple sclerosis in both men and women. Mult Scler 2012; 18(9): 1334-1336.

[45] Hedström AK, Bomfim IL, Barcellos L, et al. Interaction between adolescent obesity and HLA risk genes in the etiology of multiple sclerosis. Neurology 2014; 82(10): 865-872.

[46] Langer-Gould A, Beaber BE.Childhood obesity and risk of pediatric multiple sclerosis and clinically isolated syndrome. Neurology 2013; 80(6): 548-552.

[47] Sioka C, Fotopoulos A, Georgiou A, et al. Body composition in ambulatory patients with multiple sclerosis. J Clin Densitom 2011; 14: 465-470.

[48] Lambert CP, Lee Archer R, Evans WJ. Body composition in ambulatory women with multiple sclerosis. Arch Phys Med Rehabil 2002; 83:1559-1561.

[49] Emamgholipour S, Eshaghi SM, Hossein-Nezhad A, et al. Adipocytokine profile, cytokine levels and Foxp3 expression in multiple sclerosis: a possible link to susceptibility and clinical course of disease. PLoS ONE 2013; 8(10): e76555.

[50] Lumeng CN, Saltiel AR. Inflammatory links between obesity and metabolic disease. J Clin Invest 2011; 121(6): 2111-2117.

[51] Sumarac-Dumanovic M, Stevanovic D, Ljubic A, Jorga J, Simic M, Stamenkovic-Pejkovic D, Starcevic V, Trajkovic V, Micic D. Increased activity of interleukin-23/interleukin-17 proinflammatory axis in obese women. Int J Obes (Lond). 2009 Jan;33(1): 151-6. doi: 10.1038/ijo.2008.216.

[52] Brucklackner-Waldert V, Sturner K, Kolster M, et al. Phenotypical and functional characterization of T helper 17 cells in multiple sclerosis. Brain 2009; 132: 3329-3341.

[53] Lassmann H. Multiple sclerosis: is there neurodegeneration independent from inflammation? J Neurol Sci 2007; 259: 3-6.

[54] Kerchensteiner M, Hohlfeld R. Multiple sclerosis: neuro-immune cross-talk in acute and progressive stages of the disease. In: Kilpatrick T, Ransohoff RM, Wesselingh S. (eds.) Inflammatory Disease of the Central Nervous System. Cambridge University Press; 2010.

[55] Michelson D, Stone L, Galliven N, et al. Multiple sclerosis is associated with alterations of hypothalamo-pituitary-adrenal axis functions. J Clin Endocrinol Metab 1994; 79(3): 848-853.

[56] Minagar A, Alexander SJ. Blood-brain barrier disruption in multiple sclerosis. Mult Scler J 2003; 9 (6): 540-549.

[57] Haltia LT, Viljanen A, Parkkola R, et al. Brain white matter expansion in human obesity and the recovering effect of dieting, J Clin Endocrinol Metab 2007; 92(8): 3278-3284.

[58] Thaler JP, Yi Chun-Xia, Schur EA, et al. Obesity is associated with hypothalamic injury in rodents and humans. J Clin Invest 2012; 122(1): 153-162.

[59] Deiulius JA. MicroRNAs as regulators of metabolic disease: pathophysiologic significance and emerging role as biomarkers and therapeutics. Int J Obes 2016; 40: 88-101.

[60] Sondergaard HB, Hesse D, Krakauer M, et al. Differential microRNA expression in blood in multiple sclerosis. Mult Scler 2013; 19:1849-1857.

[61] Waschbisch A, Atiya M, Linker RA, et al. Glatiramer acetate treatment normalizes deregulated microRNA expression in relapsing remitting multiple sclerosis. PloS One 2011; 6: e24604.

[62] Du C, Liu C, Kang J, et al. MicroRNA miR-326 regulates Th-17 differentiation and is associated with the pathogenesis of multiple sclerosis. Nat Immunol 2009; 10: 1252-1259.

[63] Liu S, Yang Y, Wu J. TNFα-induced up-regulation of miR-155 inhibits adipogenesis by down-regulating early adipogenic transcription factors. Biochem Biophys Res Commun 2011; 414: 618-624.

[64] Ma X, Zhou J, Zhong Y, et al. Expression, regulation and function of MicroRNAs in multiple sclerosis. Int J Med Sci 2014; 11(8): 810-818.

[65] Lopez-Ramirez MA, Wu D, Pryce G, et al. MicroRNA-155 negatively affects blood-brain barrier function during neuroinflammation. FASEB J 2014; 28(6): 2551-2565.

[66] Junker A, Krumbholz M, Eisele S, et al. MicroRNA profiling of multiple sclerosis lesions identifies modulators of the regulatory protein CD47. Brain 2009; 132(Pt12): 3342-3352.

[67] Olsson T, Zhi WW, Hôjeberg B, et al. Autoreactive T lymphocytes in multiple sclerosis determined by antigen-induced secretion of interferon-gamma. J Clin Invest 1990; 86(3): 981-985.

[68] Levine TB, Levine AB. Metabolic Syndrome and Cardiovascular Disease. 1st ed. Philadelphia: Elsevier Inc.; 2006, p. 121-137.

[69] Sievers C, Hoffmann F, Fontoura P, et al. Effect of natalizumab on microRNA expression in B-lymphocytes of relapsing-remitting multiple sclerosis patients. Mult Scler 2010; 16: 197-352.

[70] Steiner DF, Thomas MF, Hu JK, et al. MicroRNA-29 regulates T-box transcription factors and interferon-gamma production in helper T cells. Immunity 2011; 35: 169-181.

[71] Harauz G, Ishiyama N, Hill CM, et al. Myelin basic protein - diverse conformational states of an intrinsically unstructured protein and its roles in myelin assembly and multiple sclerosis. Micron 2004; 35: 503-542.

[72] Kim MS, Pak YK, Jang PG, et al. Role of hypothalamic Foxo1 in the regulation of food intake and energy homeostasis. Nat Neurosci 2006; 9: 901-906. doi:10.1038/ nn1731

[73] Moscarelo MA, Wood DD, Ackerley C, et al. Myelin in multiple sclerosis is developmentally immature. J Clin Invest 1994; 94:146-154.

[74] John GR. Multiple sclerosis: re-expression of a developmental pathway that restricts oligodendrocyte maturation. Nat Med 2002; 8: 1115-1121.

[75] Mendes-da Silva C, Lemes SF, Baliani T da S, et al. Increased expression of Hes 5 protein in Notch signaling pathway in the hippocampus of mice offspring of dams fed a high-fat diet during pregnancy and suckling. Int J Dev Neurosci 2015; 40: 35-42.

[76] Moscarello MA, Mastronardi FG, Wood DD. The role of citrullinated proteins suggests a novel mechanism in the pathogenesis of multiple sclerosis. Neurochem Res 2007; 32: 251-256.

[77] Mastronardi FG, Noor A, Wood DD. Peptidyl argininedeiminase 2 CpG island in multiple sclerosis white matter is hypomethylated. J Neurosci Res 2007, 85: 2006-2016.

[78] Chrast R, Saher G, Nave K-A, et al. Lipid metabolism in myelinating glial cells: lessons from human inherited disorders and mouse models. J Lipid Res 2011; 52: 419-434.

[79] Bourre JM, Pascal G, Durand G, et al. Alteration in the fatty acid composition of rat brain cells (neurons, astrocytes, and oligodendrocytes) and of subcellular fraction

(myelin and synaptosomes) induced by a diet devoid of n-3 fatty acids. J Neurochem 1984; 43: 342-348.

[80] Bassett SA, Barnett MPG. The role of dietary histone deacetylases (HDACs) inhibitors in health and disease. Nutrients 2014; 6: 4273-4301.

[81] Yan K, Cao Q, Reilly CM, et al. Histone deacetylase 9 deficiency protects against effector T cell-mediated systemic autoimmunity. J Biol Chem 2011; 286: 28833-28843.

[82] Inkster B, Strijbis EMM, Vounou M, et al. Histone deacetylase gene variants predict brain volume changes in multiple sclerosis. Neurobiol Aging 2013; 34: 238-247.

[83] Tegla CA, Azimzadeh P, Adrian-Albescu M, et al. SIRT1 is decreased during relapses in patient with multiple sclerosis. Exp Mol Pathol 2014; 96(2): 139-148.

[84] D'Addario C, Di Francesco A, Pucci M, et al. Epigenetic mechanisms and endocannabinoid signalling. FEBS J 2013; 280: 905-917.

[85] Gynther P, Toropainen S, Matilainen JM, et al. Mechanism of 1alpha,25-dihydroxyvitamin D(3)-dependent repression of interleukin-12B. Biochim Biophys Acta 2011;1813: 810-818.

[86] Joshi S, Pantalena LC, Liu XK, et al. 1,25- Dihydroxyvitamin D (3) ameliorates Th17 autoimmunity via transcriptional modulation of interleukin-17A. Mol Cell Biol 2011; 31: 3653-3669.

Chapter 9

Cognitive Deficits and Neuropsychological Assessment in Multiple Sclerosis

Alena Javůrková, Denisa Zimová,
Katarína Tomašovičová and Jaroslava Raudenská

Additional information is available at the end of the chapter

http://dx.doi.org/10.5772/63968

Abstract

The aim of this chapter was to introduce the contents of neuropsychological assessment in multiple sclerosis, which should include the functional evaluation of cognitive domains, the psychopathology of personality, levels of depression, and the assessment of psychosocial aspects and quality of life with multiple sclerosis. Further, the most commonly used neuropsychological diagnostics are described. The chapter hopes to draw attention to the importance of neuropsychological assessment which should be a part of neurological diagnostics and therapy, including rehabilitation and psychotherapy.

Keywords: neuropsychology, multiple sclerosis, cognitive deficit, neuropsychiatry, neurorehabilitation

1. Introduction

Multiple sclerosis (lat. sclerosis multiplex) is a chronic disease of the central nervous system caused by the damage of the myelin sheath. The symptoms of the disease depend on the location of the damage in the nervous system and can vary: optic neuritis, paresthesia, motor symptoms (spasticity), impairment of cranial nerves, oculomotor disorders, cerebellar disorders, vertigo, urinary disorders, defecation, sexual dysfunctions, fatigue, depression, cognitive disorders, and paroxysmal symptoms. Multiple sclerosis is the most common cause of chronic neurological disabilities in young adults. The onset of the disease is usually between the ages of 20 and 40. Its prevalence is higher among women. The highest susceptibility to the disease is among Caucasians; the geographic gradient of the incidence increases together with the distance from the equator. Genetic predisposition plays a role.

1.1. Types of the disease

Four types of the disease are recognized according to their clinical course. In the early years of the disease, the most common type is relapsing-remitting MS (RRMS), occurring in 80–85% of patients and characterized by attacks and remissions. If a previous attack left no neurological deficit, remissions may be completely asymptomatic at the beginning of the disease. Half of these patients develop into the stage of secondary progression (SPMS) during the first 10 years of the disease's progression. This stage is characterized by a gradual increase in neurological deficits that are already irreversible, with both the presence and absence of relapses that are not as dramatic as in the remitting stage. The relapsing-progressive (RPMS) form of the disease is characterized by an increased neurological deficit also evident between the relapses; it is thus prognostically the most unfavorable form of the disease. The primary progressive (PPMS) form affects about 10–15% of patients and is characterized by a gradual increase in neurological deficit. This form occurs more frequently among males and with a later onset of the disease [1].

In the relapsing-remitting forms, approximately 20–30% of patients continue working following their first attack. It is uncommon for patients in the early stages of this form of MS to be physically disabled or to have noticeable alternations in terms of dementia. It is primarily the progressive form of MS, developing at a later age that tends to pose more difficulty in the cognitive domains, compared to the remitting one. Patients with the spinal form of the disease have trouble mostly with motor skills and mobility. This form often occurs in the primary progressive form. Cognitive deficits include impaired attention. The typical cognitive domains impaired in the cerebral forms of MS are described below. Psychosocial and maladaptive problems are described in the case report.

1.1.1. Case report 1

A woman of 47 years reported the first symptoms of MS (optic neuritis and paresthesia) at the age of 17; later, the attacks recurred about once a year; the problems worsened after two child deliveries. Therefore, she did not breastfeed her children, for which she blames herself for until today. She underwent an abortion 2 years after the second birth due to the above-mentioned difficulties, then was psychiatrically treated, and still has feelings of guilt. The diagnosis of MS was definitely confirmed about 4 years ago. The patient has since been considerably anxious, unreconciled with the diagnosis, dominated by hostility and distrust of the medical staff (the disease was not diagnosed correctly). MRI scans of the brain and spinal cord showed multiple demyelinating lesions or plaques in the white matter. Nobody in the family had MS. She was entitled to disability pension and has been taking antidepressants for 4 years, based on the psychiatrist's indication of anxiety and depressive problems. Formerly, she worked as a teacher. She feels very tired after only about a 3–4 km walk. She is married, has two adult sons, and lives with her family. When she learned about MS, she was overtaken by fear of dying and felt mentally ill, and thus stopped working. She did not observe any difficulties with cognition. Gradually, a panic anxiety developed; when she wakes up, she feels scared, but this

http://dx.doi.org/10.5772/63968

panic is also present while traveling; family members take her everywhere by car. The patient is recommended to systematic cognitive-behavioral psychotherapy.

2. Cognitive functions and MS

The most characteristic feature of cognitive dysfunction in MS is the slowing down of processing speed [2]. Another often affected domain is long-term episodic memory and attention (alternating and maintained). Less frequent but significant cognitive disorders include disorders of executive functions (especially abstract and conceptual reasoning and problem-solving) [3].

2.1. Outline of basic neuropsychological techniques

Due to the high incidence of cognitive disorders in patients with MS, the adequate evaluation and diagnosis of such deficits is of great importance. Their existence is often under diagnosed during an ordinary neurological examination. Various tests are used to identify these.

One of the most significant neuropsychological studies of MS patients was carried out by Rao [4]. The Brief Repeatable Battery (BRB) for neuropsychological impairment in MS [5] was created based on a set of highly sensitive tests, with a few modifications. The BRB tests were chosen with regard to time restrictions, and so the administration of the entire battery lasts only about 40–45 min. It contains the following subtests: The Paced Auditory Serial Addition Test (PASAT); The Symbol Digit Modalities Test (SDMT) measuring attention, visual accuracy, and executive functions; The Selective Reminding Test (SRT) measuring verbal memory and delayed recall periods; The Spatial Recall Test (SPART) measuring visuospatial memory and delayed recall; and The Word List Generation (WLG) measuring verbal fluency. The battery has 15 versions and is thus, despite its longer duration, the most commonly used battery for the longitudinal monitoring of patients with MS. Clinical research supports the high sensitivity of the battery. Its abbreviated version with 3 subtests has been under verification recently.

For cognitive screenings, Beatty [6] developed the Screening Examination for Cognitive Impairment (SEFCI) neuropsychological battery, which proved to confirm cognitive deficits typical of MS in a comparative study (duration 22 min) with other time-consuming neuropsychological batteries. It does not have variants and is thus not suitable for longitudinal observations. The study compared the battery with the Neuropsychological Screening Battery for Multiple Sclerosis (NPSBMS) for which the administration period lasted 31 min. Both batteries identified significantly more patients with cognitive impairment in MS than the Mini-Mental State Exam (MMSE) [7]. The Multiple Sclerosis Functional Composite (MSFC) is a score used in clinical studies, measuring the function of the lower limb—timed walk, upper limb function (nine-hole peg test), and cognitive function (PASAT) [8, 9].

In 2001, the battery Minimal Assessment of Cognitive Function in MS (MACFIMS) [10] was created with respect to neglected domains (higher cognitive functions and spatial processing), and its reliability and validity has been verified in several studies. The MACFIMS battery includes the following tests: Controlled Oral Word Association Test (COWAT); Judgement of Line Orientation Test (JLO); California Verbal Learning Test, Second edition (CVLT-II); Brief Visuospatial Memory Test-Revised (BVMT-R); Paced Auditory Serial Addition Test (PASAT); Symbol Digit Modalities Test (SDMT); and the Sorting Test from the Delis-Kaplan Executive Function System (D-KEFS). However, the MACFIMS battery is limited by time constraints and for its need to be carried out by an experienced neuropsychologist. For this reason, a shorter battery of cognitive tests has recently been designed. This consists of three subtests from the MACFIMS battery and may be administered by neuropsychological workers without training —International Brief Cognitive Assessment for Multiple Sclerosis—BICAMS [11]. It is suitable for use in routine clinical practices in centers with no neuropsychologist to administrate the MACFIMS. The BICAMS screening battery consists of three tests that are included in the MACFIMS battery: SDMT, CVLT-II (the first five experiments), BVMT-R (the first three trials).

2.2. Cognitive domains and their examination

Cognitive deficits observed within MS can have almost any composition [12]; a typical profile shows impairment of processing speed, memory, and often of executive skills as well [2].

2.2.1. Intellectual skills

Over the past two decades, numerous studies using neuropsychological assessment showed that approximately half the patients exhibit some degree of cognitive impairment. We also know that cognitive disorders may occur at any time during the illness and are not bound to the presence of physical disorders [13]. Generally, a substantial variability of cognitive impairments in MS in terms of their gravity and types has been described. Although approximately 10% of MS patients have severe problems that display extensive impairment even when measuring overall intelligence, the vast majority (90%) of patients is affected only mildly to moderately [14]. It should be emphasized that patients with MS as a group display a relatively small decline on intelligence measures, and overall dementia is rare in MS [13]. Cognitive deficits in MS are usually more focal than generalized. Verbal IQ, therefore, often remains intact during the first signs of MS [4].

2.2.2. Visuomotor skills, visuospatial skills, and attention

Visual disorders including diplopia, reduced color discrimination, blurred vision, and transient blindness, and motor symptoms such as limb weakness, spasticity, incoordination, or a combination of all the problems, as well as sensory disorders including numbness or paresthesia, contribute to the alteration of visuomotor skills in neuropsychological examinations. Deficits of visual attention in MS patients significantly influence their level of visuomotor skills. When evaluating visual attention, it is thus necessary to take into account the visual disorders. For example, test results in automatic attention (reaction time) and focused attention may be in norm in terms of errors, but the patient completes them in a longer period of time. In contrast, controlled attention and divided attention are often deficient [15].

http://dx.doi.org/10.5772/63968

2.2.3. *Memory and learning*

Long-term memory is related to the learning and retrieval of new information. Patients with MS often have difficulties with memory—the prevalence is reported between 40 and 65%. The most common verbal memory tests are tasks in which the patient learns a wordlist [16]. Visuospatial memory, too, is affected in patients with MS [13]. Patients with MS have significant abnormalities of the hippocampal functional connectivity, even before spatial memory impairment is apparent [17]. Patients with MS in the initial stages of the disease display a relatively intact short-term memory and learning ability, measured by tests of memory skills. More patients experience problems in recalling new material, while recognition is rarely altered.

2.2.4. *Verbal ability and executive functions*

Executive functions are related to planning and goal-directed behavior. Drew and colleagues [18] reported a series of executive dysfunctions—including disinhibition, poor fluency, and an inability to shift sets. Overall, 17% of their sample of MS patients displayed this kind of deficit. Language functions typically remain intact in MS; however, some minor deficits in understanding were demonstrated. Weakened sentence comprehension has been associated with slower information processing. Deficits in semantic memory and visual processing were also observed [19].

Overall verbal skills in patients with MS are usually preserved for a long time, depending on premorbid mental performance, flexibility, and vocabulary; a low level of verbal fluency is observed. Dysarthria or problems with articulation are more prevalent in speech. The best and longest preserved of all verbal skills is naming. Recalling information from long-term memory, vocabulary, and conceptual reasoning are often normal. If these abilities are altered, it is usually the result of a generalized deterioration, or of the patient having low levels of premorbid education and of cognitive reserve. Some studies have found lower levels of conceptual reasoning in patients with chronic progressive MS. A more detailed examination of verbal and oral skills is possible with a complex speech assessment.

Cognitive impairment in MS, however, does not correlate with the degree of physical disability (Expanded Disability Status Scale EDSS Kurtzke [20]); some studies showed a correlation with disease duration, yet other studies did not prove this. The impairment of cognitive functions correlates positively with some MRI abnormalities—mostly concerning atrophy, ventricular dilatation, and the total volume of impaired white matter on W T2 lesion load. The sites of predilection are areas of the corpus callosum, and extensive demyelination further affects circuits linking the prefrontal and subcortical areas. Large confluent periventricular lesions are also typical. As a whole, the huge variability in cognitive impairment may depend on many factors, such as the patient's age, sex, age at disease onset, level of education, and cognitive reserve [3]. Dysexecutive and prefrontal behavioral syndromes in a patient with a cerebral, relapsing–remitting form are illustrated in the following case report.

2.3. Case report 2

A woman of 54 years was treated for MS and migraine for 15 years. A cognition and personality assessment was recommended by a neurologist for her memory problems. MRI of the brain showed unique plaque lesions in the white matter, predominantly in the right frontal lobe; the spinal cord was not affected. There has been improvement when comparing MRI scans, the lesions were less apparent. The patient was entitled to a full disability pension 10 years ago. She was a skilled saleswoman. She has been married for 35 years; her sons are adults. There is no report of MS in the family. She commutes to a psychiatric clinic where antidepressants are prescribed. She is oriented in contact, talkative, often gets lost, and exhibits signs of the prefrontal syndrome. Memory problems have occurred for a longer period, approximately 10 or even more years. She misplaces thing and then cannot find them, someone talks about something and she does not know about it, and she does not remember old information. She also experiences sudden interruptions of activities when she goes off to do another one, although she had not planned it; it is impulsive. She experiences confusions in her mind; she wanted something and suddenly does not know what she was thinking about. It troubles her. She "masks" these difficulties in front of her family and friends. Headaches occur daily. Neuropsychologically, it is mainly attention that is impaired, and the generalized deterioration of intellect is also striking, considering her education. It is possible to explain the problems behaviorally, mainly through the prefrontal behavioral and dysexecutive syndromes, which might be related to the largest findings of plaques in the frontal lobes. Cognitive behavioral therapy and training of cognitive functions was advised.

3. The course of cognitive deficit

Studies on large MS patient samples have shown that the range of cognitive impairment prevalence in MS is between 40 and 70% and appears in all stages and types of the disease (which also includes the clinically isolated syndrome—CIS) [21]. It seems that observations carried out for long enough are able to show cognitive impairment in progressive stages [22]. Several studies have confirmed the relationship between the dysexecutive syndrome and frontal lesions, and others have focused on deficits in interhemispheric transfer (i.e., disconnection syndrome) in the atrophy of the corpus callosum.

The course of a cognitive deficit without progression but with behavioral disorders is illustrated in the following case report.

3.1. Case report 3

A 43-year-old man with the relapsing-remitting form, treated for MS for 18 years, was initially assessed due to problems with memory, concentration, exhaustion, and no sexual appetite. An MRI scan of the brain showed small plaque lesions subcortically, compared with no progression found on MRI scans 4 years ago. The patient had been treated with interferons for 3 years. He is left-handed, a skilled auto-mechanic, has his own workshop at home, and works

http://dx.doi.org/10.5772/63968

17 h a day. He has been married for 22 years, has two children and "does not get on well" with his wife, and he admits to extramarital relations. They are currently in a divorce proceeding. The main problem is with his erection. Neuropsychologically, no striking impairment of cognitive domains was found, and only anxiety and a conflictive family environment were found. Marriage counseling, a sexologist, and conflict solving were recommended. The patient refused the proposed recommendations and increasingly adopted strange and promiscuous behaviors; he forced his wife and their children to move out of the house. He was incapable of rational thinking; he explained the promiscuity as a verification of his sexual functions. A 1-year follow-up neuropsychological assessment showed no impairment of cognitive domains and intellect, but a psychiatric examination was recommended due to paranoid thinking and aggressiveness.

On the contrary, a rapid development of cognitive deficits into dementia can be seen in the following case report.

3.2. Case report 4

A 42-year-old woman diagnosed with chronic progressive MS for 10 years was treated by interferons for 6 years. At the time of her visit, eye problems are dominant for the first time; she uses a white cane. She also experiences hearing difficulties, but does not complain about memory at all. A former governess, now entitled to full disability pension, divorced, with two children, both studying, not in contact with her ex-husband. Her mother and brother help her mostly, but the patient feels dependent and helpless. According to an MRI scan of the brain, periventricular plaque lesions are apparent in the white matter of both hemispheres. There has been a slight progression of plaque and atrophy when compared to an MRI from 4 years ago. The initial psychological examination suggested a multi-domain impairment, a decrease of more than 2 SDs (verbal mnestic and visual skills, construction, executive functioning), with severe anosognosia. The performance may have been influenced by her impaired visual and auditory perception. Two years later, she comes fundamentally oriented, and the right eye is blind. The outcome of the examination is a multi-domain cognitive disorder; cognitive abilities are significantly impaired across the whole profile.

4. Cognitive abilities and imaging methods

Magnetic resonance imaging (MRI) is used as one of the basic methods for diagnostics, visualization, and monitoring of the inflammatory lesion dynamics in the brain and spinal cord. The first MRI studies in patients with MS were published in 1981. It was found that inflammatory lesions occur 5–10 times more than MS clinical attacks. Commonly used images for the diagnosis of MS are those in which lesions of hyperintense signal of size from 1 mm to several cm are apparent, located in the white matter of both hemispheres, mostly in the cerebral ventricles, as well as in the brain stem, medulla, cerebellum, and upper cervical spinal cord. If the radiologist wants to depict the active lesions, he/she applies gadolinium. The range of lesions visible in this way does not correlate with clinical disability as it is not known whether the lesion is currently in the stage of reparation or destruction.

The only areas described as hypodensities ("black holes") are areas where a loss of axons, thus the definitive loss of tissue, has occurred. The typical brain damage in the white matter in MS patients is clearly associated with a loss of axons [23]. Loss of axons is also a natural sign of brain aging, and its verification is only possible postmortem.

Recent neuropsychological studies especially use functional magnetic resonance imaging (fMRI) to assess the plasticity of functional cognitive deficits in patients with MS. The method consists of recording the activation of brain areas during the presentation of various simple neuropsychological tests. Compensatory mechanisms of cognitive functions already in the early stages of chronic MS are described. The results of fMRI scans in a group of MS patients with mild cognitive impairment and a healthy control group were compared. The functional activation areas of the brain were completely distinct during the presentation of the verbal naming test in each group (in MS patients in the frontal part of the right cortex and in the left Brodmann's area, and in the right cingulate gyrus in the healthy group). The functional reorganizations of motor functions are also described in fMRI assessments of MS patients, when compared to healthy subjects. MS patients with mild cognitive deficits assessed by neuropsychological tests were presented with auditory memory tests during an fMRI and were found to display heightened activity in different areas. Patients with greater neuropsychological deficits were found to exhibit lower activation of brain areas during the fMRI assessment, which probably supports the theory of adaptive mechanisms resulting from neural disorganization or inhibition associated with MS [24]. It is therefore also possible to explain the unproven relationship between the extent of morphological findings of gliosis and plaques in the white matter, and the severity and location of neuropsychological deficits in terms of this plasticity of neuropsychological functions. The range of specific cognitive deficits, such as memory disorders, reduced processing speed, and attention disorders, can be better explained by the cortical gray matter lesions (lesions and atrophy) than subcortical white matter lesions [25]. It has been shown that neocortical atrophy is associated with impaired verbal memory, visual episodic and working memory, verbal fluency, attention/concentration, and processing speed [26]. It is also possible that the neocortical atrophy is further responsible for slight personality changes, such as euphoria, that are seen in MS patients [27]. The left frontal atrophy occurs in patients with impaired verbal/auditory memory, while the right frontal atrophy is associated with impaired visual episodic and working memories. The medial temporal cortex atrophy is associated with a decrease in processing speed and impaired episodic and verbal memories. The most important within the subcortical gray mater are atrophy, structural changes, and an altered metabolism of the thalamus, which are associated with the impairment of many cognitive domains [28]. Generally, it can be concluded that the cognitive impairment observed in MS patients is caused by inflammatory lesions and a widespread loss of gray matter. Although it is not possible to define the neuropsychological profile of MS patients as strictly "cortical" or "subcortical", it seems that it is the disruption of the cortical gray matter which determines the degree and nature of cognitive dysfunction. Instead of the term subcortical dementia, often associated with a severe multi-domain cognitive impairment, the term multiple disconnection syndrome is also used for cognitive deficits in MS [29].

5. Neuropsychiatric aspects of MS

Cognitive and affective disorders in MS have largely been ignored for many years, yet they occur in 5% of the patients early in the disease, while in its advanced stages, this can be up to 70% of cases. MS is associated with a variety of behavioral changes. These may be associated with emotional disorders and cognitive distortions and may often overlap. The prevalence of depression is at least 50%; it is often manifested in parallel with the MS attack, and suicidal tendencies may occur. The causes of depression are probably neuropathological changes associated with the limbic system, neuroendocrinological, and psychoneuroimmunological changes, responses to life change, or a side effect of MS therapy (especially corticosteroids). The prevalence of bipolar disorders in MS is approximately 15%, and the prevalence of anxiety disorders in MS is about 36%. The occurrence of bipolar disorder and psychosis in MS is twice as common as in the general population, and the so-called pseudobulbar affectation (involuntary emotional expression disorder) affects one in ten patients. It is likely that the interruption of frontolimbic and temporolimbic connections plays a role in the pathogenesis of euphoria. Euphoric patients tend to have higher EDSS and a significantly more impaired cognition, including anosognosia. The incidence of euphoria is lower (approximately 2%) than is described in the older literature, thanks to an earlier diagnosis and treatment of MS. Symptoms of depression do not correlate with neurological findings or with disease severity, as measured by the sum of symptoms of physical disability and cognitive dysfunction [30]. However, depression positively correlates with subjective experience of stress, memory deficits, and with age in elderly patients over 65 years of age, in patients with the chronic progressive form and in patients with a predominance of spinal distortion. The neuropsychological assessment should therefore, in addition to cognitive domains, also include assessments of emotional alterations, especially depression and anxiety scales (e.g., methods HAD–Hospital Anxiety and Depression Scale, BDI-II) and their development over time [31].

Other changes in patients with MS, particularly changes in values and attitudes, progress together with the psychosocial adjustment and are mostly associated with the subjective perception of a physical handicap, but do not correlate with the duration of MS or other demographic indicators. Specific quality of life with MS questionnaires is used to measure the quality of life in these patients, such as the MSQOL-54 [32], which measures 12 subscales: physical function, role limitations—physical, role limitations—emotional, pain, emotional well-being, energy, health perceptions, social function, cognitive function, health distress, overall quality of life, and sexual function.

The Multi-domain battery Multiple Sclerosis Quality of Life Inventory (MSQLI) contains 10 scales, both generic and specific to MS [33]; some scales also have a shortened version: Health Status Questionnaire (SF-36), Modified Fatigue Impact Scale (MFIS), MOS Pain Effects Scale (PES), Sexual Satisfaction Scale (SSS), Bladder Control Scale (BLCS), Bowel Control Scale

(BWCS), Impact of Visual Impairment Scale (IVIS), Perceived Deficits Questionnaire (PDQ), Mental Health Inventory (MHI), and MOS Modified Social Support Survey (MSSS). The scales can also be presented individually.

6. Multi-disciplinary MS treatment

6.1. Cognitive disorders therapy in MS

Pharmacotherapy for cognitive impairment in MS is currently the subject of intense research. First and foremost, a preventive effect of early initiation and immunomodulatory therapy, in association with the possible development of cognitive disorders, is assumed. The primary point is to prevent axonal loss and the development of atrophy. Very few randomized trials have been carried out so far. Acetylcholinesterase inhibitors have currently been examined, through only with questionable or entirely negative results. No effective pharmacological treatment for cognitive disorders in MS has yet been found [34]. The pharmacological manipulation of depression is also significant, however, and should always be combined with psychotherapy in MS patients. Moreover, depression can be enhanced by a variety of bio-psychosocial factors, such as reduced work performance or increased neurological symptoms.

6.2. Neuropsychological rehabilitation and the cognitive deficit psychotherapy

Kalb and Reitman [35] report the so-called cognitive rehabilitation as the basic therapy for cognitive deficits. They present two approaches: The first is to restore functions, such as through direct training and exercising of skills that are altered in neuropsychological tests (this approach, however, has a limited benefit in improving daily activities in MS patients) and the second approach is more compensatory, and closer to current neuropsychology, with its desire to improve a function through substitution, that is, the individual use of residual cognitive abilities in order to improve the quality of life through behavioral and cognitive therapy. The first approach is based on a more experimental approach, while the second is more clinical. It concerns creating an individual plan, "customized" for each patient.

This plan is based on neuropsychological assessment and interviews with the patient and their family. The evidence for the efficacy of cognitive rehabilitation in MS is, unfortunately, quite limited and contradictory. Memory rehabilitation studies suggest that individualized computer programs focused on patient-specific difficulties could be most effective. The most beneficial in the rehabilitation of executive functions is perhaps a direct instruction by a therapist, that is, paper and pencil method. The main problem of cognitive training in MS remains to be particularly its unavailability for patients and their often low motivation. It is therefore very important to maintain employability of patients for as long as possible and motivate them toward mental activity.

For these purposes, teams of multi-disciplinary experts work with people with MS, where a neurologist, psychologist, psychiatrist, speech therapist, occupational therapist, physiotherapist, and a psychotherapist cooperate in complex, holistic, all-day programs, based on cognitive as well as emotional, behavioral, and physiological changes. Even though it is impossible to increase one's premorbid IQ and brain volume, we can work on cognitively stimulating leisure activities. It is also very important to motivate the patient to lead an active life that includes adherence to the prescribed pharmacotherapy, but also an active attitude toward physiotherapy, psychotherapy, and cognitive training. It is the combination of physiotherapy and cognitive training that has the correct effect on the neurogenesis and formation of new synapses.

The specific model of psychosocial support for patients with MS at different levels, which has the characteristics of a cognitive-behavioral supportive therapy and family therapy, includes [35]: (1) psychoeducation, that is, education leading to the understanding of the disease, explanation of adaptive coping strategies; (2) diagnostics/treatment of emotional or cognitive problems; (3) family intervention, that is, how to organize family support for members with MS for adaptive coping with the illness; (4) work support for MS patients, that is, to work productively in a field for as long as they are able and interested, and vice versa, to stop working if necessary; (5) individual psychosocial assistance to individuals with MS. In addition to professional psychotherapy, a support group of people with the same disease, but also of family, friends, possibly a cultural-social or religious community, is appropriate.

6.3. Disability, employability, and MS

The organization of care for MS patients is similar around the world. A patient with a benign course of the disease is usually checked by a neurologist twice a year; more complicated patients are consulted in centers for MS that are a part of most university neurological clinics. In the case of a more severe disability, it is advisable to contact social services or long-term care. Neuropsychological approaches, however, show that employability can also be predicted by a short battery of tests that focuses on relevant domains, such as the aforementioned battery BICAMS [36]. The issue of employment restrictions, disability, work, and life disability due to MS is illustrated in the following case report.

6.3.1. Case report 5

A doctor, surgeon specialist, formerly a chief physician, 50 years old, with remitting MS. MRI scans revealed the cerebrospinal form with multiple plaques in the white matter of the brain and spinal cord; the demyelinating plaque findings are unchanged for 3 years. The patient was recommended to a cognition assessment for his memory problems, was dismissed from the surgical specialty, and thus works as a GP, which does not satisfy him. He is divorced and has problems with his second wife, who is a nurse, approximately 25 years younger. The wife is hostile, blames him for the change of social status. Neuropsychologically, only his psychomotor speed and motor dexterity are slightly reduced, which exhibits moderate depression in emotional experience, not suicidal. Couples therapy was recommended to address the changes in his professional situation and partner quality of life, together with a psychiatric consultation.

7. Conclusion

This article summarizes a neuropsychologist's perspective on cognitive skills in MS. When evaluating the cognitive level of patients, the comprehensive or screening assessment should examine specific domains that may not correlate with the length of the illness, neurological objective findings, the amount of plaque on MRI scans, and the MS form or type. Cognitive disorders are a significant predictor of quality of life during all stages of MS; they reduce physical independence and the ability to perform both activities of daily life and of employment, they influence one's coping and compliance to the treatment and their rehabilitation potential. The employability of people with MS can thus be easily predicted by the severity of cognitive disorders and their premorbid cognitive reserves, rather than by physical disability. The neuropsychological assessment of cognitive functions in MS should be a part of care for patients with MS and a part of a multi-disciplinary approach to neurorehabilitation.

Acknowledgements

The authors would like to express their sincere gratitude toward Lucie Steinerova from the University of Edinburgh for helping out with the language revision.

This article is supported by Ministry of Health, Czech Republic—conceptual development of research organization, Motol University Hospital, Prague, Czech Republic, 00064203.

Author details

Alena Javůrková[1,2*], Denisa Zimová[3], Katarína Tomašovičová[4] and Jaroslava Raudenská[2,5]

*Address all correspondence to: alena.javurkova@post.cz

1 Department of Clinical Psychology, University Hospital FNKV, Prague, Czech Republic

2 Department of Nursing, 2nd Medical Faculty, Charles University, University Hospital Motol, Prague, Czech Republic

3 Department of Neurology, 3rd Medical Faculty, Charles University, University Hospital FNKV, Prague, Czech Republic

4 Department of Psychology, Faculty of Arts, Charles University, Prague, Czech Republic

5 Department of Clinical Psychology, University Hospital Motol, Prague, Czech Republic

References

[1] Weinshenker BG, Bass B, Rice GP, Noseworthy J, Carriere W, Baskerville J, Ebers GC: The natural history of multiple sclerosis: a geographically based study I. Clinical course and disability. Brain. 1989;112(Pt1):133–146. doi: 10.1093/brain/112.1.133

[2] DeLuca J, Chelune GJ, Tulsky DS, Lengenfelder J, Chiaravalloti ND: Is speed of processing or working memory the primary information processing deficit in multiple sclerosis? J Clin Exp Neuropsychol. 2004;26(4):550–562. doi: 10.1080/13803390490496641

[3] Benedict RH, Zivadinov R: Risk factors for and management of cognitive dysfunction in multiple sclerosis. Nat Rev Neurol. 2011;7(6):332–342. doi: 10.1038/nrneurol.2011.61

[4] Rao SM, Leo GJ, Bernardin L, Unverzagt F: Cognitive dysfunction in multiple sclerosis. I. Frequency, patterns, and prediction. Neurology. 1991;41(5):685–691.doi: 10.1212/WNL.41.5.685

[5] Rao SM: A Manual for the Brief, Repeatable Battery of Neuropsychological Tests in Multiple Sclerosis. New York: National Multiple Sclerosis Society; 1991

[6] Beatty WW, Paul RH, Wilbanks SL, Hames KA, Blanco CR, Goodkin DE: Identifying multiple sclerosis patients with mild or global cognitive impairment using the Screening Examination for Cognitive Impairment (SEFCI). Neurology. 1995;45(4):718–723. doi: 10.1212/WNL.45.4.718

[7] Aupperle RL, Beatty WW, Shelton Fde N, Gontkovsky ST: Three screening batteries to detect cognitive impairment in multiple sclerosis. Mult Scler. 2002;8:382–389. doi: 10.1191/1352458502ms832oa

[8] Rudick R, Antel J, Confavreux C, Cutter G, Ellison G, Fischer J, Lublin F, Miller A, Petkau J, Rao S, Reingold S, Syndulko K, Thompson A, Wallenberg J, Weinshenker B, Willoughby E: Recommendations from the national multiple sclerosis society clinical outcomes assessment task force. Ann Neurol. 1997;42: 379–382. doi: 10.1002/ana.410420318

[9] Rudick RA, Cutter G, Baier M, Fisher E, Dougherty D, Weinstock-Guttman B, Mass MK, Miller D, Simonian NA: Use of the multiple sclerosis functional composite to predict disability in relapsing MS. Neurology. 2001; 56(10):1324–1330. doi: 10.1212/WNL.56.10.1324

[10] Benedict RH, Fischer JS, Archibald CJ, Arnett PA, Beatty WW, Bobholz J, Chelune GJ, Fisk JD, Langdon DW, Caruso L, Foley F, LaRocca NG, Vowels L, Weinstein A, DeLuca J, Rao SM, Munschauer F: Minimal neuropsychological assessment of MS patients: a consensus approach. Clin Neuropsychol. 2002;16(3):381–397. doi: 1385-4046/02/1603-381

[11] Langdon DW, Amato MP, Boringa J, Brochet B, Foley F, Fredrikson S, Hämäläinen P, Hartung HP, Krupp L, Penner IK, Reder AT, Benedict RH: Recommendations for a Brief

International Cognitive Assessment for Multiple Sclerosis (BICAMS). Mult Scler. 2012;18(6):891–898. doi: 10.1177/1352458511431076

[12] Prakash RS, Snook EM, Lewis JM, Motl RW, Kramer AF: Cognitive impairments in relapsing-remitting multiple sclerosis: a meta-analysis. Mult Scler. 2008;14(9):1250–1261. doi: 10.1177/1352458508095004

[13] Langdon DW: Cognition in multiple sclerosis. Curr Opin Neurol. 2011;24(3):244–249. doi: 10.1097/WCO.0b013e328346a43b

[14] Patti F: Cognitive impairment in multiple sclerosis. Mult Scler. 2009;15(1):2–8. doi: 10.1177/1352458508096684

[15] Beatty WW: Assessment of cognitive and psychological functions in patients with multiple sclerosis: considerations for databasing. Mult Scler. 1999;5(4):239–243. doi: 10.1177/135245859900500408

[16] Stegen S, Stepanov I, Cookfair D, Schwartz E, Hojnacki D, Weinstock-Guttman B, Benedict RH: Validity of the California Verbal Learning Test-II in multiple sclerosis. Clin Neuropsychol. 2010;24(2):189–202. doi: 10.1080/13854040903266910

[17] Roosendaal SD, Hulst HE, Vrenken H, Feenstra HE, Castelijns JA, Pouwels PJ, Barkhof F, Geurts JJ: Structural and functional hippocampal changes in multiple sclerosis patients with intact memory function. Radiology. 2010;255(2):595–604. doi: 10.1148/radiol.10091433

[18] Drew M, Tippett LJ, Starkey NJ, Isler RB: Executive dysfunction and cognitive impairment in a large community-based sample with multiple sclerosis from New Zealand: a descriptive study. Arch Clin Neuropsychol. 2008;23(1):1–19. doi: 10.1016/j.acn.2007.09.005

[19] Laatu S, Revonsuo A, Hämäläinen P, Ojanen V, Ruutiainen J: Visual object recognition in multiple sclerosis. J Neurol Sci. 2001;185(2):77–88. doi: 10.1016/S0022-510X(01)00461-0

[20] Kurtzke JF. Rating neurologic impairment in multiple sclerosis: an expanded disability status scale (EDSS). Neurology. 1983;33(11):1444–1452. doi: 10.1212/WNL.33.11.1444

[21] Potagas C, Giogkaraki E, Koutsis G, Mandellos D, Tsirempolou E, Sfagos C, Vassilopoulos D: Cognitive impairment in different MS subtypes and clinically isolated syndromes. J Neurol Sci. 2008;267(1–2):100–106. doi: 10.1016/j.jns.2007.10.002

[22] Denney DR, Sworowski LA, Lynch SG: Cognitive impairment in three subtypes of multiple sclerosis. Arch Clin Neuropsychol. 2005;20(8):967–981. doi: 10.1016/j.acn.2005.04.012

[23] Evangelou N, Konz D, Esiri MM, Smith S, Palace J, Matthews PM: Regional axonal loss in the corpus callosum correlates with cerebral white matter lesion volume and

distribution in multiple sclerosis. Brain. 2000;123 (Pt 9):1845–1849. doi: 10.1093/brain/123.9.1845

[24] Mainero C, Caramia F, Pozzilli C, Pisani A, Pestalozza I, Borriello G, Bozzao L, Pantano P: fMRI evidence of brain reorganization during attention and memory tasks in multiple sclerosis. Neuroimage. 2004; 21(3): 858–867. doi: 10.1016/j.neuroimage.2003.10.004

[25] Calabrese M, Rinaldi F, Grossi P, Gallo P: Cortical pathology and cognitive impairment in multiple sclerosis. Expert Rev Neurother. 2011;11(3):425–432. doi: 10.1586/ern.10.155

[26] Batista S, Zivadinov R, Hoogs M, Bergsland N, Heininen-Brown M, Dwyer MG, Weinstock-Guttman B, Benedict RH: Basal ganglia, thalamus and neocortical atrophy predicting slowed cognitive processing in multiple sclerosis. J Neurol. 2012; 259(1):139–146. doi: 10.1007/s00415-011-6147-1

[27] Benedict RH, Hussein S, Englert J, Dwyer MG, Abdelrahman N, Cox JL, Munschauer FE, Weinstock-Guttman B, Zivadinov R: Cortical atrophy and personality in multiple sclerosis. Neuropsychology. 2008;22(4):432–441. doi: 10.1037/0894-4105.22.4.432

[28] Benedict RH, Ramasamy D, Munschauer F, Weinstock-Guttman B, Zivadinov R: Memory impairment in multiple sclerosis: correlation with deep grey matter and mesial temporal atrophy. J Neurol Neurosurg Psychiatry. 2009;80(2):201–206. doi: 10.1136/jnnp.2008.148403

[29] Calabrese P, Penner IK: Cognitive dysfunctions in multiple sclerosis–a "multiple disconnection syndrome"? J Neurol. 2007;254 Suppl 2:II18–II21. doi: 10.1007/s00415-008-0901-z

[30] Feinstein A: Neuropsychiatric syndromes associated with multiple sclerosis. J Neurol. 2007;254 Suppl 2:II73–II76. doi: 10.1007/s00415-008-0901-z

[31] Javůrková A, Amlerová J, Raudenská J: Long-term observation of cognitive, emotional and behavioral changes in patient with multiple sclerosis—a case report (In Czech). Cesk Slov Neurol N. 2014;77(4):501–504

[32] Vickrey BG, Hays RD, Harooni R, Myers LW, Ellison GW: A health-related quality of life measure for multiple sclerosis. Qual Life Res. 1995;4(3):187–206.

[33] Fischer JS, LaRocca NG, Miller DM, Ritvo PG, Andrews H, Paty D: Recent developments in the assessment of quality of life in multiple sclerosis (MS). Mult Scler. 1999;5(4):251–259. doi: 10.1177/135245859900500410

[34] Patti F, Leone C, D'Amico E: Treatment options of cognitive impairment in multiple sclerosis. Neurol Sci. 2010;31(Suppl 2):S265–S269. doi: 10.1007/s10072-010-0438-7

[35] Kalb , R, Reitman, N: Multiple Sclerosis: A model of Psychosocial Support [Internet]. 2012. http://www.nationalmssociety.org/NationalMSSociety/media/MSNationalFiles/Brochures/Book-A-Model-of-Psychosocial-Support.pdf

[36] Benedict RH, Cookfair D, Gavett R, Gunther M, Munschauer F, Garg N, Weinstock-Guttman B: Validity of the minimal assessment of cognitive function in multiple sclerosis (MACFIMS). J Int Neuropsychol Soc. 2006;12(4):549–558

Chapter 10

Social Cognition Impairments in Patients with Multiple Sclerosis and Comparison with Imaging Studies, Disease Duration and Grade of Disability

Valentina Ignatova, Lyudmila Todorova and
Jivko Surchev

Additional information is available at the end of the chapter

http://dx.doi.org/10.5772/63465

Abstract

Cognitive impairments in multiple sclerosis (MS) are heterogeneous and their rate varies between 43% and 70%. A less studied aspect of cognition is social cognition, which is not a uniform theoretical construct. It includes emotion perception, prosody, empathy, theory of mind (ToM) and assessment of mood. In addition to progressive physical disability, social cognitive impairments are a reason for job loss in 24–80% of patients with MS, increased divorce rate, dissolution of partnerships and social communication difficulties.

Social cognitive impairments are the result of disruptions in the mentalization network at the neuroanatomical, neurochemical and/or genetic level, which can lead to malfunctions in the dopaminergic–serotoninergic system and to compromising the development of neuroanatomical targets within the network. The wide dissemination of demyelinating lesions and cortical thinning typical of patients with MS often lead to anatomic and functional disorders of the above-mentioned specific brain structures. A correlation has been established among specific cortical areas involved in emotion identification from facial expression (right and left fusiform face area, frontal eye), emotion processing (right entorhinal cortex) and socially relevant information (left temporal pole). The most active brain region involved in social cognitive processing is the medal frontal cortex (MFC), which is described as the brain's social cognitive center. During performance of various sociocognitive tasks for mental state attribution, common areas of increased activation in the medial prefrontal gyrus and the temporoparietal junctions are registered bilaterally, while the area of the medial prefrontal cortex (the paracingulate cortex) is the only region uniquely activated by the performance of ToM.

Most MRI studies of patients with MS found a correlation between the cognitive and/or affective disorders, on the one hand, and lesion localization, total lesion load, or cerebral atrophy, on the other. A significant correlation was also reported between abnormal activities in specific cortical zones on fMRI, on the one hand, and clinical manifestation, conventional MRI findings and behavioral changes, on the other. Altered patterns of brain activity were found in all clinical phenotypes of MS, including when cognitive abilities were intact and/or restored, social cognitive dysfunction in MS actually affects all stages of the disease and all types of clinical course. The cortical plastic changes are a dynamic phenomenon that can be modulated by external factors. This phenomenon would facilitate the mapping of individual strategies for adequate treatment and rehabilitation of each patient.

Keywords: social cognition, multiple sclerosis, empathy, theory of mind, mentalization, emotional perception, faux pas, disability, social brain, imaging studies

1. Introduction

Multiple sclerosis (MS) is a chronic inflammatory autoimmune degenerative disease of the central nervous system (CNS) leading to both physical and neuropsychological disability. These two types of impairment may occur simultaneously or independently [1]. Until now the focus of scientific research has predominantly been on the physical disablement in patients with MS and its impact on their quality of life. Over the last few decades, researchers have shown an increasing interest in mood disorders, behavior and cognition in this disease.

Cognitive impairments in MS are heterogeneous [2] and their rate varies between 43% and 70% [3–5]. They are in an independent form of disability and make the performance of routine daily activities difficult, sometimes impossible. Up to now studies have mostly been conducted on impairments in the main cognitive domains such as memory, attention and executive functions. A less studied aspect of cognition is social cognition, which is not a uniform theoretical construct. It includes emotion perception, prosody, empathy, theory of mind (ToM) and assessment of mood [6, 7]. Findings in MS show disturbance not only in emotion recognition from facial expressions but in the whole area of general emotion processing. The connection between cognitive decline and impaired social cognitive skills in MS remains debatable.

Social cognitive dysfunction in MS actually affects all stages of the disease and all types of clinical course. Such disturbances are reported even in clinically isolated syndrome (CIS). Relatively, little is known about the evolution of cognitive deficits in MS, especially about those manifested in the early stages of the disease [8].

The frequency of social cognition impairments and the nature of pathological changes in the brain in patients with MS are reasonable grounds for seeking a relationship between deteriorated mentalization and findings from imaging/functional brain studies. Studies looking for a correlation between cognitive decline and MRI changes (lesion volume, lesion load, cortical thinning) are still at an early stage. This also applies to studies seeking to detect functional changes in specific brain areas responsible for the performance of relevant sociocognitive tasks. Additional data from future research in this field are needed for better understanding of social cognition impairments [9].

http://dx.doi.org/10.5772/63465

In addition to progressive physical disability, social cognitive impairments are a reason for job loss in 24–80% of patients with MS [10, 11], increased divorce rate, dissolution of partnerships [12] and social communication difficulties. Furthermore, these disturbances restrict the career development and social life of patients. This calls for a multidisciplinary approach in research and concurrent assessment of the physical, neuropsychological and social aspects of disability in MS.

The main objective is to evaluate the frequency and degree of social cognition impairments in patients with MS based on systematic analysis of advanced scientific research and to outline scientific trends in the field.

2. Methods

We conducted advanced search based on the following key words in different combinations: "social cognition", "multiple sclerosis", "empathy", "theory of mind (ToM)", "faux pas", "mentalization", "emotional perception", "disability", "social brain" and "imaging studies". The selection was made by two independent reviewers who retrieved relevant scientific works (original articles, book chapters, systematic reviews) published in English from electronic database (PubMed, MEDLINE). The search period was unrestricted. The following inclusion criteria were determined: (1) subjects, suffering from multiple sclerosis; (2) assessment of social cognition abilities; and (3) brain imaging findings and impaired social cognition. Case report articles were excluded. A relationship between social cognition skills, physical disability and duration of the disease was searched. We also checked up the bibliography of the related sources and included the relevant articles. We also checked up the bibliography of the related sources and included the relevant articles. We selected six books, seven book chapters, 43 scientific reviews, 86 original articles, one thesis, two conference papers and one manual regarding social cognition and/or MS. Finally, we retrieved two book chapters, 10 scientific reviews, 32 research studies, one thesis and two conference papers on the current topic "social cognition" in MS. Meta-analysis was not suitable for summarizing of the results due to methodological heterogeneity between reviewed studies. Quantitative assessment of the relevant data was conducted. Different points of views, as well as controversies within the scientific field, were presented. We highlighted key results, determined importance of social cognition impairments for quality of life in patients with MS and outlined a framework of research trends.

3. What is social cognition?

Numerous attempts to define social cognition have been made. In early 1994, Thomas M. Ostrom collected more than 100 definitions and accepted conceptual orientation in information processing in the context of cognitive psychology as the core of social cognition. According to him, the sociocognitive approach is based on the belief that constructs relevant to cognitive performance and processing are fundamental to understanding all human responses regardless of whether these responses are social or unsocial in nature. This basic definition has been supplemented and updated over time. Augoustinos et al. accept that social cognition is not a theory per se but an approach or perspective strongly influenced by the methods and concepts of cognitive psychology [13].

In 1980s, scientific research postulated that humans store and give meaning to complex social information by simplifying and organizing this information in understandable cognitive structures called schemata. The schemata theory implies that we use the same mental structures for the selection and processing of incoming information from the surrounding social environment. Schemata are based on the general expectations from experience (socialization) and allow the prediction and control of social interactions. This theory is applied to the following four key zones: person schemata, self-schemata, role schemata and event schemata [14]. The categorization process is borrowed from cognitive psychology. It includes the identification of stimuli, their grouping as part of a category similar to other parts in the same category and differentiating them from the components of other categories. It is fundamental to perception, thought, language and actions. In the 1990s, the concept was further developed with the assumption that categorization may present not only average abstraction but also a number of specific and concrete cases or samples found in this category. According to Mead and Vygotsky, intrapersonal processes originate and are modeled after interpersonal processes.

Social cognition is a level of mental capacity developed over the evolution process for successful adaptation to the social environment. The basic domains of social cognition are empathy and ToM.

Empathy is the natural ability to understand the emotions and feelings of others regardless of whether one is directly participating in a given situation, viewing photos, reading a book, listening to a story or just imagining. It refers to the phenomenological experience of compassion [15]. The term "empathy" comes from the German word Einfühlung translated by Titchener as "feeling into" [16, 17]. Empathy includes an intuitive feeling of having something in common with others which relies on socially shared emotional experience, cognitive mechanisms of perspective taking, the ability to maintain a self-other distinction during interpersonal interaction. The cognitive aspect of empathy is also defined as empathy accuracy [18].

ToM, also called mentalization, was described as a cognitive component of empathy by Baron-Cohen in 2003 [19, 20]. ToM is viewed as a specific capacity of the mind to understand ourselves and others in terms of mental states. It is based on "reading the thoughts and emotions" of others through analyzing their facial expressions and other behavioral signs [21, 22]. ToM provides the opportunity for establishing a connection between internal conditions manifested through expressions, gestures, signals and internal states of mind. The capacity to recognize the emotions, intentions and thoughts of others can be regarded as an important component of a broader set of skills called social competence or social intelligence.

More recent studies have explored ToM in two aspects—cognitive ToM (the ability to understand the intentions of others – 'cold') and affective ToM (the ability to infer others' emotional states – 'hot') [23]. The affective component of ToM requires empathy. According to Ickes, "everyday mind reading" [24] is not a skill that needs to be learned. However, one develops it in the course of life experience. In addition to personality traits, at least three types of mind-reading accuracy tests need to be examined, that is, the ability to assess someone in terms of the following: (1) mental state (both affective and nonaffective), (2) behavior, and (3) roles, identity and/or condition [25]. Emotion recognition is perhaps the most thoroughly investigated and best known of all mind-reading tasks.

The contemporary neurobiological ToM model includes both neuroanatomic and neurochemical levels of specificity. In this model, cortical and subcortical zones are functionally organized so as to ensure the expression of cognitive and affective mental states for both self and others. According to this model, the cognitive and affective aspects of ToM are based on dissociable but interacting prefrontal networks. The cognitive ToM network includes primarily the dorsomedial prefrontal cortex, the dorsal anterior cingulate cortex (ACC) and the dorsal striatum, while the affective ToM network comprises mainly the ventromedial and orbitofrontal cortices, the ventral anterior cingulate cortex, the amygdala and the ventral striatum. The ability to distinguish the mental condition for self from that for others is based on different brain representations within the mentalizing network and is modulated by the functional interaction between the dorsal and ventral systems for attention and selection in the temporoparietal junction and the anterior cingulate cortex.

The functioning of ToM depends on the integrity of the dopaminergic and serotonergic systems, which are primarily involved in the process of comprehension of mental states. Social cognitive impairments are the result of disruptions in the mentalization network at the neuroanatomical, neurochemical and/or genetic level, which can lead to malfunctions in the dopaminergic–serotoninergic system and to compromising the development of neuroanatomical targets within the network [26]. ToM abilities are variably influenced, depending on the type of pathology in the functioning of the mentalization network.

It is presumed that there are two systems involved in belief processing in humans: implicit ToM (iToM) and explicit ToM (eToM). The iToM system builds a hypothesis empirically in the absence of awareness. It is supposedly available from birth [27]. The eToM system is associated with thinking, control and awareness of the approach in mental state recognition. It responds and develops in the first years of life. Little is known about the connection between implicit and explicit processing of social cognition [28]. It is assumed that they are largely independent.

Social cognition comprises two levels relating to all its domains. The first level includes quick, relatively routine cognitive processing which is largely automatic, implicit and can occur without awareness. At the higher level, these processes are slow, flexible and explicitly require exertion of mental effort [28].

4. Clinical assessment of social cognition in patients with MS

Research on social cognition is experimental and focuses on intra-individual mental processing. Studies on emotional and cognitive impairments in patients with MS are based on different test batteries. Mental schemata are used for focusing attention and facilitating information encoding and retrieval.

Empathy can be regarded as a set of interrelated constructs including social competence, self-assessment, emotion and sensitivity to others [29]. Therefore, there is no universal tool objectively assessing empathy in all its aspects. In a recent review of empathy measurement tools [30], 1147 citations were used to select 50 articles describing 36 empathy tests, eight of which demonstrated satisfactory reliability, internal consistency and validity.

The empathy quotient is most often determined through self-assessment questionnaires. Interpersonal empathy is usually studied by applying the Hogan Empathy Scale (HES) [31], the Toronto Empathy Questionnaire (TEQ) and the 50 Item Interpersonal Skills Questionnaire (50 IISQ). The affective component of empathy can be assessed through the Questionnaire Measure of Emotional Empathy (QMEE), while the cognitive component is more precisely determined through HES. The Balanced Emotional Empathy Scale (BEES), developed by Mehrabian, evaluates responders' reaction to the mental state of others [32].

The instrument most often used for determining the level of self-empathy is Neff's self-compassion scale, which assesses self-kindness, common humanity and mindfulness [33]. The measurement of compassionate or altruistic love toward different targets through the Compassionate Love Scale (CLS) provides additional information about the perception of close others and all of humankind [34]. The Empathy Construct Rating Scale (ECRS) can test the ability to understand accurately the feelings of others through careful listening, thus checking whether the subject properly understands what others experience.

More complex information regarding compassion to self and others is provided by Baron-Cohen and Wheelwright in The Empathy Quotient, which measures cognitive empathy, emotional reactivity and social skills [35] and most of all in the Interpersonal Reactivity Index (IRI), which allows measuring of multidimensional individual empathy differences [36].

Recently, tests with nonverbal stimuli have also been applied to the evaluation of empathy. They are commonly used in patients with autism and aphasia but are also an important complement to self-assessment questionnaires, because they contribute to the greater objectivity of overall empathy assessment. Nonverbal tests provide additional information on the empathy quotient through analyzing what feelings and thoughts are inferred from facial expressions in pictures. Most often they are based on a series of photographs which depict people with different mental and emotional charge, thus measuring the cognitive and affective components of empathy. The most frequently used ones are the multifaceted empathy test (MET) [37], the visual recognition test, the Florida Affect Battery (FAB) and Ekman and Friesen's black and white stimulus set. The results of these tests minimize subjectivity in the patient's self-assessment [38].

ToM, as a key aspect of social cognition, requires greater cognitive effort for slower and more explicit processing. In general, ToM tests are classified into three groups: attribution of epistemic mental states, attribution of intention and attribution of affective mental states [39]. They are based on verbally or visually delivered information, and in recent years, ToM movies have been developed for increasing test sensitivity and approximating the demands of everyday life social cognition [40]. Verbal tests, such as "Strange Stories" and "Faux Pas Recognition", require interpretation of auditory information for grasping false belief and deception based on short stories with social context similar to real situations. Such tasks could be accompanied by pictures. Decoding complex emotions from voice is measured by "Reading the Mind in the Voice" [41] and the "Voice Emotion Identification Test" [42] and prediction of intentions and emotions—by "Reading the Mind in the Eyes" [43] and the "Facial Symbol Test", [44] which are sensitive indicators of the socioperceptual component involved in the immediate recognition of mental states [45]. Even more informative is the "Cambridge Mind-reading Face Voice Battery", [46] which combines verbal and dynamic visual stimuli.

ToM cartoons assess the ability to understand emotions and intentions by interpreting graphic design images and/or cartoon strips. Some of these use jokes involving false beliefs [47], and others combine representations of mental and physical states [48]. The following are some video tasks appropriate for ToM assessment in patients with MS: conversations and insinuations (C&I) [49], the social inference-enriched subtest of the TASIT, containing video-taped social interactions in which lies and sarcasm are presented [50], the Face Puzzle—for measuring the explicit and implicit aspects of facial emotion recognition, the social cue recognition test [51] and the videotape emotion identification test [52].

In the comprehensive evaluation of social cognitive skills in patients with MS, it is necessary to take into account the level of general cognition, personal characteristics, such as individual perspective, idiosyncrasies, purpose and attitudes [53], as well as a possible genetic modulation of individual empathic ability [54].

So far ToM research has used small groups of patients with MS and a narrow range of cognitive tasks. The fact that there is no unified neuropsychological battery for the assessment of social cognitive impairments should also be taken into account. For the reasons outlined earlier, it is difficult to generalize on their results for the entire MS population, numbering about 1.3 million worldwide, as well as to reach definitive conclusions

5. Impairment of social cognitive abilities in patients with MS

Social cognition is considered a main determinant of the functional outcome in many psychiatric and neurologic degenerative diseases, including MS. Social cognitive impairments have been registered even in the first clinical episode prior to conversion to MS.

Decreased empathy was reported in patients with MS (cohort of 34 MS subjects) compared to healthy controls of the same age and education level ($p < 0.01$) [55]. These results were obtained from a study by Benedict et al., which is the first of its kind. It matched self-reports of patients with MS on their level of empathy against external evaluation by informants. The authors found large discrepancies between the responses from the two groups—the scores obtained from patients were significantly higher ($p < 0.01$) than those of the informants. Personal abnormalities, such as elevated neuroticism, agreeableness and conscientiousness, were also registered in the patients. The authors emphasize the predictive role of executive control over the manifestation of these anomalies and suggest frontal lobe syndrome [55]. Ten years later,

Kraemer et al. also revealed a significantly lower level of empathy in patients with MS assessed by self-rating questionnaire ($p < 0.02$). A study of Banati et al. registered a higher level of empathy, attributed by ambulatory MS subjects to themselves by using self-assessment questionnaire. The patients ($n = 40$) showed 14 times better empathizing abilities to themselves compared to control individuals ($p < 0.05$) [56]. Ot self-compassion mechanisms suppress anxiety and negative thinking [57]. When self-compassion is lowered, mild symptoms of depression and anxiety could escalate into more severe ones.

A systematic review of 72 studies provides evidence of worse adjustment in MS, which is associated with emotional stress and specific emotionally focused coping strategies in these patients. The authors stress the need for further research in this direction because of insufficient evidence on the relation between adjustment outcomes and level of cognition, interaction with others, disease symptoms, social support obtained [58].

Significantly reduced self-perception in different subcategories was established in patients with MS as compared to healthy controls with similar demographic characteristics. Perception of emotional and social functioning (including global health perception) is impaired but mental characteristics are preserved [59].

Incorrect recognition of emotional information during the daily activities of patients with MS hinders the performance of social cognitive skills [60]. Alexithymia, the impaired ability to verbalize emotions due to violation of their processing, might have a significant impact on self-perception, emotion regulation, behavior control and interaction with others in these patients [61]. Alexithymia is a personal construct, characterized by subclinical inability to identify and describe the emotions in the self [62]. It is a common finding in patients with MS and further hinders social cognition [63], making them nonempathic and ineffective in emotional responding [64]. For example, in a study comparing 40 MS patients with the same number of normal volunteers, Montreuil and Petropoulo registered alexithymia in 50% of the patients and only in 9% of controls [65]. No correlation was found between alexithymia, on the one hand, and cognitive impairment, mood disorders and disease duration in MS patients, on the other. However, MRI studies established a significant connection between alexithymia and atrophy of the posterior part of corpus callosum [66]. This result supports the hypothesis of interhemispheric transfer dysfunction in patients with alexithymic MS [67].

One of the most sensitive indications of social cognition impairment, in particular in MS, is the difficulty in facial expression recognition [68, 69]. Most MS research detects a deficiency in emotional facial expression recognition. Beatty studied patients with MS and established impaired identification not only of facial affect, but also of neutral facial expressions [60]. Testing this ability in patients with MS again (cohort of 22 patients with MS and 11 healthy controls), Krause et al. detected unequivocal emotion recognition deficits in patients with MS who had shown no difficulties in face identification. In line with current findings, these impairments were most common in the recognition of unpleasant facial emotions, while deficits in the recognition of happy expression were not observed. Furthermore, the reaction times to happy facial expressions were significantly faster ($p < 0.001$) compared to that to negative emotional expressions. One reason may be that it is usually easier to recognize a happier facial expression, and consequently, these impairments can be better compensated for

[70]. Based on specific tests for perception from facial photographs, Philips expanded and supplemented the currently available data with the conclusion that MS leads to an impaired ability for processing emotional information from both static and dynamic images [71]. However, differences in emotion recognition are discreet and subtle, and according to some researchers, correlate significantly with cognitive functioning, suggesting a global deficiency in the speed of information processing [50]. Despite some variability in findings, several contemporary studies support the thesis that ToM impairments are independent from neuropsychological functioning in adult patients with MS [49, 56]. A correlation between impaired emotional perception and the physiological and social aspects of quality of life was found in MS [71]. Some studies have shown a correlation between the inability to recognize facial emotions from presented photographs and alexithymia [72–74].

In a study of patients with MS in 2003, which was the first of its kind, Beatty revealed affective prosody comprehension deficits not due to a hearing loss, cognitive decline, aphasia or depression (47 patients, 19 demographic controls). MRI studies of these patients did not detect a connection between affective prosody violations and the size of the corpus callosum or lesion load [75].

Empathy reflects the ability to infer and share the emotional state of others, therefore it is strongly related to ToM [76]. ToM (mentalization) refers to the perception of the mental condition of ourselves and others, which may serve for understanding and predicting their behavior [77].

ToM disorders are often detected in patients with MS. Their ability to read thoughts is reduced due to their impaired decoding of nonverbal signs such as facial expressions, gestures, gaze fixation and comprehensive processing of abstract verbal information.

The first study assessing ToM abilities in patients with MS was conducted in 2009 by Henry et al. [45], who applied both a test for basic recognition of emotional facial expressions and ToM tests (27 patients with MS and 30 controls). The "Reading the Mind in the Eyes" test (belonging to ToM tests) allowed the differentiation of more complex emotional states often associated with social relationships (e.g., attraction or repulsion, friendly or hostile attitude, noticing or ignoring the tested). The authors found impaired recognition of anger and fear in patients with MS but did not establish intergroup differences between subjects and controls in the recognition of surprise, sadness, disgust and happiness. A significant correlation was registered between dealing successfully with facial emotion recognition and ToM tasks. For both groups, a statistical correlation was discovered between the level of coping and executive control.

In the same year, Ouellet arrived at the conclusion that patients with MS suffering from cognitive deficits tend not to recognize the mental state of others unlike MS patients with preserved cognition (15 cognitively intact and 26 cognitively impaired patients) [49], while Henry (64 patients with relapsing-remitting MS (RRMS), 30 controls) [78] and Pöttgen (45 patients with MS, 45 healthy controls) [21] found that ToM deficits in MS appear independently of the well-known cognitive deficits. Emotion recognition impairments were more pronounced in patients with MS than impairments in thought and intention recognition [21, 79].

More errors of interpretation and lower total scores were reported in patients with MS when using nonverbal tests [56]. Subjects performed worse than controls ($p < 0.05$) at the facial symbol test (FST) [80].

In their pilot study, Genova et al. used a dynamic sociocognitive task—The Awareness of Social Inference Test (TASIT)—and established an impaired ability in patients with MS to interpret and understand lies and sarcasm. These impairments correlated with severe cognitive disorders in information processing speed, working memory, learning and memory and with premorbid IQ [50].

Charvet et al. devoted their scientific work on social cognition in patients with MS, which has debuted in childhood. The authors reported significantly worse results of the pediatric onset MS patients ($n = 28$) compared to those of healthy peers ($n = 32$) in the following three domains of social cognition: facial affect recognition ($p = 0.008$), detection of social faux pas ($p = 0.009$), perspective taking ($p = 0.06$) [81].

5.1. Social cognition impairments in different clinical subtypes of MS

Studies exploring the relatedness of social cognition impairments to clinical subtypes of MS are still insufficient. The available data indicate significant variation in the degree of cognitive impairment among individual phenotypes of the disease.

5.1.1. Clinically isolated syndrome (CIS)

In 2010, Jehna et al. conducted a study in which they established significant slower speed of emotional facial expression processing in patients with CIS compared to healthy persons ($p < 0.01$). They suggested storage of facial emotion recognition based on the lack of significant differences in the number of correct answers. Since response time is an indicator of cognitive processing speed, the authors interpreted these results as evidence of general delay in information processing in MS [80].

5.1.2. Relapsing-remitting multiple sclerosis (RRMS)

Patients with RRMS demonstrated significantly lower levels of empathy toward others and fantasy compared to healthy subjects [82]. An earlier study by Beatty conducted in 1989 with MS patients assessed their ability to identify facial affect by viewing photographs depicting basic emotional states. Patients with RRMS fulfilled these tasks properly [60]. The findings of a new study, conducted by Kraemer et al. in 2013, with a homogeneous cohort of 25 patients with RRMS in the early stages of the disease (less than two years' duration) and with low levels of disability Expanded Disability Status Scale- <2 (EDSS <2) showed significantly worse results in affective prosody comprehension in MS subjects compared to the same number healthy controls. Patients gave less accurate solutions to "discrimination of affective prosody" and more incorrect responses in the subtest "matching of affective prosody to facial expression" for the emotion "anger". Paradoxically, regarding the emotion "fear" they showed better results than controls [6]. Gleichgerrcht et al found that MS subjects (patients $n = 38$; controls n

http://dx.doi.org/10.5772/63465

= 38) had significantly higher self-oriented personal distress ($p < 0.01$) and higher levels of alexithymia compared to controls [82].

So far the only available study in patients with MS examining the cognitive and affective components of ToM separately is that of Roca et al. from 2014. Using faux pas and executive function tests in 18 RRMS patients with low grade of disability, Roca et al. found deficits in the cognitive component of ToM in the presence of a stored affective component. Such dissociation between the cognitive and affective components of ToM has also been reported in other neurological and psychiatric disorders [83].

5.1.3. Primary progressive MS (PPMS)

Patients with primary progressive MS (PPMS) have experienced considerable difficulties in identifying the emotions of others, as well as their own emotions. Patients from this subgroup gave lower results in faux pas tasks compared to RRMS patients [84].

5.1.4. Secondary progressive multiple sclerosis (SPMS)

Patients with secondary progressive MS (SPMS) are significantly more alexithymic compared to healthy controls [61]. Beatty's study in 1989 revealed that the patients with chronic progradient MS experienced difficulties in the discrimination of facial affect and neutral faces, unlike those with RRMS. Error analysis demonstrated that patients had the same difficulties in depicting each of the represented seven emotional states without serious errors in indicating their polar opposites [60]. Current studies have not shown abnormal identification of neutral faces by subjects with SPMS. In patients with this subtype, lower accuracy has been reported in performing tasks for perception of fear, surprise, anger and sadness [61], while difficulties in identifying disgust and happiness were not reported. Compared to healthy controls, patients took less time in recognizing fear and surprise, while detecting anger and sadness took them longer.

A retrospective longitudinal review with 1845 MS patients, 351 of whom with chronic progradient multiple sclerosis (CPMS), 636 — with RRMS and 858 — with mixed or nonspecific MS, compared to 265 healthy individuals registered worse results in patients with CPMS than in RRMS patients at the Benton Facial Recognition Test (BFRT) [85].

5.2. Social cognition impairments depending on MS duration

A positive correlation was detected between duration of MS and level of empathy, that is, the greater the duration of the disease, the lower the empathy quotient [55, 56, 86]. Banati et al. found profoundly increasing of the empathizing quotient (p 0.03) among patients with short-term MS ($n = 40$) compared to controls ($n = 35$). In addition, Pakenham and Cox in longitudinal study of 388 persons with MS and 232 caregivers registered positive correlation between the time since diagnosis and compassion/empathy ($p < 0.01$), mindfulness ($p < 0.01$) and personal growth ($p < 0.01$). Contrarily, other studies found a significant decrease in the empathy level in patients with MS who are still in the early stages of the disease and with a low degree of disability compared to healthy subjects. The authors explain the unrealistic self-assessment results of most subjects with the greater impairment of ToM skills and partly with the higher emotional stress they were experiencing [22, 86].

In 2010, Banati et al. found more prominent ToM deficits in patients with longer disease duration ($p = 0.05$) [56]. In some research, the duration of the disease did not correlate with the emotional and cognitive scores from nonverbal tests [80], while Kraemer reported positive correlation between impaired social cognitive skills and executive function deficits in the early stages of the disease in fully ambulatory patients [6].

5.3. Social cognition impairments in MS depending on the grade of physical disability

Paradoxically, patients with more severe physical disorders relatively often show a higher level of empathy compared to controls and patients with mild neurological deficits. A positive correlation was found between the difficulty in emotional facial expression recognition and the degree of disability [44]. Patients with a higher grade of disability demonstrated greater difficulties in affective prosody recognition [75]. More interpretation errors and lower scores were reported for patients with MS when nonverbal tests were used [56]. With deterioration of the disability the results from ToM verbal tests also get worse [87]. In a study of Jehna, EDSS scores did not correlate significantly with scores from emotion recognition tests or with results from FST in MS subjects (sample of 20 patients: CIS $n = 12$, RRMS = 7, SPMS = 1) [80]. Results from other recent studies indicate that the severity of the disease (respectively the degree of physical disability) does not correlate with the degree of impaired emotion recognition or with the psychological and social aspects of the quality of life [71, 88]. Therefore, some researchers consider social cognition as a separate domain of cognition which could independently affect the quality of life of the individual, in particular, that of patients with MS. Based on the extensive review of the literature available, we can conclude that social cognition impairments in these patients require further in-depth research.

6. Social brain

Leslie Brothers was one of the first scientists talking about the social brain, using proof from studies in nonhuman animals [89]. Later Prinz created the common coding theory, according to which perception and actions rely on common codes [90]. The discovery of the so-called "mirror neurons" within the premotor and parietal cortices [91], activated while an action directed to the object is performed and while an action is perceived by the object [92, 93], became a basis for extensive research on the so-called social brain [91].

The discovery of social cognitive impairments in patients with MS presupposes brain damage. The difficulty in facial expression identification is among the most sensitive indicators for social cognition impairments. It is supposed that a disconnection mechanism due to white matter lesions and cortical thinning of specific brain zones causes a cognitive decline. This worsens the processing of emotions and the decoding of mental states from facial expressions. Functional MRI study, conducted by Jehna et al., provides evidence of altered functional brain processing in the posterior cingulate cortex and precuneus during emotion recognition in subjects with MS (sample of 15 patients and 15 healthy individuals) [88]. Abnormalities in face encoding and recognition vary in different stages of MS. Patients with CIS experience increased recruitment of the posterior visual areas. In patients with RRMS, the thalamus, parahippocampal gyrus and right anterior cingulum are more activated than in patients with CIS and SPMS. In SPMS, an increased recruitment in the frontal areas is also registered. Significant correlation has been described between the above-mentioned abnormal activations, on the one hand, and clinical symptoms, conventional MRI findings and behavioral disorders, on the other [94].

It is considered that mentalization is carried out by a large network of functionally related neurons [26]. A correlation has been established among specific cortical areas involved in emotion identification from facial expression (right and left fusiform face area, frontal eye), emotion processing (right entorhinal cortex) and socially relevant information (left temporal pole) [95]. According to a model of Ross and Mesulam, affective prosody comprehension could be related to the right-sided perisylvian region, whose structure is similar to the language areas in the left hemisphere [96]. Later studies have suggested an involvement of the basal ganglia and prefrontal cortex (PFC) [97, 98]. Alexithymia may be associated with deactivation and activation of the anterior cingulate cortex (ACC) in response to highly negative and respectively highly positive emotional stimuli [72].

The most active brain region involved in social cognitive processing is the medal frontal cortex (MFC) [99, 100], which is described as the brain's social cognitive center. This region is activated during tasks requiring self-knowledge and reflection, person perception and attribution of intentions. It is supposed that von Economo neurons [101] serve as a relay tract from the frontoinsular and anterior cingulate cortices (responsible for fast intuitive processes) to parts of the frontal and temporal cortices (associated with making slower conscious decisions), thus playing an important role in ToM [102]. It was discovered that damage to the VM frontal lobe plays a crucial role in the existence of a higher level of social cognition: social reasoning [69].

Individuals with bilateral damage of the orbitofrontal cortex show a decline in their ability to attribute higher-order mental states to other people from stories. In particular, they fail to detect faux pas during functional imaging study. Emotion recognition tasks establish priority activation of Brodman Area 47 (orbital area) compared to activation of the medial orbitofrontal region [103]. Tissue loss in BA47 correlates with the inability to recognize negative emotions [104].

It is reported that sections of the left medial prefrontal cortex also contribute significantly to understand the mental state of others [105] or to reasoning about the beliefs and intentions of others [106]. Functional MRI studies demonstrate activation of the amydgala during attribution of mental states and intentions to other people by viewing pictures of their eyes [107].

The wide dissemination of demyelinating lesions and cortical thinning typical of patients with MS often lead to anatomic and functional disorders of the above-mentioned specific brain structures. A subsequent disconnection mechanism leads to a cognitive decline [108]. Single-photon emission computed tomography (SPECT) studies in cognitively impaired patients with MS registered a deficiency of brain perfusion, mainly in the frontal and temporal lobe of the left hemisphere [109]. Positron emission tomography (PET) in these patients registered both global and regional reduction of cerebral glucose metabolism [110, 111]. An increase in the white matter lesion load, especially in the insula, precentral gyrus, prefrontal and temporal cortices, reduces the effectiveness of large-scale brain structural networks in patients with MS, which leads to cognitive deficits [108]. Functional MRI studies point to a positive correlation between the degree of activation of certain cerebral zones during performance of specific cognitive tasks and lesion load. These findings support the notion that increased cortical activity in patients with MS occurs as a result of axonal damage related to MS activity and aims to limit the clinical impact of structural damage [112].

According to Krause et al., the orbitoinsular cluster, which includes the ventral lateral prefrontal cortex (VLPF) and parts of the anterior insula, is crucial to deficits in emotional perception in patients with MS [70], which is one of the most sensitive indications of impaired social cognition. Functional MRI studies have indicated that after initial activation of the early visual fields visual stimuli are selectively processed in a specific region of the fusiform gyrus, the fusiform face area (FFA) and the facial part of the superior temporal sulcus (fSTS) [113]. FFA is activated mostly with invariable traits, which is possibly related to person identification [70, 113], while fSTS activation is more often associated with variable aspects related to the eyes, spoken speech and expression of emotions and intentions [114–116]. The high-level visual temporal cortex projects to a small proportion of amygdala neurons whose answers are relatively selectively modulated by viewing faces compared to other visual stimuli. Functional MRI research has proved that the amygdala is critical for emotion recognition from facial expression, especially with negative emotions, such as fear [117, 118]. The amygdala is involved in the automatic focusing of attention for detecting emotional stimuli and filtering emotionally relevant information through the signs perceived [119, 120]. Thus, it participates in making more complex social decisions in humans [121]. There is evidence that bilateral amygdala damage leads to severely impaired ability for the recognition of fear through facial expression [118, 122]. A study by Jehna et al. provided proof for functional differences between patients with MS and healthy controls concerning the perception of neutral and emotional facial expressions of anger and disgust. These differences were found relatively early in the course of the disease, even in the absence of behavioral differences between subjects and controls. Since the functional changes registered in the occipital areas of patients with MS during recognition of nonemotional faces are usually associated with face processing, the authors explain the excessive activation of the posterior cingulate and precuneus during emotion processing as an additional attentive requirement [88].

As regards the ability to simulate the emotional state of others, the anterior insula, functionally connected to the ventrolateral prefrontal cortex (VLPFC), shows reduced activation in subjects experiencing problems in facial emotion recognition [123]. More difficult cognitive tasks lead to higher activation of the more lateral regions of ventrolateral prefrontal cortex (VLPFC) [70, 124].

During performance of various sociocognitive tasks for mental state attribution, common areas of increased activation in the medial prefrontal gyrus and the temporoparietal junctions are

http://dx.doi.org/10.5772/63465

registered bilaterally, while the area of the medial prefrontal cortex (the paracingulate cortex) is the only region uniquely activated by the performance of ToM tasks [47].

A hypothesis has been developed for explaining social cognition via three related but distinct dimensions of anatomical and functional brain organization [124]. It states that the medial-lateral dimension connects the medial prefrontal cortex (MPFC) (emotional aspects of mental state attribution and emotions) to the lateral prefrontal cortex (LPFC), associated with visuospatial centers supporting externally generated representations (cognitive aspects of mental state attribution and emotions) [125, 126]. The midline posterior-anterior dimension links the "first-order" perceptual substratum for the flow of socioemotional processing (superior temporal sulcus), the posterior insula and the middle ACC to the anterior insula and MPFC, where it is presented again with increased complexity [99, 127] and results in awareness and explicit judgments of affective mental states. The third dimension is the projection from ventral regions of the frontal midline involved mainly in stimulus-driven processes (amygdala, striatum and OFC) to dorsal regions supporting monitoring and reflective processes (dorso-medial and lateral prefrontal cortex) [124, 126]. This means that mental state attributions are supported by various neural structures depending on the type of sociocognitive task and processing demands.

Most MRI studies of patients with MS found a correlation between the cognitive and/or affective disorders, on the one hand, and lesion localization [128], total lesion load [129] or cerebral atrophy, on the other [129, 130]. A significant correlation was also reported between abnormal activities in specific cortical zones on fMRI, on the one hand, and clinical manifestation, conventional MRI findings and behavioral changes, on the other [94]. However, a study of voxel-based lesion symptom mapping did not reveal a significant connection of the total lesion volume to the degree of emotional recognition or to the activation of specific cortical areas during task performance. A statistically significant relationship was discovered between lesions in the left temporal periventricular white matter and decreased accuracy in dealing with cognitive tests, which points to a disturbance in information transmission from the temporal visual processing areas to the frontal regulation areas [70, 131].

Altered patterns of brain activity were found in all clinical phenotypes of MS, including when cognitive abilities were intact and/or restored [112, 132, 133]. However, such research is still insufficient. A recent fMRI study of different forms and stages of MS reported results from performance of face encoding and recognition [94]. In patients with CIS an increased recruitment of the posterior visual area, where face perception and encoding is processed, was revealed. The result was interpreted as an adaptive response of cerebral reorganization for compensating sociocognitive functioning in the early stages of the demyelinating disease. In patients with RRMS, an increased activation of the thalamus, parahippocampal gyrus and right anterior cingulum was reported. In patients with SPMS, an increased recruitment of the frontal fields, associated with higher cognitive functions, was registered. The findings suggest disadaptation and inadequate coping with cognitive tasks in a social context as the disease progresses. MRI findings show that in different clinical subtypes of MS the decreased cortical recruitment often correlates with increased T2 lesion load [112, 134].

Functional MRI studies in patients with MS prove that cortical plastic changes are a dynamic phenomenon that can be modulated by external factors. Unfortunately, fMRI studies of social cognitive abilities are still scarce, especially in patients with MS. Accumulation of data from future studies will allow early registering of the specifics of morphological and functional brain changes. This would facilitate the mapping of individual strategies for adequate treatment and rehabilitation of each patient.

7. Discussion

People are profoundly social creatures, and therefore, successful social communication is crucial to their satisfactory lifestyle. The quality of this communication depends on their ability to detect emotional and cognitive processes in others and to understand their own internal state. These two features of social cognition—affective and mental—are the basis for empathy and ToM (mentalization). During social interactions, these different levels of social cognitive response are highly intertwined and each is influenced by the other.

Between 40% and 70% of patients with MS are affected by cognitive impairments [5], which are linked to a significant decline in activities of daily living. Despite the rapidly growing amount of research establishing frequent social cognitive deficits in such patients, there is still no statistics on the frequency of this type of disturbances. We set ourselves the goal of providing an overview of studies in this scientific area and contributing, through summarizing the results, to a better understanding of the specifics of social cognitive disorders and the way they determine the functional outcome and quality of life of patients with MS. We also made attempts at discussing controversies, discovering outstanding issues and outlining a framework for future research.

A wide range of literary sources report that the pathology of white matter in MS has the potential not only to disrupt the basic parameters of cognitive functions but also to hinder important social perception skills. The accumulated data suggest that the neuronal processes of ToM and empathy are performed in different brain networks which partially overlap [56]. No significant controversies exist concerning the pathophysiological significance of altered brain activation patterns in MS [112]. Rather, various studies complement the knowledge on functional processing in specific brain areas responsible for the different aspects of social cognition. Common activation areas include the medial prefrontal cortex, the temporoparietal junction and the temporal poles. ToM stimuli lead to increased activation of the lateral orbitofrontal cortex, the middle frontal gyrus, the cuneus and the superior temporal gyrus, while empathy is associated with enhanced activations of the paracingulate, the anterior and posterior cingulate and the amygdale [135]. A more pronounced global and regional cortical atrophy in the left hemisphere, which is a frequent finding in MS [136], suggests more severe ToM deterioration. However, no studies have been conducted yet of the functional relation between empathy and ToM in MS.

Pathways composed of white matter, which have a key role in coordinating the information flow between different regions of gray matter of the brain, are particularly vulnerable in MS

[108]. Patients with lesions located in the ventromedial prefrontal cortex demonstrate selective deficits in affective ToM. Lesions in the inferior frontal gyrus are associated with extremely impaired empathy and emotion recognition [137].

ToM tests based on verbal and nonverbal stimuli not only serve for clinical evaluation of social cognitive impairments, but are also at the core of studying the functional anatomy of ToM in fMRI research [47]. The MPFC, associated with mentalizing tasks, activates whenever the person is attending to certain states of the self or others. The MPFC is equally active when the person is engaged in true beliefs, knowledge of the world based on past experience applied to the current situation, and partially in personal observations and behavioural predictions (STS) [48] There is increasing evidence of functional cortical changes in the early stages of MS, even after a single clinical episode [138, 139], when expansion and recruitment of additional cortical fields as common compensation of brain damage are registered [112].

The ability to decode specific facial emotions and ToM skills, which largely determines social communication in the real world, was first studied in MS patients in 2009 by Henry et al. For the first time, researchers presented clear evidence of increased difficulties in both aspects of emotion understanding, as well as in mental state attribution. Although the authors realized that their research was limited due to the lack of study of structural brain changes, their data were the first to establish a correlation between cognitive capacities and important aspects of emotion perception [45].

The diffuse demyelination and atrophy of both gray and white matter typical of MS lead to pronounced deficits in empathy and ToM. While white matter lesion load accounts only for some cognitive deficits in MS, this type of disorders can be better explained through pathological processes affecting gray matter, which are revealed in very early stages of the disease [140–142]. A significant positive correlation was established between neocortical volume and cognitive damage in patients with RRMS [143], as the gray matter atrophy occurring faster than white matter atrophy and, as recent research indicates, probably playing a central role in the emerging and deepening of cognitive deficits [144].

New technologies can help maximize our ability to assess cerebral integrity in MS. Regardless of the rapid development of imaging technology for detecting the earliest possible morphological abnormalities in MS, the focus of research has primarily been on the physical disability and/or general cognition. Unfortunately, the study of social cognition still remains outside the scope of such type of research. We strive to contribute to a better understanding of the neurobiological correlates of social cognitive deficits, hoping in this way to provide opportunities for future research to develop medicinal and therapeutic strategies for modifying the pathological brain processes involved in these deficits. This would increase the level of empathy and ToM skills in patients with MS and could also facilitate their successful social adaptation.

On the other hand, morphological damage in MS is highly variable both with regard to the load, location and size of demyelinating lesions and in relation to individual global and regional cortical thinning. The particular phenotype of MS introduces additional specific features of brain damage. This explains the heterogeneity of social cognition impairments in terms of their severity and regarding the predominant disturbance of certain social cognitive domains. According to Henry, while testing empathy and ToM skills, it is also recommended to perform in parallel direct mapping of underlying MS-related neuropathology for detecting a link between structural brain pathology and social cognitive impairments. Pöttgen established a deficient ability to reason about the mental state of others (ToM) and to have insight into the emotional stages and feelings of others (empathy) in the early stages of RRMS [21, 22], even in patients who have no substantial neuropsychological deficits. Emotional prosody comprehension may also be disrupted in the early stages of RRMS [6]. It is argued that this is the earliest social cognitive impairment in patients with MS. Deteriorated emotional perception at this early stage can create a difficulty in perceiving nuances, such as sarcasm, irony and sincerity, which may lead to interpersonal problems. To confirm these observations, international research with larger groups of patients is required. Data from this study indicate that one year after diagnosing a patient with CIS and RRMS, they experience diminished power of attention and memory speed, which is related to a capacity for fewer working hours, fatigue, depression and may have a negative impact, as opposed to self-efficacy, which affects working hours positively. The level of ToM abilities and their relation to the above-mentioned consequences have not been followed up.

Information on social cognition impairments and different forms of MS is still scarce. The main controversies that we encountered in the course of reviewing the material on the topic are about how the grade of disturbance of social cognition skills relates to the state of general cognition, on the one hand, and to the grade of physical disability and/or the duration of the disease, on the other. These issues remain disputable due to the small size of patient cohorts and the lack of homogeneity within the groups of conducted studies. Moreover, the majority of studies on social cognition skills in MS assess the patients' social cognitive skills at a given point without following up on their development over time. This prevents us from making conclusions about their dynamics during the course of the disease or taking into account the effect of a therapeutic and/or rehabilitation approach. Extensive long-term follow-up studies with well-defined inclusion criteria, consistent sample characteristics and a wide range of clinical and imaging measurements could establish which domains of ToM change in the course of the disease, in what way and at to what extent.

We devoted a lot of time to reviewing studies on social cognition also in other neurodegenerative and mental diseases. We were impressed with the extensive research in skills for interpersonal problem solving, for recognizing social cues, for detecting situational characteristics and for solving situation connection tasks. Our opinion is that a similar approach towards social cognitive impairments in MS would throw additional light on the objective evaluation of the patient's dealing with real situations in a social context. Even studies on the relation between social cognition disturbances and functional outcome define this relation in general terms, without specifying which domains of social cognition should refer to which functional outcome domains. Resolving these issues in the MS field is a challenge for scientists requiring uniform strategies, long-term follow-up, creativity and interdisciplinary cooperation among researchers.

Two longitudinal studies in schizophrenia provide evidence for the predictive role of emotional perception in the functional outcome at a later point in time [145, 146]. Their findings support the causal relationship between social cognition and functional outcome, which gives us good grounds for drawing attention to the opportunity for similar long-term studies in patients with MS. Surprisingly, despite the chronic nature of MS, which affects young people and inevitably disables them both physically and neuropsychologically, psychotherapeutic or psychoeducational programs are still widely lacking for MS, while being successfully implemented for other neuropsychiatric diseases associated with social cognition deficiency, such as alcoholism, schizophrenia, autism, Parkinson's disease and depression [22].

Irrespective of the limitations of most studies, they share the unanimous opinion that social cognition impairments in MS are a common finding in the early stages of the disease and are characterized by clinical significance. Functional MRI often objectifies deteriorations within the mentalizing network before structural brain disorders are detected. The cortical reorganization reported in these studies may serve as an objective marker for follow-up over time. Unfortunately, fMRI is not yet a routine method of examination due to the high cost, study complexity and lack of unified standards of interpretation.

8. Conclusion

Social cognitive impairments are a common finding in patients with MS and are often manifested at the initial stages of the disease. Both empathy and ToM deficits, regardless of physical disability, lead to psychosocial consequences such as failure to achieve life goals, limitations to employment and leisure activities, inadequacy in social relationships and daily activities [58, 61]. The preservation of a better quality of life in patients with MS requires special attention to the above mentioned aspects of the disease. Timely recognition of the deficit and adequate rehabilitation of social cognition would help patients enjoy a fulfilling social life for a longer time.

Author details

Valentina Ignatova[1*], Lyudmila Todorova[2] and Jivko Surchev[3]

*Address all correspondence to: valyaig@abv.bg

1 National Heart Hospital-MHAT, Clinic of neurology, Sofia, Bulgaria

2 Institute of Biophysics and Biomedical Engineering, Bulgarian Academy of Sciences, Sofia, Bulgaria

3 Medical University of Sofia, Department of Neurosurgery, St Ivan Rilski University Hospital, Clinic of Neurosurgery, Sofia, Bulgaria

References

[1] Chiaravalloti N, DeLuca J. Cognitive impairment in multiple sclerosis. Lancet Neurol. 2008;7:1139–1151.

[2] Langdon DW. Cognition in multiple sclerosis. Curr Opin Neurol. 2011;24:244–249.

[3] Pelosi L, Geesken JM, Holly M, Hayward M, Blumhardt LD. Working memory impairment in early multiple-sclerosis. Evidence from an event-related potential study of patients with clinically isolated myelopathy. Brain. 1997;120:2039–2058.

[4] Piras MR, Magnano I, Canu ED, et al. Longitudinal study of cognitive dysfunction in multiple sclerosis: neuropsychological, neuroradiological, and neurophysiological findings. J Neurol Neurosurg Psychiatry. 2003;74:878–885.

[5] DeLuca G, Yates R, Beale H, Morrow S. Cognitive impairment in multiple sclerosis: clinical, radiologic and pathologic insights. Brain Pathol. 2015;25:79–98.

[6] Kraemer M, Herold M, Uekermann J, et al. Perception of affective prosody in patients at an early stage of relapsing-remitting multiple sclerosis. J Neuropsychol. 2013;7(1): 91–106.

[7] Santiesteban I, White S, Cook J, Gilbert SJ, Heyes C, et al. Training social cognition: from imitation to theory of mind. Cognition. 2012;122:228–235.

[8] Amato MP, Zipoli V, Portaccio E. Multiple sclerosis-related cognitive changes: a review of cross-sectional and longitudinal studies. J Neurol Sci. 2006;245(1–2):41–46.

[9] Dulau C. Social cognition and multiple sclerosis. In: Brochet B, editor. Neuropsychiatric symptoms of inflammatory demyelinating diseases. Switzerland: Springer International Publishing; 2015. p. 213–226. DOI: 10.1007/978-3-319-18464-7-15

[10] Julian LJ, Vella L, Vollmer T, Hadjimichael O, Mohr DC. Employment in multiple sclerosis. J Neurol. 2008;255(9):1354–1360.

[11] Rao SM, Ellington L, Nauertz T, et al. Cognitive dysfunction I n multiple sclerosis. II. Impact of employment and social functioning. Neurology. 1991;41:692–696.

[12] Burgess M, editor. Multiple sclerosis: theory and practice for nurses. London: Whurr; 2002.

[13] Augoustinos M, Walker I, Donaghue N, editors. Social cognition: an integrated introduction. 3rd ed. Thousand Oaks, Calif: Sage; 2014.

[14] Fiske ST, Taylor SE, editors. Social cognition. 2nd ed. New York: McGraw-Hill; 1991.

[15] Decety J, Jackson PL. The functional architecture of human empathy. Behav Cogn Neurosci Rev. 2004;3(2):71–100.

[16] Titchener E, editor. Experimental psychology of the thought process. New York: Macmillan; 1909.

[17] Wispé L. History of the concept of empathy. In: Eisenberg N, Strayer J, editors. Empathy and its development. Cambridge: Cambridge University Press; 1987.

[18] Ickes W, editor. Empathic accuracy. New York: Guilford; 1997.

[19] Samson AC. The influence of empathizing and systemizing on humor processing: theory of mind and humor. Humor. 2012;25(1):75–98.

[20] Baron-Cohen S, Richler J, Bisarya D, Gurunathan N, Wheelwright S. The systemizing quotient: an investigation of adults with Asperger Syndrome or high-functioning autism, and normal sex differences. In: Frith U, Hill E, editors. Autism: mind and brain. Oxford: Oxford University Press; 2003. p. 161–186.

[21] Pöttgen J, Dziobek I, Reh S, Heesen C, Gold SM. Impaired social cognition in multiples clerosis. J Neurol Neurosurg Psychiatry. 2013;84(5):523–528.

[22] Kraemer M, Herold M, Uekermann J, Kis B, Wiltfang J, Daum I, Dziobek I, Berlit P, Diehl R, Abdel-Hamid M. Theory of mind and empathy in patients at an early stage of relapsing remitting multiple sclerosis. Clin Neurol Neurosurg. 2013;115:1016–1022.

[23] Brothers L, Ring B. A neuroethological framework for the representation of minds. J Cogn Neurosci 1992;4:107–118.

[24] Ickes W, editor. Everyday mind reading: understanding what other people think and feel. Amherst, NY: Prometheus Books; 2003.

[25] Davis MH, Kraus LA. Personality and empathic accuracy. In: Ickes W, editor. Empathic accuracy. New York: The Guilford Press; 1997. p. 144–168.

[26] Abu-Akel A, Shamay-Tsoory S. Neuroanatomical and neurochemical bases of theory of mind. Neuropsychologia. 2011;49(11):2971–2984.

[27] Apperly IA, Butterfill S. Do humans have two systems to track beliefs and belief like states? Psychol Rev. 2009;116:953–970.

[28] Frith CD, Frith U. Implicit and explicit processes in social cognition. Neuron. 2008;603(3):503–510.

[29] Davis MH. Measuring individual differences in empathy: evidence for a multidimensional approach. J Personal Soc Psychol. 1983;44:113–126.

[30] Hemmerdinger JM, Stoddart S, Lilford R. A systematic review of tests of empathy in medicine. BMC Med Educ. 2007;7:1–8.

[31] Hogan R. Development of an empathy scale. J Consult Clin Psychol. 1969;33:307–316.

[32] Mehrabian A, editor. Manual for the balanced emotional empathy scale (BEES). Available from Albert Mehrabian ed. 1130, Alta Mesa Road, Monterey, CA 93940; 2000.

[33] Neff KD. Development and validation of a scale to measure self-compassion. Self Identity. 2003;2:223–250.

[34] Sprecher S. Compassionate love for close others and humanity. J Soc Pers Relationsh. 2005;22(5):629–651.

[35] Lawrence EJ, Shaw P, Baker D, Baron-Cohen S, David A. Measuring empathy: reliability and validity of the Empathy Quotient. Psychol Med. 2004;34(05):911–920.

[36] Davis MH. A multidimensional approach to individual differences in empathy. JSAS Cat Sel Doc Psychol. 1980;10:85.

[37] Dziobek I, Rogers K, Fleck S, Bahnemann M, Heekeren HR, Wolf OT, et al. Dissociation of cognitive and emotional empathy in adults with Asperger syndrome using the Multifaceted Empathy Test (MET). J Autism Dev Disord. 2008;38:464–473.

[38] Feinstein AJ, DeLuca, Baune BT, Filippi M, Lassman H. Cognitive and neuropsychiatric disease manifestations in MS. Mult Scler Relat Disord. 2013;2(1):4–12.

[39] Stone VE, Baron-Cohen S, Calder A, Keane J, Young A. Acquired theory of mind impairments in individuals with bilateral amygdala lesions. Neuropsychologia. 2003;41:209–220.

[40] Dziobek I, Fleck S, Kalbe E, Rogers K, Hassenstab J, Brand M, Kessler J, Woike JK, Wolf OT, Convit A. Introducing MASC: a movie for the assessment of social cognition. J Autism Dev Disord. 2006;36:623–636.

[41] Rutherford MD, Baron-Cohen S, Wheelwright S. Reading the mind in the voice: a study with normal adults and adults with Asperger syndrome and high functioning autism. J Autism Developmental Disord. 2002;32:189–194.

[42] Kerr SL, Neale JM. Emotion perception in schizophrenia: specific deficit or further evidence of generalized poor performance? J Abnorm Psychol. 1993;102:312–318.

[43] Vellante M, Baron-Cohen S, Melis M, et al. The "Reading the Mind in the Eyes" test: systematic review of psychometric properties and a validation study in Italy. Cogn Neuropsychiatr. 2013; 18(4):326-354

[44] Scherer P, Penner IK, Rohr A, et al. The faces symbol test, a newly developed screening instrument to assess cognitive decline related to multiple sclerosis: first results of the Berlin Multi-Centre FST Validation Study. Mult Scler. 2007;13:402–411.

[45] Henry JD, Phillips LH, Beatty WW, McDonald S, Longley WA, Joscelyne A, et al. Evidence for deficits in facial affect recognition and theory of mind in multiple sclerosis. J Int Neuropsychol Soc. 2009;15(2):277–285.

[46] Golan O, Baron-Cohen S. Systemizing empathy: teaching adults with Asperger syndrome or high-functioning autism to recognize complex emotions using interactive multimedia. Dev Psychopathol. 2006;18:591–617.

[47] Gallagher HL, Happe F, Brunswick N, Fletcher PC, Frith U, Frith CD. Reading the mind in cartoons and stories: an fMRI study of 'theory of mind' in verbal and nonverbal tasks. Neuropsychologia. 2000;38:11–21.

[48] Frith U, Frith CD. Development and neurophysiology of mentalizing. Phil Trans R Soc Lond B. 2003;358:459–473.

[49] Ouellet J, Scherzer PB, Rouleau I, Me'tras P, Bertrand-Gauvin C, Djerroud N, et al. Assessment of social cognition in patients with multiple sclerosis. J Int Neuropsychol Soc. 2010;1:287–296.

[50] Genova H, Cagna C, Chiaravalloti N, DeLuca J, Lengenfelder J. Dynamic assessment of social cognition in individuals with multiple sclerosis: a pilot study. J Int Neuropsychol Soc. 2016;22(1):83–88.

[51] Ihnen GH, Penn, DL, Corrigan PW, Martin J. Social perception and social skill in schizophrenia. Psychiatry Res. 1998;80:275–286.

[52] Kee KS, Kern, RS, Green MF. Perception of emotion and neurocognitive functioning in schizophrenia: what's the link? Psychiatry Res. 1998;81:57–65.

[53] Taselli S, et al. The microfoundations of organizational social networks: a review and an agenda for future research. J Manag. 2015;41(5):1361–1387.

[54] Gong P, Liu J, Li S, Zhou X. Dopamine beta-hydroxylase gene modulates individuals' empathic ability. Soc Cogn Affect Neurosci. 2014;9:1341–1345.

[55] Benedict RHB, Priore RL, Miller C, et al. Personality disorder in MS correlates with cognitive impairment. J Neuropsychiatry Clin Neurosci. 2001;13:70–76.

[56] Banati M, Sandor J, Mike A, et al. Social cognition and theory of mind in patients with relapsing-remitting multiple sclerosis. Eur J Neurol. 2010;17:426–433.

[57] Raes F. Rumination and worry as mediators of the relationship between self-compassion and depression and anxiety. Personal Individ Differ. 2010;48:757–761.

[58] Dennison L, Moss-Morris R, Chalder T. A review of psychological correlates of adjustment in patients with multiple sclerosis. Clin Psychol Rev. 2009;29:141–153.

[59] Mostert S, Kesselring J. Effects of a short-term exercise training program on aerobic fitness, fatigue, health perception and activity level of subjects with multiple sclerosis. Mult Scler. 2002;8:161–168.

[60] Beatty WW, Goodkin DE, Weir WS, Staton RD, Monson N, Beatty PA. Affective judgements by patients with Parkinson's disease or chronic progressive multiple sclerosis. Bull Psychon Soc. 1989;27:361–364.

[61] Prochnow D, Donell J, Schafer R, Jorgens S, Hartung HP, et al. Alexithymia and impaired facial affect recognition in multiple sclerosis. J Neurol. 2011;258:1683–1688.

[62] Sifneos PE. The prevalence of 'alexithymic' characteristics in psychosomatic patients. Psychother Psychosom. 1973;22(2):255–262.

[63] Petropoulo H, Montreuil M, Truelle Jl, Lyon-Caen O, et al. Étude émotionnelle et cognitive de 40 patients attaints de sclérose en plaques récente. In: Atelier de conjoncture: développement, fonctionnement: perspective historico-culturelle. Société Française de Psychologie; 13–14 octobre; Paris. 2002.

[64] FeldmanHall O, Dalgleish T, Mobbs D. Alexithymia decreases altruism in real social decisions. Cortex. 2012;49:899–904.

[65] Montreuil M, Petropoulo H. Humeur et émotions dans la sclérose en plaques. Neuropsy News. 2003;2:91–96.

[66] Pelletier J, Montreuil M, Habib M, Ali Cherif A, et al. Alexithymia and multiple sclerosis: alteration of interhemispheric transfer. Eur J Neurol. 1996;3:63.

[67] Montel S, Bungener C. Les troubles de l'humeur et des émotions dans la sclérose en plaques: une revue de la littérature. Rev Neurol Mood and emotional disorders in Multiple Sclerosis: a literature review(Paris). 2007;163:27–37.

[68] Said CP, Haxby JV, Todorov A. Brain systems for assessing the affective value of faces. Philos Trans R Soc Lond B Biol Sci. 2011;366(1571):1660–1670.

[69] Adolphs R. Social cognition and the human brain. Trends Cogn Sci. 1999;3:469–479.

[70] Krause M, Wendt J, Dressel A, Berneiser J, Kessler C, Hamm AO, Lotze M. Prefrontal function associated with impaired emotion recognition in patients with multiple sclerosis. Behav Brain Res. 2009;205(1):280–285.

[71] Phillips LH, Henry JD, Scott C, Summers F, Whyte M, Cook M. Specific impairments of emotion perception in multiple sclerosis. Neuropsychology. 2011;25(1):131–136.

[72] Kano M, Fukudo S, Gyoba J. Specific brain processing of facial expressions in people with alexithymia: an H215O-PET study. Brain. 2003;126:1474–1484.

[73] Parker JDA, Taylor GJ, Bagby RM. Alexithymia and the recognition of facial expressions of emotion. Psychother Psychosom. 1993;59:197–202.

[74] Lane RD, Sechrest L, Riedel R, Shapiro DE, Kaszniak AW. Pervasive emotion recognition deficit common to alexithymia and the repressive coping style. Psychosom Med. 2000;62:492–501.

[75] Beatty WW, Orbelo DM, Sorocco KH, Ross ED. Comprehension of affective prosody in multiple sclerosis. Mult Scler. 2003;9:148–153.

[76] Chakrabarti B, Baron-Cohen S. Empathizing: neurocognitive developmental mechanisms and individual differences. Prog Brain Res. 2006;156:403–417.

[77] Premack D, Woodruff G. Does the chimpanzee have a theory of mind? Behav Brain Sci. 1978;4:515–526.

[78] Henry A, Tourbah A, Chaunu MP, et al. Social cognition impairments in relapsing–remitting multiple sclerosis. J Int Neuropsychol Soc. 2011;17:1122–1131.

[79] Phillips LH, Beatty WW, et al. Evidence for deficits in facial affect recognition and theory of mind in multiple sclerosis. J Int Neuropsychol Soc. 2009;15:277–285.

[80] Jehna M, Neuper C, Petrovic K, Wallner-Blazek M, Schmidt R, Fuchs S. An exploratory study on emotion recognition in patients with a clinically isolated syndrome and multiple sclerosis. Clin Neurol Neurosurg. 2010;112(6):482–484.

[81] Charvet LE, Cleary RE, Vazquez K, et al. Social cognition in pediatric-onset multiple sclerosis (MS). Mult Sclr J. 2014;20:1478–1484.

[82] Gleichgerrcht E, Tomashitis B, Sinay V. The relationship between alexithymia, empathy and moral judgment in patients with multiple sclerosis. Eur J Neurol. 2015;22(9):1295–1303.

[83] Roca M, Manes F, Gleichgerrcht E, Ibáñez A, González de Toledo ME, Marenco V, Bruno D, Torralva T, Sinay V. Cognitive but not affective theory of mind deficits in mild relapsing-remitting multiple sclerosis. Cogn Behav Neurol. 2014;27(1):25–30.

[84] Dulau C. Existe-t-il vraiment une atteinte de la cognition sociale dans la sclerose en plaques? [thesis]. Hum Health Pathol. 2014. Available from: <dumas-01089147>

[85] Zakzanis KK. Distinct neurocognitive profiles in multiple sclerosis subtypes. Arch Clin Neuropsychol. 2000;15:115–136.

[86] Pakenham KI, Cox S. The dimensional structure of benefit finding in multiple sclerosis and relations with positive and negative adjustment: a longitudinal study. Psychol Health. 2009;24:373–393.

[87] Berneiser J, Wendt J, Grothe M, et al. Impaired recognition of emotional facial expressions in patients with multiple sclerosis. Mult Scler Relat Disord. 2014;3(4):482–488.

[88] Jehna M, Langkammer C, Wallner-Blazek M, et al. Cognitively preserved MS patients demonstrate functional differences in processing neutral and emotional faces. Brain Imaging Behav. 2011;5(4):241–251.

[89] Brothers L. The social brain: a project for integrating primate behaviour and neurophysiology in a new domain. Concepts Neurosci. 1990;1:27–51.

[90] Prinz W. Perception and action planning. Eur J Cogn Psychol. 1997;9:129–154.

[91] Rizzolatti G, Craighero L. The mirror neuron system. Annu Rev Neurosci. 2004;27:169–172.

[92] Gallesse V, Metzinger T. Motor ontology: the representational reality of goals, actions and selves. Philos Psychol. 2003;13(3):365–388.

[93] Gallesse V, Fadiga L, Fogassi L, Rizzolatti G. Action recognition in the premotor cortex. Brain. 1996;119:593–609.

[94] Vacchi L, Rocca M, Riccitelli GC, Rodegher M. Processing face encoding in multiple sclerosis: a fMRI investigation (P6. 134). Neurology. 2015 April 6;84(14 Supplement):P6.134.

[95] Mike A, Strammer E, Aradi M, Orsi G, Perlaki G, Hajnal A, et al. Disconnection mechanism and regional cortical atrophy contribute to impaired processing of facial expressions and theory of mind in multiple sclerosis: a structural MRI study. PloS One. 2013 Dec 13;8(12):e82422.

[96] Ross ED, Mesulam MM. Dominant language functions of the right hemisphere? Prosody and emotional gesturing. Arch Neurol. 1979;36:144–148.

[97] Buchanan TW, Lutz K, Mirzazade S, Specht K, Shah NJ, Zilles K, Jancke L. Recognition of emotional prosody and verbal components of spoken language: an fMRI study. Cogn Brain Res. 2000;9:227–238.

[98] Abdel-Hamid M, Lehmkamper C, Sonntag C, Juckel G, Daum I, Brune M. Theory of Mind in schizophrenia: the role of clinical symptomatology and neurocognition in understanding other people's thoughts and intentions. Psychiatry Res. 2009;165:19–26.

[99] Amodio DM, Frith CD. Meeting of minds: the medial frontal cortex and social cognition. Nat Rev Neurosci. 2006;7(4):268–277.

[100] Fiske ST, Markus HR. Facing social class: how societal rank influences interaction. New York, NY: Russell Sage Foundation, 2012.

[101] Von Economo C, Koskinas G, editors. Die Cytoarchitectonik der Hirnrinde des erwachsenen Menschen.Berlin, Springer: 1925.

[102] Allman JM, Watson KK, Tetreault NA, Hakeem AY. Intuition and autism: a possible role for Von Economo neurons. Trends Cogn Sci. 2005;9:367–373.

[103] Steele JD, Lawrie SM. Segregation of cognitive and emotional function in the prefrontal cortex: a stereotactic meta-analysis. Neuroimage. 2004;21:868–875.

[104] Rosen HJ, Wilson MR, Schauer GF, et al. Neuroanatomical correlates of impaired recognition of emotion in dementia. Neuropsychologia. 2006;44:365–373.

[105] Stone VE, Baron-Cohen S, Knight RT. Frontal lobe contributions to theory of mind. J Cogn Neurosci. 1998;10:640–656.

[106] Goel V, et al. Modeling other minds. Neuro Report. 1995;6:1741–1746.

[107] Baron-Cohen S, et al. Social intelligence in the normal and autistic brain: an fMRI study. Eur J Neurosci. 1999;11:1891–1898.

[108] He Y, Dagher A, Chen Z, Charil A, Zijdenbos A, Worsley K, Evans A. Impaired small-world efficiency in structural cortical networks in multiple sclerosis associated with white matter lesion load. Brain. 2009;132(12):3366–3379.

http://dx.doi.org/10.5772/63465

[109] Paulesu E, Perani D, Fazio F, et al. Functional basis of memory impairment in multiple sclerosis: a [18F]FDG PET study. NeuroImage. 1996;4:87–96.

[110] Blinkenberg M, Rune K, Jensen CV, et al. Cortical cerebral metabolism correlates with MRI lesion load and cognitive dysfunction in MS. Neurology. 2000;54:558–564.

[111] Penner IK, Opwis, Kappos L . Relation between functional brain imaging, cognitive impairment and cognitive rehabilitation in patients with multiple sclerosis. J Neurol. 2007;254(2):II53–II57.

[112] Pantano P, Mainero C, Caramia F. Functional brain reorganization in multiple sclerosis: evidence from fMRI studies. J Neuroimaging. 2006;16:104–114.

[113] Kanwisher N, Yovel G. The fusiform face area: a cortical region specialized for the perception of faces. Philos Trans R Soc Lond B Biol Sci. 2006;361:2109–28.

[114] Allison T, Puce A, McCarthy G. Social perception from visual cues: role of the STS region. Trends Cogn Sci. 2000;4:267–278.

[115] Thompson JC, Hardee JE, Panayiotou A, Crewther D, Puce A. Common and distinct brain activation to viewing dynamic sequences of face and hand movements. Neuroimage. 2007;37(3):966–973.

[116] Esterman M, Yantis S. Perceptual expectation evokes category-selective cortical activity. Cereb Cortex. 2010;20(5):1245–1253.

[117] Morris JS, et al. A differential neural response in the human amygdala to fearful and happy facial expressions. Nature. 1996;383:812–815.

[118] Adolphs R, et al. Impaired recognition of emotion in facial expressions following bilateral damage to the human amygdala. Nature. 1994;372:669–672.

[119] Vuilleumier P, Pourtois G. Distributed and interactive brain mechanisms during emotion face perception: evidence from functional neuroimaging. Neuropsychologia. 2007;45:174–194.

[120] Adolphs R, Spezio M. Role of the amygdala in processing visual social stimuli. Prog Brain Res. 2006;156:363–378.

[121] Buchel C, Morris J Dolan RJ, Friston KJ. Brain systems mediating aversive conditioning: an event-related fMRI study. Neuron. 1998;20:947–957.

[122] Young AW, Aggleton JP, Hellawell DJ, Johnson M, Broks P, Hanley JR. Face processing impairments after amygdalotomy. Brain. 1995;118(Pt 1):15–24.

[123] Singer T, Seymour B, O'Doherty J, Kaube H, Dolan RJ, Frith CD. Empathy for pain involves the affective but not sensory components of pain. Science. 2004;303:1157–1162.

[124] Olsson A, Ochsner KN. The role of social cognition in emotion. Trends Cogn Sci. 2008;12:65–71.

[125] Lieberman MD. Social cognitive neuroscience: a review of core processes. Annu Rev Psychol. 2007;58:259–289.

[126] Ochsner KN et al. Reflecting upon feelings: an fMRI study of neural systems supporting the attribution of emotion to self and other. J Cogn Neurosci. 2004;16:1746–1772.

[127] Burgess PW, et al.. The gateway hypothesis of rostral prefrontal cortex (area 10) function. Trends Cogn Sci. 2007;11:290–298.

[128] Reischies FM, Baum K, Nehrig C, Schorner W. Psychopathological symptoms and magnetic resonance imaging findings in multiple sclerosis. Biol Psychiatry. 1993;33:676–678.

[129] Bobholz JA, Rao SM, Lobeck L, et al. fMRI study of episodic memory in relapsingremitting MS: correlation with T2 lesion volume. Neurology. 2006;67:1640–1645.

[130] Lazeron RH, Boringa JB, Schouten M, et al. Brain atrophy and lesion load as explaining parameters for cognitive impairment in multiple sclerosis. Mult Scler. 2005;11:524–531.

[131] Cavada C, Company T, Tejedor J, Cruz-Rizzolo RJ, Reinoso-Suarez F. The anatomical connections of the macaque monkey orbitofrontal cortex. A review. Cereb Cortex. 2000;10:220–242.

[132] Audoin B, Ibarrola D, Ranjeva JP, et al. Compensatory cortical activation observed by fMRI during a cognitive task at the earliest stage of MS. Hum Brain Mapp. 2003;20:51–58.

[133] Staffen W, Mair A, Zauner H, et al. Cognitive function and fMRI in patients with multiple sclerosis: evidence for compensatory cortical activation during an attention task. Brain. 2002;125:1275–1282.

[134] Lee M, Reddy H, Johansen-Berg H, et al. The motor cortex shows adaptive functional changes to brain injury from multiple sclerosis. Ann Neurol. 2000;47:606–613.

[135] Völlm BA, Taylor AN, Richardson P, Corcoran R, Stirling J, McKie S, et al. Neuronal correlates of theory of mind and empathy: a functional magnetic resonance imaging study in a nonverbal task. Neuroimage. 2006;29(1):90–98.

[136] Narayana PA, Govindarajan KA, Goel P, et al. Regional cortical thickness in relapsing remitting multiple sclerosis: a multi-center study. NeuroImage Clin. 2012;2:120–131.

[137] Shamay-Tsoory SG, Aharon-Peret J, Perry D. Two systems for empathy: a double dissociation between emotional and cognitive empathy in inferior frontal gyrus versus ventromedial prefrontal lesions. Brain. 2009;132:617–627.

[138] Pantano P, Iannetti GD, Caramia F, et al. Cortical motor reorganization after a single clinical attack of multiple sclerosis. Brain. 2002;125:1607–1615.

http://dx.doi.org/10.5772/63465

[139] Rocca MA, Mezzapesa DM, Falini A, et al. Evidence for axonal pathology and adaptive cortical reorganization in patients at presentation with clinically isolated syndromes suggestive of multiple sclerosis. Neuroimage. 2003;18:847–855.

[140] Amato MP, Bartolozzi ML, Zipoli V, Portaccio E, Mortilla M, Guidi L, Siracusa G, Sorbi S, Federico A, De Stefano N. Neocortical volume decrease in relapsing-remitting MS patients with mild cognitive impairment. Neurology. 2004;63(1):89–93.

[141] Lazeron RH, Langdon DW, Filippi M, van Waesberghe JH, Stevenson VL, Boringa JB, Origgi D, Thompson AJ, Falautano M, Polman CH, et al. Neuropsychological impairment in multiple sclerosis patients: the role of (juxta)cortical lesion on FLAIR. Mult Scler. 2000;6(4):280–285.

[142] Rovaris M, Filippi M, Minicucci L, Iannucci G, Santuccio G, Possa F, Comi G. Cortical/subcortical disease burden and cognitive impairment in patients with multiple sclerosis. AJNR Am J Neuroradiol. 2000;21(2):402–408.

[143] Amato MP, Ponziani G, Siracusa G, Scorbi S. Cognitive dysfunction in early-onset multiple sclerosis: a reappraisal after 10 years. Arch Neurol. 2001;58:1602–1606.

[144] Pirko I, Lucchinetti CF, Sriram S, Bakshi R. Gray matter involvement in multiple sclerosis. Neurology. 2007;68:634–642.

[145] Brekke JS, Kay DD, Kee KS, Green MF. Biosocial pathways to functional outcome in schizophrenia. Schizophr Res. 2005;80:213–225.

[146] Kee KS, Green MF, Mintz J, Brekke JS. Is emotion processing a predictor of functional outcome in schizophrenia? Schizophr Bull. 2003;29:487–497.

Sex Hormones and Multiple Sclerosis

Anastasiya G. Trenova

Additional information is available at the end of the chapter

http://dx.doi.org/10.5772/63630

Abstract

Experimental and clinical data about the influence of sex hormones on the course of multiple sclerosis (MS) grow rapidly during the past two decades. Estrogens, progesterone, and androgens have been shown to ameliorate experimental autoimmune encephalomyelitis (EAE) in animals, and pregnancy in women is associated with a dramatic reduction in disease activity. Immunomodulatory and neuroprotective properties of sex hormones are the most probable underlying mechanisms, creating a background for testing similar hormonal treatments in humans. Several pilot studies in this field present promising results, but larger trials are necessary to identify the adverse events and to estimate precisely the place of sex steroids in multiple sclerosis therapeutic strategies.

The objective of this chapter is to summarize the recent advances in the research about the effects of sex steroids in EAE and MS and to create a ground for the development of more powerful treatments in the future.

Keywords: EAE, immune modulation, multiple sclerosis, neuroprotection, sex hormones

1. Introduction

Gender differences, observed in many aspects of autoimmune diseases, also concern multiple sclerosis (MS) to a high degree. Experimental and clinical data have suggested a role of sex hormones in the pathogenesis of MS and disclose additional therapeutic possibilities.

Initially, empirical observations, such as female prevalence in susceptibility to MS, differences in the clinical presentation between men and women, and the effect of pregnancy on the course of the disease drew attention on the effects of sex hormones in the development of the pathological process in MS. Female gender is now regarded as an independent risk factor for the development of the disease, with female:male ratio 3:1, and even higher (3.2:1) in subjects with MS onset before age 20 [1, 2]. Despite this incidence, women do not have poorer prognosis than men, suggesting a biological mechanism underlying these divergences. Pregnancy, the most potent disease-modifying factor in MS, is a physiological condition characterized with significant hormonal and immunological changes, which raises the idea that sex hormones are implicated in some aspects of the autoimmune process. Many of these observations have been confirmed and elaborated in experimental autoimmune encephalomyelitis (EAE).

The purpose of this chapter is to provide an updated, summarized overview of currently published scientific information about the role of sex hormones in the pathogenesis and clinical course of multiple sclerosis and to outline the perspectives to use this knowledge for control of the disease activity.

An advanced search was conducted, based on the following key words in different combinations: "multiple sclerosis", "experimental autoimmune encephalomyelitis", "sex hormones", "pregnancy", "cytokines", "estriol", "estradiol", "progesterone", "testosterone", disability", and "MRI". The relevant scientific works (original articles, book chapters, and systematic reviews) published in English, in electronic database (PubMed, MEDLINE, and Medscape) have been retrieved and summarized. The search period was unrestricted. The following inclusion criteria have been determined: (1) subjects, suffering from multiple sclerosis; (2) studies on EAE; (3) assessment of sex hormones and cytokines; (4) brain imaging findings in relation to hormonal concentrations. Case report articles were excluded. A relationship between the concentrations of sex hormones, cytokines, physical disability, and the course of the disease has been searched.

2. Sex hormones and the immune system

Many differences have been identified between men and women with respect to the immune responses. In general, women show higher immunoglobulin levels, but lower activity of cell-mediated immune reactions than men [3]. These differences result in the effects of two major groups of biological factors: endocrine (sex hormones) and genetic (X-chromosome) [4]. Unique immunological peculiarities are observed in women during pregnancy.

Sex hormones affect the immune system in various ways. Immune cells, such as T and B lymphocytes, monocytes, macrophages, natural killer (NK) cells, dendritic cells (DC), express receptors for sex hormones although the lymphoid cells are not their main target. Estrogen effects are mediated through two isoforms of estrogen receptors (ER)—ERα and ERβ. Two isoforms have been identified for the progesterone receptor (PR) as well—PRA and PRB, while androgen receptor has no variants and binds both testosterone and 5α- dihydrotestosterone [5–8].

The regulation of T helper 1 (Th1)-type cytokine production by estrogens, appears to be dose dependent. Some authors report increased production of IFN-γ and IL-2 by low, "physiolog-

http://dx.doi.org/10.5772/63630

ical" doses of estrogens, while others find them unchanged [9, 10]. Biphasic secretion of TNF-α has also been described, with stimulation by low doses and inhibition by high doses of estrogens [11]. Increased production of IL-4 by T lymphocytes has been registered after incubation with progesterone [12].

Studies on Th2 cytokine production (IL-4 and IL-10) do not reveal any effect of estrogens in normal conditions. No differences have been found between fertile and postmenopausal women in regard to IL-4 levels [13–15]. No differences in IL-10 production have been detected between women and men [10]. On the other hand, an enhancing effect of estrogen on IL-10 production has been found in T lymphocytes from patients with MS, suggesting potentially different regulatory pathways in autoimmune diseases [16, 17]. Consistent with these findings are the results from experiments, showing that estradiol at 10–100 nM inhibits lipopolysaccharide (LPS)-induced TNF-α production from human peripheral blood mononuclear cells (PBMCs) but is stimulatory in the absence of LPS. These data illustrate the importance of cellular context for the effect of estrogens on T cells—cytokine secretion [18].

In vitro, naïve T cells stimulated with CNS autoantigens in the presence of testosterone produce higher levels of IL-5 and IL-10, but decreased levels of IFN-γ [19]. Testosterone can also reduce the in vitro production of proinflammatory cytokines, such as TNF-α and IL-1β by human macrophages and monocytes [20, 21].

Concentrations of IL-1β producing monocytes have been found higher in men than in women [10]. The influence of estrogens on IL-1 production from monocytes and macrophages seems to be biphasic as well. Progressive inhibition of IL-1 transcription with increasing concentrations of estrogen and progesterone has been described in cultured peripheral monocytes [22]. The study conducted by Kramer et al. [23] demonstrated that 17-β-estradiol can mediate release of IL-1, IL-6, and TNF-α from activated monocytes and/or macrophages through modulation of CD16 expression, with low doses being stimulatory for CD16-expression and cytokine secretion, respectively. Clear evidence for dose-dependent effects of estrogens on cytokine secretion was revealed by Matalka [24]. At preovulatory concentrations, estradiol significantly enhanced IFN-γ, IL-12, and IL-10 secretion from stimulated whole blood cells. Concentrations, similar to those in pregnancy, have caused increased production of IL-10 and reduced IL-12, IFN-γ levels and IFN-γ/IL-10 ratio. In the same concentration, estradiol has been shown to increase IL-10 secretion and decrease expression of TNF-α mRNA in proteolipid protein (PLP)-activated peripheral blood mononuclear cells isolated from healthy subjects [17].

During pregnancy, ovarian secretion of female sex hormones gradually reaches the peak of physiological levels. At the same time, a shift from Th1 toward Th2-type immune responses is observed. Marzi et al. [25] have studied the antigen and mitogen-stimulated cytokine production by PBMC obtained from healthy women during pregnancy and postpartum, and has established decreased secretion of IL-2 and IFN-γ, and increased IL-4 and IL-10 expression in the last trimester of pregnancy [25]. Another study in healthy pregnant women has found reduced serum levels of IL-12 and TNF-α together with high estrogen and progesterone levels during pregnancy compared with puerperium [26]. Similar changes have been observed in pregnant women with MS [27].

Hormonal influences on the function of B lymphocytes have been assessed by the analysis of immunoglobulin levels. Higher immunoglobulin levels in women than in men are a part of the sex differences in immune responses [3, 4]. Kanda et al.'s [28] study has shown that estrogens increase IgG and IgM production in both males and females directly, and through a potentiating effect of IL-10, released from monocytes [28]. The effect of testosterone appears to be opposite, as it inhibits IgM and IgG production both directly and indirectly by reducing the production of IL-6 by monocytes [29].

Progesterone and estrogens have been shown to influence the activity of NK cells. Increased activity of these cells has been reported in postmenopausal women and men compared with fertile females in the luteal phase of the cycle [30]. Partially in line with these data are the results from experiments, investigating the direct effect of sex hormones on NK cells activity. High-dose estrogen elicits a suppressive effect, whereas progesterone, testosterone, and estrogen at physiological concentrations have no effect in vitro on established cell lines [31, 32].

There are evidence for estrogen impact on DC functions. Exposure of the immature cells to estrogen has increased their IL-6, IL-8, and MCP-1 production, but most importantly, has enhanced their capacity to stimulate T lymphocytes [33–35]. Another study has revealed the ability of estrogen to enhance DC proinflammatory cytokine production in animal models [36].

These findings demonstrate that the interactions between sex hormones and the immune system are extremely complex and variable during different physiological states. The dependence of hormonal effects on the concrete cellular context and local cytokine milieu suggests that some specifics might be present in pathological conditions and especially in autoimmune diseases.

3. Influence of gender and sex hormones on EAE

EAE, the most widely used animal model for MS, shares many common characteristics with the disease in humans regarding the gender and sex hormone impact on susceptibility and clinical presentations.

In the relapsing SJL murine model, EAE has the same sex bias as MS, with males being less susceptible to the disease than females [37–40]. The difference may result partially from the protective effect of testosterone in male mice. This hypothesis is supported by studies demonstrating that testosterone depletion via castration increases disease susceptibility [41]. In agreement with this are the results of Voskuhl et al. [42], showing greater severity of EAE when autoreactive T cells used for induction, were extracted from female experimental animals. Thus, the immunological processes leading to T-cell priming and induction of the immune response appear to be much stronger in female mice. Some strains of mice (C57BL/6, NOD, B10.Pl, and PL/J) do not show female prevalence in susceptibility [43, 44]. These data, together with the findings of Palaszynski et al. [45], showing that effects of androgen removal depend upon genetic factors, highlight the other key point—genetic background of gender differences in EAE and MS [45].

Very interesting results about differences between genders in the clinical course of EAE have been found by Smith et al. [40]. Both male and female SJL mice had chronic relapses, but the relapses in females were more distinct and severe than those in males, which had more gradual onset and milder clinical changes. Although male animals were relatively resistant to clinical disease in comparison to female animals, once a severe disease occurred, the older age group retained substantial clinical disease with more rapid accumulation of chronic neurological deficits [40]. In other strains, B10.Pl and PL/J, male mice have shown more severe disease than females [44]. Genetic differences, modifying the effect of hormonal status on the clinical course could account for the strain-specific disparities.

Pregnancy, the condition with the highest physiological levels of female sex hormones estriol and progesterone, makes experimental animals less susceptible to EAE. Numerous studies using rats, rabbits, guinea pigs, and SJL mice have confirmed that pregnancy reduces the incidence of the disease and/or delays the day of onset [46–50]. Data about clinical improvement of EAE during pregnancy are also highly consistent [42, 49–52]. Earlier studies could not find any histopathological differences between virgin and pregnant mice with EAE [49, 50], but a succeeding investigation found reduced CNS demyelination and cell infiltration during late pregnancy in animals with preinduced EAE [51]. Later on, an elegant experiment of Haghmorad et al. [52] has confirmed that pregnancy-induced alleviation of clinical manifestations is accompanied by reduced CNS demyelination and cell infiltration. Important information about the mechanisms underlying the amelioration of the disease activity is provided by examinations of the immunological changes related to pregnancy. Langer-Gould et al. [49] have found that serum obtained from mice in late pregnancy inhibits the proliferative response and IL-2 production of proteolipid protein p139-151-specific T cells [49]. In the study of McClain et al. [50] mice immunized during pregnancy produced less TNF-α and IL-17, and displayed an increased number of IL-10-secreting cells within the CD11b+, CD11c+, CD19+, and CD4+/CD25+ populations. Another study has confirmed suppressed production of IL-17 and TNF-α in cells from pregnant mice, compared to virgin controls with EAE [51]. Enhanced production of anti-inflammatory cytokines in splenocytes and increased percentage of Th2 and Treg cells in pregnant animals have been found by Haghmorad et al. [52]. Real-time PCR for transcription factors and related cytokines of Th1, Th2, Th17, and Treg cells in the CNS of the same animals have shown reduced expression levels of Th1 and Th17 transcription factors, and decreased Th1 and Th17 cytokines including IFN-γ, TNF-α, IL-17, and IL-23. The authors conclude that pregnancy and pregnancy levels of estrogen ameliorate the EAE by favoring Treg and Th2 differentiation in the CNS.

Since estrogens and progesterone concentrations increase progressively during pregnancy, the EAE model was used to determine whether elevation in levels of a certain hormone might be responsible for disease improvement. Two estrogens, estradiol and estriol, are increased during pregnancy. Although estradiol is present at much lower, fluctuating levels in nonpregnant fertile women and female mice, estriol is synthesized by the fetal placenta and is absent in nonpregnant states [53].

The effectiveness of both estrogens in different doses has been tested for suppressing EAE activity. Numerous studies have demonstrated reduction in the clinical severity of active and/

or adoptive EAE by estrogen treatment (17-β-estradiol or estriol) in different strains of mice (SJL, C57BL/6, B10.PL, and B10.RIII) [54–62]. Clinical amelioration has been achieved when estriol is used at doses producing serum levels that are physiologic during pregnancy. Estradiol has to be administered at doses, fivefold higher than in pregnancy in order to induce the same degree of disease protection, suggesting estriol is more potent to control EAE [54]. Now it is widely accepted that high doses of estrogens are protective. Data about the effects of low doses are divergent to some degree. Some authors have found that ovariectomy of female mice worsens EAE [58], whereas others have not observed any significant influence [42]. A study by Bebo et al. [56] has shown that both hormones in low doses reduce the ability of activated T-cells to induce EAE, but their administration after the onset of the disease does not decrease the severity of the clinical manifestations.

Histopathologically, the beneficial effect of estrogens is expressed by reduced leukocyte infiltration, demyelination, and neuronal damage in CNS, suggesting immunomodulatory and neuroprotective properties of sex steroids [57, 61–64]. Kim et al. [54] have found significantly increased production of IL-10 in cultured splenocytes obtained from estriol-treated animals [54]. Decreased number of TNF-α producing T lymphocytes in CNS and spleen suspension as a consequence of 17-β-estradiol administration has been demonstrated by Ito et al. [65]. Subramanian et al. [62] have observed a tendency toward reduced secretion of IFN-γ, TNF-α, and IL-6 from activated T lymphocytes along with decreased incidence and severity of EAE under ethinyl-estradiol treatment. The latter has also suppressed the migration of encephalitogenic T cells into the CNS through downregulation of chemokines. In addition, estrogen treatment has been shown to induce certain regulatory T cells and to impair the ability of dendritic cells to present antigen [58, 59, 66, 67]. Mature dendritic cells have been shown to decrease expression of TNF-α, IFN-γ, and IL-12 mRNA with estradiol treatment, and T cells, cocultured with dendritic cells that have been pretreated with estradiol, showed a shift from Th1 to Th2 cytokine production [59]. Estriol exerts a similar effect on DC. Estriol-treated dendritic cells exhibit decreased IL-23, IL-6, IL-12 mRNA expression and an increased secretion of the immunoregulatory cytokines TGF-β and IL-10 [68]. B cells also appear to be involved in estradiol's protective effects in EAE. Removal of B cells from EAE mice has abrogated its protective effects [69]. B cells from estradiol treated mice have shown increase in IL-10 production [70]. Although both ERs are expressed in the immune system and the CNS, studies using ERα-deficient mouse strains have shown that clinical protection from EAE by estradiol and estriol depends on signaling through ERα [60, 61]. Anti-inflammatory effects of estrogens are also proven to be mediated by ERα. Treatment with ERα-selective ligand has induced favorable changes in autoantigen-specific cytokine production in the peripheral immune system (decreased TNF-α, IFN-γ, and IL-6, with increased IL-5 production), and has reduced CNS white matter inflammation and demyelination in EAE [71]. These findings are confirmed by the studies of Tiwari-Woodruff et al. [64] and Gold et al. [72]. In addition to these peripheral effects, Garidou et al. [73] have found that ERα-mediated regulation of CNS microglial cells is important for amelioration of the disease.

Along with the impact on the immune responses, estrogens exert a direct neuroprotective effect. Treatment with estrogen has decreased glutamate- and TNF-α-induced apoptosis and preserved electrophysiologic function in neurons [74–76]. Estrogen treatment has protected oligodendrocytes from cytotoxicity and has accelerated oligodendrocyte process formation [67, 77–79]. Tiwari-Woodruff et al. [64] have shown that neuroprotective effects of estrogens are mediated predominantly through the ERβ pathway. ERβ ligand treatment has promoted recovery during the chronic phase of EAE, reduced demyelination, preserved axon numbers in white matter, and decreased neuronal abnormalities in gray matter [80].

Progesterone is also considered capable of influencing pathological processes in EAE. Earlier studies have shown no effect or even augmentation of disease severity under progesterone treatment [55, 81]. These results contradict the well-documented amelioration of EAE by late pregnancy, when the highest physiological concentrations of female sex hormones are observed. Recent studies resolve these discrepancies. Pretreatment with progesterone has been shown to decrease disease severity and reduce axonal damage and demyelination [82, 83]. Yates et al. [84] have examined the treatment potential of the hormone, administered after the induction of EAE. Progesterone treated animals have shown reduced peak disease scores and cumulative disease indices, compared to the placebo group. The immunomodulatory effect of the hormone has been demonstrated by decreased secretion of pro-inflammatory cytokines IL-2 and IL-17, and increased production of anti-inflammatory IL-10, in addition to increased numbers of CD19+ cells and CD8+ cells. Inhibited Th1- and enhanced Th2-type immune responses by progesterone have been previously reported by Piccinni et al. [12], Drew and Chavis [85], Miyaura et al. [86], Hughes et al. [87], and De Leon-Nava et al. [88]. Neuroprotective properties of the hormone have also been evidenced in different experiments [89, 90]. Yu et al. [91] have shown that progesterone can promote successful remyelination in EAE. The results of the study using progesterone receptor agonist Nestorone for treatment of chronic EAE are promising. In addition to the decreased clinical manifestations and enhanced motor behavior in experimental animals, increased cell proliferation and doublecortin positive neuroblasts in the hippocampus have been found. Increased number of GABA-ergic interneurons and attenuated number of Iba1+ microglia/macrophages have also been observed. These data suggest possible activation of neurogenesis through progesterone signaling [92].

Kipp et al. [93] have studied the effect of estrogen and progesterone, given separately or in combination, on cuprizone-induced demyelination in C57B1/6 mice. Concomitant administration of cuprizone with either estrogen or progesterone reduced myelin loss when compared with the control animals. Simultaneous treatment with both hormones resulted in almost complete prevention of demyelination, suggesting mutual increase in their effects.

The clear detrimental effect of orchiectomy in EAE and the female prevalence in humans with MS has led to investigations of androgens' impact on the course of the disease. Foster et al. [94] have found decreased levels of this hormone in male mice during EAE relapse. Either testosterone or 5-α-dihydrotestosterone (which does not convert to estrogen) have been used for treatment of EAE. Both of them have shown protective effect in gonadally intact males of SJL and C57BL/6 strains [95]. Dihydrotestosterone has been effective in reducing the severity of chronic EAE in Dark Agouti rats (an experimental model showing a protracted relapsing EAE). Decreased gliosis and inflammation in the spinal cord has also been observed [96]. These results are in line with previous findings of Dalal et al. [97] who reported a less severe course of EAE in dihydrotestosterone treated female SJL mice. MBP-specific T lymphocytes, derived from dihydrotestosterone-implanted females, have produced significantly higher levels of IL-10 than those from the placebo group. Bebo et al. [19] have demonstrated that testosterone reduces encephalitogenicity of myelin-reactive T cells: EAE induced by the adoptive transfer of androgen-treated T cell lines is less severe than disease induced with untreated T cell lines. In addition, decreased production of IFN-γ and increased secretion of IL-10 has been found in androgen-selected T cell lines compared to untreated cell lines. Taken together these data suggest different mechanisms of disease protection between endogenous physiological testosterone and exogenous supraphysiological androgen treatment. The study of Matejuk et al. [98] has demonstrated age-dependent differences in response to androgen therapy, with no protective effect of testosterone against EAE in middle-age males and almost complete resistance to the disease of young animals. These same authors found that testosterone inhibited proliferation of myelin oligodendrocyte glycoprotein 35–55-specific T cells and secretion of TNF-α and IFN-γ in young males, supporting the immunomodulatory properties of androgens.

There are evidence for direct neuroprotective effects of androgens. Testosterone has been shown to protect neuronal cell lines from oxidative stress and against β-amyloid toxicity induced cell death [99–101]. Experimental data suggest that neuroprotective properties of androgens are at least partially mediated through influence on expression of neurotrophic factors such as BDNF [102].

4. Clinical evidence for the effects of sex hormones on disease course

The onset of MS typically takes place during the childbearing period of life. It is well known that pregnancy has a strong influence on disease activity [103]. The effect of pregnancy in women with MS is in agreement with the experimental data, presented earlier in this chapter. A 70% decline in the relapse rate during the last trimester compared to prepregnancy period has been found in the largest study conducted by a French research group—the PRIMS study (pregnancy in multiple sclerosis). A rebound effect has been observed after delivery, with significantly increased frequency of relapses. However, the overall one-year effect (pregnancy + puerperium) on the relapse rate was neutral (the increase during the first three months of puerperium was balanced by the reduction during pregnancy) [104]. A number of earlier prospective studies with a smaller sample size have reported similar results [105–107]. A meta-analysis of 22 reports on pregnancy in MS has confirmed the overall effect of pregnancy and puerperium on disease activity [108].

The results of MRI studies are highly corresponding to the clinical observations. A small study has followed two patients with MS throughout pregnancy using MRI and showed similar reduction of MRI activity during the course of pregnancy and activation in the postpartum phase [109]. A consequent larger observation of Paavilainen et al. [110] has found a significant increase in the number of T2 lesions and DWI-positive lesions as well as in the total lesion load measured from FLAIR images after delivery, compared to the scans performed during pregnancy. The majority of the active postpartum scans have been performed within 5 weeks of delivery, indicating that MS disease activation commonly takes place at a very early postpartum period. Interesting findings in the same study are the active lesions, observed in two patients at 35–37 gestational weeks, when blood estriol concentration begins to decline as a result of placental ageing. Consequently, the loss of high estriol concentrations might be one of the underlying mechanisms for an increase in MS activity after delivery.

The amelioration of MS in the last trimester of pregnancy is thought to be induced mainly by higher concentrations of estriol, estradiol, and progesterone, but human choriongonadotropin, human placental lactogen, prolactin, cortisol, 1,25-dihydroxyvitamine D3, α-fetoprotein, pregnancy-associated glycoprotein, blocking antibodies, and cytokines secreted by the feto-placental complex can also be involved. Pregnancy tends to suppress the immune system of the mother to prevent rejection of the semiallogeneic fetus [111]. "Physiological immune suppression" with change in the type of immune responses and cytokine production is regarded as one of the underlying mechanisms [112]. One of the important changes is the shift from Th1- to Th2-type of immune reactions [25, 27]. Langer-Gould et al. [113] have found a decline in IFN-γ producing CD4+ T cells during pregnancy but no increase postpartum. An increase in the level of Treg and Th2 populations and a decrease in Th1 and Th17 cells are typical for normal pregnancy [114–117]. The increase in Tregs has been shown to be mediated through the effects of estradiol on the immune system [118]. The total number of NK cells is reduced during pregnancy, both among patients with MS and among controls, before increasing again after delivery [119]. One study has correlated the postpartum relapses with an increased level of IL-8 in the first trimester [120]. Reduced HLA-G gene expression has been observed in the postpartum situation in all patients with MS but in none of the healthy controls. Decreased soluble HLA-G level has been associated with increased relapse status [121]. As the HLA-G CD4 T cells have suppressive properties and are characterized as a new regulatory T cell population, it can be hypothesized that reduced HLA-G expression contributes to the increased postpartum relapse frequency [103].

Menstrual cycle is another physiological state in women, associated with a specific fluctuation in serum sex hormones. Several studies have registered worsening of the neurological signs just before or during the menstrual bleeding in a majority of the patients, and in some women with MS the onset of all relapses was in the same phase of the menstrual cycle [122–125]. The precise mechanisms for these fluctuations are unclear but decrease in female sex hormones levels is highly probable.

Investigations on the serum concentrations of sex hormones in fertile women with MS have revealed relatively high incidence of disturbances. These findings are in accordance with disruption of estrus cycle homeostasis, observed in SJL/J mice with EAE [126]. One study found abnormally low serum concentrations of estradiol and/or progesterone in one or both phases (exacerbation or remission) of the disease in 60% of the patients and the levels of hormones significantly increased during clinical remission. Presence of hormonal abnormalities was associated with higher concentrations of TNF-α and IFN-γ, suggesting a suppressive effect of estradiol and progesterone on proinflammatory cytokine secretion. Less severe residual neurological deficit (in remission) was registered in patients with normal hormonal status which could be attributed to additional neuroprotective effects of female sex hormones [127]. Another study has registered hormonal disturbances in 56% of women with MS and abnormal hormonal pattern correlated with the intensity of MRI pathology [128].

Little data are available about the impact of hormonal decline during menopause on the course of MS. Smith and Studd [129] have found increased disability in 54% of menopausal women with MS and Holmquist et al. [130] have reported worsening of MS symptoms related to menopause in 40% of the patients.

Onset of MS in men (age 30–40) usually occurs later in life than in women, coinciding with the age at which serum testosterone levels normally begin to decline [53]. Examination of serum testosterone concentrations has shown divergent results. Abnormally low levels have been found by Wei and Lightman [131] in 24% of male MS patients with primary or secondary progressive MS. Foster et al. [94] have observed the same disturbance in all four men (three with relapsing-remitting and one with secondary progressive MS) with sexual dysfunctions. On the contrary, male patients with relapsing-remitting MS, studied by de Andrés et al. [132] have presented elevated testosterone blood concentrations compared to the healthy controls and a tendency toward reduction during the relapse phase. The small sample size may account for these contradictory results, suggesting that larger studies are needed for more detailed examination of hormonal status and its relation to disease activity in MS. A recent longitudinal study, comprising 96 male patients with MS or clinically isolated syndrome, has found hypogonadal status (testosterone levels below the lower limit of normal) in 39% of the subjects. A negative age-adjusted correlation between total testosterone and EDSS has been revealed and higher baseline testosterone levels have been associated with less cognitive decline, measured by SDMT during longitudinal follow-up [133].

Gender differences are observed not only in susceptibility and clinical manifestations but also in brain damage characteristics. A study in a large cohort of MS patients has shown that men are prone to develop less inflammatory, but more destructive brain lesions than women [134]. Intracortical lesions are more frequent in men [135]. The relationship between sex hormone levels and tissue damage has been explored in MS. A MRI study of disease activity during different phases of the menstrual cycle has shown significant correlation between progesterone/17β-estradiol (PEL) ratio in the luteal phase and the number of gadolinium-enhanced CNS lesions [136, 137]. Another study has found a significantly higher number of Gd-enhanced lesions in women with abnormally low testosterone levels. In men, estradiol concentration has correlated with the volume of T1 lesions and the contrast-enhanced T2 lesions [138]. These data provide evidence that sex hormones modulate the development of brain tissue damages and repair in MS. Luchetti et al. [139] have extended the research in gender differences of steroid synthesis and signaling in the brains of MS patients. They have studied gene expression of these pathways and of inflammatory cytokines in MS lesions and normal-appearing white matter of male and female patients and controls. In MS lesions in males, local upregulation of aromatase (an enzyme involved in estrogen biosynthesis), ERβ, and TNFmRNA has been found; whereas in females, local upregulation of 3β-hydroxysteroid-dehydrogenase (a progesterone synthetic enzyme), and of progesterone receptor has been detected. Aromatase and ERαmRNA levels have positively correlated with that of TNF in primary cultures of

http://dx.doi.org/10.5772/63630

human microglia and astrocytes. Together these findings may represent contributing factors to gender differences in the brain damages and the course of MS, and suggest much more intricate interactions between CNS, endocrine and immune system.

5. Future perspectives

Promising results of testosterone, estrogens and progesterone in EAE have initiated pilot studies in humans, in which sex hormones are used separately or in combination with each other or with another immunomodulatory drug.

The first clinical study using sex hormones in women with MS has been performed with oral estriol 8 mg/day, given for 6 months to 10 patients (six with a relapsing-remitting course and four with a secondary progressive course). In the relapsing-remitting patients, the trial has been extended after a 6-month posttreatment period with a 4-month retreatment period, during which estriol has been given in combination with progesterone. Estriol treatment has decreased gadolinium enhancing lesion numbers and volumes on MRI, significantly increased production of IL-5 and IL-10 and decreased secretion of TNF-α. When estriol administration was stopped, MRI-lesions increased to pretreatment levels, but after treatment reinstitution, they significantly decreased again [140, 141].

Female sex hormones, given in addition to interferon-β therapy, have reduced the number of relapses and delayed progression of disability [142].

Larger, placebo controlled, clinical trials of estrogens in MS are ongoing. These include a multicenter placebo controlled trial of estriol in combination with glatiramer acetate (ClinicalTrials.gov: NCT00451204) and a trial, examining the potential of estradiol and progestin to prevent postpartum relapses—POPART'MUS trail (NCT00127075) [112, 143].

Ten male patients with relapsing-remitting MS have been treated with testosterone 100 mg/day via transdermal application for 12 months. Improvement of cognitive performance and slowing of brain atrophy, as measured by MRI, have been observed under testosterone treatment. Immunological changes consisted of decreased production of IL-2 and increased production of TGFβ1, BDNF, and PDGF-BB from PBMCs [144, 145].

The main expected adverse event about these high-dose hormonal treatments is the increased risk of malignancies. Data in the literature demonstrate that breast and uterine endometrial cancer are both mediated through ERα. Treatment with an ERβ ligand has shown neuroprotective effect in EAE and can be explored as a potential therapeutic strategy in multiple sclerosis [64]. On the other side, testosterone replacement is widely used in aging and hypogonadal men and there is no clear evidence that higher levels of circulating testosterone, within the physiological range, are linked to an increased risk of prostate cancer [80].

The variations in the susceptibility and in the clinical course of MS reflect the differences in immune responses between the genders. Now it is widely accepted that these differences are partially due to the impact of sex hormones. Estrogens, progesterone and androgens change the cytokine secretion and interactions between immune cells and through this suppress the disease activity. Their direct neuroprotective properties enhance the amelioration of EAE and MS. Several pilot clinical trials using sex steroids as treatment agents in MS patients established positive results and need to be confirmed and expanded in larger cohorts.

In conclusion, a large amount of evidence about the influence of sex hormones on the pathological processes in MS has been accumulated. Although they are not a primary pathogenic factor, immunomodulatory and neuroprotective effects of sex steroids provide opportunities for development of new disease-modifying strategies.

Author details

Anastasiya G. Trenova

Address all correspondence to: atrenova@yahoo.com

Department of Neurology, Medical University-Plovdiv, Plovdiv, Bulgaria

References

[1] Koch-Henriksen N, Sorensen PS. The changing demographic pattern of multiple sclerosis epidemiology. Lancet Neurol 2010;9:520–532.

[2] Swanton JK, Fernando KT, Dalton CM Miszkiel KA, Altmann DR, Plant GT, Thompson AJ, Miller DH. Early MRI in optic neuritis: the risk for clinically definite multiple sclerosis. Mult Scler 2010;16:156–165.

[3] Coyle PK. Women's issues. In: Bruks JS, Johnson KP. Multiple sclerosis: diagnosis, medical management and rehabilitation. New York: Demos; 2000. p. 505–513.

[4] Oertelt-Prigione S. The influence of sex and gender on the immune response. Autoimmun Rev 2012;11(6–7):A479–A485.

[5] Gelmann EP. Molecular biology of the androgen receptor. J Clin Oncol 2002;20:3001–3015.

[6] Kovats S. Estrogen receptors regulate an inflammatory pathway of dendritic cell differentiation: mechanisms and implications for immunity. Horm Behav 2012;62(3): 254–262.

[7] Kovats S. Estrogen receptors regulate innate immune cells and signaling pathways. Cell Immunol 2015;294(2):63–69.

[8] Tan IJ, Peeva E, Zandman-Goddard G. Hormonal modulation of the immune system —a spotlight on the role of progestogens. Autoimmun Rev 2015;14(6):536–542.

[9] Girón-González JA, Moral FJ, Elvira J, García-Gil D, Guerrero F, Gavilán I, Escobar L. Consistent production of a higher TH1:TH2 cytokine ratio by stimulated T cells in men compared with women. Eur J Endocrinol 2000;143:31–36.

[10] Bouman A, Schipper M, Heineman MJ, Faas MM. Gender difference in the non-specific and specific immune response in humans. Am J Reprod Immunol 2004;52:19–26.

[11] Correale J, Arias M, Gilmor W. Steroid hormone regulation of cytokine secretion by proteolipid protein-specific CD4+ T cell clones isolated from multiple sclerosis patients and normal control subjects. J Immunol 1998;161:3365–3374.

[12] Piccinni MP, Giudizi MG, Biagiotti R, Beloni L, Giannarini L, Sampognaro S, Parronchi P, Manetti R, Annunziato F, Livi C, et al. Progesterone favors the development of human T helper cells producing Th2-type cytokines and promotes both IL-4 production and membrane CD30 expression in established Th1 cell clones. J Immunol 1995;155:128–133.

[13] Kamada M, Irahara M, Maegawa M, Ohmoto Y, Murata K, Yasui T, Yamano S, Aono T. Transient increase in the levels of T-helper 1 cytokines in postmenopausal women and the effects of hormone replacement therapy. Gynecol Obstet Invest 2001;52:82–88.

[14] Cioffi M, Esposito K, Vietri MT, Gazzerro P, D'Auria A, Ardovino I, Puca GA, Molinari AM. Cytokine pattern in postmenopause. Maturitas 2002;41:187–192.

[15] Kumru S, Godekmerdan A, Yilmaz B. Immune effects of surgical menopause and estrogen replacement therapy in peri-menopausal women. J Reprod Immunol 2004;63:31–38.

[16] Gilmore W, Weiner L, Correale J. Effect of estradiol on cytokine secretion by proteolipid protein-specific T cell clones isolated from multiple sclerosis patients and normal control subjects. I Immunol 1997;158(1):446–451.

[17] Javadian A, Salehi E, Bidad K, Sahraian MA, Izad M. Effect of estrogen on Th1, Th2 and Th17 cytokines production by proteolipid protein and PHA activated peripheral blood mononuclear cells isolated from multiple sclerosis patients. Arch Med Res 2014;45(2): 177–182.

[18] Asai K, Hiki N, Mimura Y, Ogawa T, Unou K, Kaminishi M. Gender differences in cytokine secretion by human peripheral blood mononuclear cells: role of estrogen in modulating LPS-induced cytokine secretion in an *ex vivo* septic model. Shock 2001;16:340–343.

[19] Bebo BF Jr, Schuster JC, Vandenbark AA, Offner H. Androgens alter the cytokine profile and reduce encephalitogenicity of myelin-reactive T cells. J Immunol 1999;162:35–40.

[20] D'Agostino P, Milano S, Barbera C, Di Bella G, La Rosa M, Ferlazzo V, Farruggio R, Miceli DM, Miele M, Castagnetta L, Cillari E. Sex hormones modulate inflammatory mediators produced by macrophages. Ann N Y Acad Sci 1999;876:426–429.

[21] Liva SM, Voskuhl RR. Testosterone acts directly on CD4+ T lymphocytes to increase IL-10 production. J Immunol 2001;167:2060–2067.

[22] Polan ML, Loukides J, Nelson P, Carding S, Diamond M, Walsh A, et al. Progesterone and estradiol modulate interleukin-1 beta messenger ribonucleic acid levels in cultured human peripheral monocytes. J Clin Endocrinol Metab 1989;69:1200–1206.

[23] Kramer PR, Kramer SF, Guan G. 17 beta-estradiol regulates cytokine release through modulation of CD16 expression in monocytes and monocyte-derived macrophages. Arthritis Rheum 2004;50:1967–1975.

[24] Matalka KZ. The effect of estradiol, but not progesterone, on the production of cytokines in stimulated whole blood, is concentration-dependent. Neuro Endocrinol Lett 2003;24:185–191.

[25] Marzi M, Vigano A, Trabattoni D, Villa ML, Salvaggio A, Clerici E, Clerici M. Characterization of type 1 and type 2 cytokine production profile in physiologic and pathologic human pregnancy. Clin Exp Immunol 1996;106(1):127–133.

[26] Elenkov IJ, Wilder RL, Bakalov VK, Link AA, Dimitrov MA, Fisher S, Crane M, Kanik KS, Chrousos GP. IL-12, TNF-alpha and hormonal changes during late pregnancy and early postpartum: implications for autoimmune disease activity during these times. J Clin Endocrinol Metab 2001;86(10):4933–4938.

[27] Al-Shammri S, Rawwoot P, Azizieh F, AbuQoora A, Hanna M, Saminathan TR, Raghupathy R. Th1/Th2 cytokine patterns and clinical profiles during and after pregnancy in women with multiple sclerosis. J Neurol Sci 2004;222(1–2):21–27.

[28] Kanda N, Tamaki K. Estrogen enhances immunoglobulin production by human PBMCs. J Allergy Clin Immunol 1999;103:282–288.

[29] Kanda N, Tsuchida T, Tamaki K. Testosterone inhibits immunoglobulin production by human peripheral blood mononuclear cells. Clin Exp Immunol 1996;106:410–415.

[30] Souza SS, Castro FA, Mendonça HC, Palma PV, Morais FR, Ferriani RA, Voltarelli JC. Influence of menstrual cycle on NK activity. J Reprod Immunol 2001;50:151–159.

[31] Ferguson MM, McDonald FG. Oestrogen as an inhibitor of human NK cell cytolysis. FEBS Lett 1985;191:145–148.

[32] Sulke AN, Jones DB, Wood PJ. Hormonal modulation of human natural killer cell activity in vitro. J Reprod Immunol 1985;7:105–110.

[33] Bengtsson AK, Ryan EJ, Giordano D, Magaletti DM, Clark EA. 17beta-estradiol (E2) modulates cytokine and chemokine expression in human monocyte-derived dendritic cells. Blood 2004;104:1404–1410.

[34] Paharkova-Vatchkova V, Maldonado R, Kovats S. Estrogen preferentially promotes the differentiation of CD11c+ CD11b(intermediate) dendritic cells from bone marrow precursors. J Immunol 2004;172:1426–1436.

[35] Kovats S, Carreras E. Regulation of dendritic cell differentiation and function by estrogen receptor ligands. Cell Immunol 2008;252:81–90.

[36] Siracusa MC, Overstreet MG, Housseau F, Scott AL, Klein SL. 17beta-estradiol alters the activity of conventional and IFN-producing killer dendritic cells. J Immunol 2008;180:1423–1431.

[37] Voskuhl RR, Pitchekian-Halabi H, MacKenzie-Graham A, McFarland HF, Raine CS. Gender differences in autoimmune demyelination in the mouse: implications for multiple sclerosis. Ann Neurol 1996;39(6):724–733.

[38] Bebo BF Jr, Schuster JC, Vandenbark AA, Offner H. Gender differences in experimental autoimmune encephalomyelitis develop during the induction of the immune response to encephalitogenic peptides. J Neurosci Res 1998;52(4):420–426.

[39] Kim S, Voskuhl RR. Decreased IL-12 production underlies the decreased ability of male lymph node cells to induce experimental autoimmune encephalomyelitis. J Immunol 1999;162(9):5561–5568.

[40] Smith ME, Eller NL, McFarland HF, Racke MK, Raine CS. Age dependence of clinical and pathological manifestations of autoimmune demyelination: implications for multiple sclerosis. Am J Pathol 1999;155(4):1147–1161.

[41] Bebo BF Jr, Zelinka-Vincent E, Adamus G, Amundson D, Vandenbark AA, Offner H. Gonadal hormones influence the immune response to PLP 139–151 and the clinical course of relapsing experimental autoimmune encephalomyelitis. J Neuroimmunol 1998;84(2):122–130.

[42] Voskuhl RR, Palaszynski K. Sex hormones in experimental autoimmune encephalomyelitis: implications for multiple sclerosis. Neurosci 2001;7(3):258–270.

[43] Okuda Y, Okuda M, Bernard CC Gender does not influence the susceptibility of C57BL/6 mice to develop chronic experimental autoimmune encephalomyelitis induced by myelin oligodendrocyte glycoprotein. Immunol Lett 2002;81(1):25–29.

[44] Papenfuss TL, Rogers CJ, Gienapp I, Yurrita M, McClain M, Damico N, Valo J, Song F, Whitacre CC. Sex differences in experimental autoimmune encephalomyelitis in multiple murine strains. J Neuroimmunol 2004;150:59–69.

[45] Palaszynski KM, Loo KK, Ashouri JF, Liu HB, Voskuhl RR. Androgens are protective in experimental autoimmune encephalomyelitis: implications for multiple sclerosis. J Neuroimmunol 2004;146(1–2):144–152.

[46] Keith AB. Effect of pregnancy on experimental allergic encephalomyelitis in guinea pigs and rats. J Neurol Sci 1978;38:317–326.

[47] Mertin LA, Rumjanek VM. Pregnancy and the susceptibility of Lewis rats to experimental allergic encephalomyelitis. J Neurol Sci 1985;68:15–24.

[48] Brenner T, Evron S, Abramsky O. Effect of experimental autoimmune encephalomyelitis on pregnancy: studies in rabbits and rats. Isr J Med Sci 1991;27:181–185.

[49] Langer-Gould A, Garren H, Slansky A, Ruiz PJ, Steinman L. Late pregnancy suppresses relapses in experimental autoimmune encephalomyelitis: evidence for a suppressive pregnancy-related serum factor. J Immunol 2002;169:1084–1091.

[50] McClain MA, Gatson NN, Powell ND, Papenfuss TL, Gienapp IE, Song F, Shawler TM, Kithcart A, Whitacre CC. Pregnancy suppresses experimental autoimmune encephalomyelitis through immunoregulatory cytokine production. J Immunol 2007;179(12): 8146–8152.

[51] Gatson NN, Williams JL, Powell ND, McClain MA, Hennon TR, Robbins PD, Whitacre CC. Induction of pregnancy during established EAE halts progression of CNS autoimmune injury via pregnancy-specific serum factors. J Neuroimmunol 2011;230(1–2): 105–113.

[52] Haghmorad D, Amini AA, Mahmoudi MB, Rastin M, Hosseini M, Mahmoudi M. Pregnancy level of estrogen attenuates experimental autoimmune encephalomyelitis in both ovariectomized and pregnant C57BL/6 mice through expansion of Treg and Th2 cells. J Neuroimmunol 2014;277(1–2):85–95.

[53] Voskuhl R, Giesser BS. Gender and reproductive issues in multiple sclerosis. In: Giesser BS. Primer on multiple sclerosis. New York: Oxford University Press Inc; 2011. p. 221–240.

[54] Jansson L, Olsson T, Holmdahl R. Estrogen induces a potent suppression of experimental autoimmune encephalomyelitis and collagen-induced arthritis in mice. J Neuroimmunol 1994;53:203–207.

[55] Kim S, Liva SM, Dalal MA, Verity MA, Voskuhl RR. Estriol ameliorates autoimmune demyelinating disease: implications for multiple sclerosis. Neurology 1999;52:1230–1238.

[56] Bebo BF Jr, Fyfe-Johnson A, Adlard K, Beam AG, Vandenbark AA, Offner H. Low-dose estrogen therapy ameliorates experimental autoimmune encephalomyelitis in two different inbred mouse strains. J Immunol 2001;166:2080–2089.

[57] Ito A, Bebo BF, Jr, Matejuk A, Zamora A, Silverman M, Fyfe-Johnson A, Offner H. Estrogen treatment down-regulates TNF-alpha production and reduces the severity of experimental autoimmune encephalomyelitis in cytokine knockout mice. J Immunol 2001;167:542–552.

[58] Matejuk A, Bakke AC, Hopke C, Dwyer J, Vandenbark AA, Offner H. Estrogen treatment induces a novel population of regulatory cells, which suppresses experimental autoimmune encephalomyelitis. J Neurosci Res 2004;77:119–126.

[59] Liu HY, Buenafe AC, Matejuk A, Ito A, Zamora A, Dwyer J, Vandenbark AA, Offner H. Estrogen inhibition of EAE involves effects on dendritic cell function. J Neurosci Res 2002;70:238–248.

[60] Liu HB, Loo KK, Palaszynski K, Ashouri J, Lubahn DB, Voskuhl RR. Estrogen receptor alpha mediates estrogen's immune protection in autoimmune disease. J Immunol 2003;171:6936–6940.

[61] Polanczyk M, Zamora A, Subramanian S, Matejuk A, Hess DL, Blankenhorn EP, Teuscher C, Vandenbark AA, Offner H. The protective effect of 17beta-estradiol on experimental autoimmune encephalomyelitis is mediated through estrogen receptor-alpha. Am J Pathol 2003;163:1599–1605.

[62] Subramanian S, Matejuk A, Zamora A, Vandenbark AA, Offner H. Oral feeding with ethinyl estradiol suppresses and treats experimental autoimmune encephalomyelitis in SJL mice and inhibits the recruitment of inflammatory cells into the central nervous system. J Immunol 2003;170:1548–1555.

[63] Polanczyk MJ, Jones RE, Subramanian S, Afentoulis M, Rich C, Zakroczymski M, Cooke P, Vandenbark AA, Offner H. T lymphocytes do not directly mediate the protective effect of estrogen on experimental autoimmune encephalomyelitis. Am J Pathol 2004;165:2069–2077.

[64] Tiwari-Woodruff S, Morales LB, Lee R, Voskuhl RR. Differential neuroprotective and antiinflammatory effects of estrogen receptor (ER)alpha and ERbeta ligand treatment. Proc Natl Acad Sci USA 2007;104:14813–14818.

[65] Ito A, Buenafe AC, Matejuk A, Zamora A, Silverman M, Dwyer J, Vandenbark AA, Offner H. Estrogen inhibits systemic T cell expression of TNF-alpha and recruitment of TNF-alpha(+) T cells and macrophages into the CNS of mice developing experimental encephalomyelitis. Clin Immunol 2002;102:275–282.

[66] Polanczyk MJ, Carson BD, Subramanian S, Afentoulis M, Vandenbark AA, Ziegler SF, Offner H. Cutting edge: estrogen drives expansion of the CD4+CD25+ regulatory T cell compartment. J Immunol 2004;173(4):2227–2230.

[67] Zhang QH, Hu YZ, Cao J, Zhong YQ, Zhao YF, Mei QB. Estrogen influences the differentiation, maturation and function of dendritic cells in rats with experimental autoimmune encephalomyelitis. Acta Pharmacol Sin 2004;25(4):508–513.

[68] Papenfuss TL, Powell ND, McClain MA, Bedarf A, Singh A, Gienapp IE, Shawler T, Whitacre CC. Estriol generates tolerogenic dendritic cells in vivo that protect against autoimmunity. J Immunol 2011;186:3346–3355.

[69] Bodhankar S, Wang C, Vandenbark AA, Offner H. Estrogen-induced protection against experimental autoimmune encephalomyelitis is abrogated in the absence of B cells. Eur J Immunol 2011;41:1165–1175.

[70] Subramanian S, Yates M, Vandenbark AA, Offner H. Oestrogen-mediated protection of experimental autoimmune encephalomyelitis in the absence of Foxp3+ regulatory T

cells implicates compensatory pathways including regulatory B cells. Immunology 2011;132:340–347.

[71] Morales LB, Loo KK, Liu HB, Peterson C, Tiwari-Woodruff S, Voskuhl RR. Treatment with an estrogen receptor alpha ligand is neuroprotective in experimental autoimmune encephalomyelitis. J Neurosci 2006;26:6823–6833.

[72] Gold SM, Manda SV, Morales LB, Sicotte NL, Voskuhl RR. Estriol treatment reduces matrix metalloprotease-9 activity in multiple sclerosis and experimental autoimmune encephalomyelitis. Mult Scler 2008;14:S29.

[73] Garidou L, Laffont S, Douin-Echinard V, Coureau C, Krust A, Chambon P, Guery JC. Estrogen receptor alpha signaling in inflammatory leukocytes is dispensable for 17beta estradiol-mediated inhibition of experimental autoimmune encephalomyelitis. J Immunol 2004;173:2435–2442.

[74] Koski CL, Hila S, Popescue T, Hoffman G. Ovarian hormones differentially effect neuron death mediated by TNF-α via expression of antiapoptotic proteins and activation of JNK1 pro-appoptotic signal cascade. Mult Scler Clin Lab Res 2002;8(1):18–19.

[75] Sribnick EA, Ray SK, Nowak MW, Li L, Banik NL. 17beta-estradiol attenuates glutamate-induced apoptosis and preserves electrophysiologic function in primary cortical neurons. J Neurosci Res 2004;76:688–696.

[76] Zhao L, Wu TW, Brinton RD. Estrogen receptor subtypes alpha and beta contribute to neuroprotection and increased Bcl-2 expression in primary hippocampal neurons. Brain Res 2004;1010:22–34.

[77] Sur P, Sribnick EA, Wingrave JM, Nowak MW, Ray SK, Banik NL. Estrogen attenuates oxidative stress-induced apoptosis in C6 glial cells. Brain Res 2003;971:178–188.

[78] Takao T, Flint N, Lee L, Ying X, Merrill J, Chandross KJ. 17beta-estradiol protects oligodendrocytes from cytotoxicity induced cell death. J Neurochem 2004;89:660–673.

[79] Cantarella G, Risuglia N, Lombardo G, Lempereur L, Nicoletti F, Memo M, Bernardini R. Protective effects of estradiol on TRAIL-induced apoptosis in a human oligodendrocytic cell line: evidence for multiple sites of interactions. Cell Death Differ 2004;11(5):503–511.

[80] Gold SM, Voskuhl RR. Estrogen and testosterone therapies in multiple sclerosis. Prog Brain Res 2009;175:239–251.

[81] Hoffman GE, Le WW, Murphy AZ, Koski CL. Divergent effects of ovarian steroids on neuronal survival during experimental allergic encephalomyelitis in Lewis rats. Exp Neurol 2001;171(2):272–284.

[82] Garay L, Gonzalez Deniselle MC, Lima A, Roig P, De Nicola AF. Effects of progesterone in the spinal cord of a mouse model of multiple sclerosis. J Steroid Biochem Mol Biol 2007;107(3–5):228–237.

[83] Garay L, Deniselle MCG, Gierman L, Meyer M, Lima A, Roig P, De Nicola AF. Steroid protection in the experimental autoimmune encephalomyelitis model of multiple sclerosis. Neuroimmunomodulation 2008;15:76–83.

[84] Yates MA, Li Y, Chlebeck P, Proctor T, Vandenbark AA, Offner H. Progesterone treatment reduces disease severity and increases IL-10 in experimental autoimmune encephalomyelitis. J Neuroimmunol 2010;220(1–2):136–139.

[85] Drew PD, Chavis JA. Female sex steroids: effects upon microglial cell activation. J Neuroimmunol 2000;111(1–2):77–85.

[86] Miyaura H, Iwata M. Direct and indirect inhibition of Th1 development by progesterone and glucocorticoids. J Immunol 2002;168:1087–1094.

[87] Hughes GC, Thomas S, Li C, Kaja MK, Clark EA. Cutting edge: progesterone regulates IFN-alpha production by plasma cytoid dendritic cells. J Immunol 2008;180(4):2029–2033.

[88] De León-Nava MA, Nava K, Soldevila G, López-Griego L, Chávez-Ríos JR, Vargas-Villavicencio JA, Morales-Montor J. Immune sexual dimorphism: effect of gonadal steroids on the expression of cytokines, sex steroid receptors, and lymphocyte proliferation. J Steroid Biochem Mol Biol 2009;113(1–2):57–64.

[89] Gonzalez SL, Labombarda F, Gonzalez Deniselle MC, Mougel A, Guennoun R, Schumacher M, De Nicola AF. Progesterone neuroprotection in spinal cord trauma involves up-regulation of brain-derived neurotrophic factor in motoneurons. J Steroid Biochem Mol Biol 2005;94(1–3):143–149.

[90] Garay L, Deniselle MC, Meyer M, Costa JJ, Lima A, Roig P, De nicola AF. Protective effects of progesterone administration on axonal pathology in mice with experimental autoimmune encephalomyelitis. Brain Res 2009;1283:177–185.

[91] Yu HJ, Fei J, Chen XS, Cai QY, Liu HL, Liu GD, Yao ZX. Progesterone attenuates neurological behavioral deficits of experimental autoimmune encephalomyelitis through remyelination with nucleus-sublocalized Olig1 protein. Neurosci Lett 2010;476(1):42–45.

[92] Garay L, Gonzalez Deniselle MC, Sitruk-Ware R, Guennoun R, Schumacher M, De Nicola AF. Efficacy of the selective progesterone receptor agonist Nestorone for chronic experimental autoimmune encephalomyelitis. J Neuroimmunol 2014;276(1–2):89–97.

[93] Kipp M, Acs P, Beyer C, Komoly A. Estrogen and progesterone treatment prevents cuprizone-induced demyelination in C57B1/6 male mice. Mult Scler Clin Lab Res 2007;13(2):149.

[94] Foster SC, Daniels C, Bourdette DN, Bebo BF Jr. Dysregulation of the hypothalamic-pituitary-gonadal axis in experimental autoimmune encephalomyelitis and multiple sclerosis. J Neuroimmunol 2003;140(1–2):78–87.

[95] Palaszynski KM, Loo KK, Ashouri JF, Liu HB, Voskuhl RR. Androgens are protective in experimental autoimmune encephalomyelitis: implications for multiple sclerosis. J Neuroimmunol 2004;146(1–2):144–152.

[96] Giatti S, Rigolio R, Romano S, Mitro N, Viviani B, Cavaletti G, Caruso D, Garcia-Segura LM, Melcangi RC. Dihydrotestosterone as a protective agent in chronic experimental autoimmune encephalomyelitis. Neuroendocrinology 2015;101(4):296–308.

[97] Dalal M, Kim S, Voskuhl RR. Testosterone therapy ameliorates experimental autoimmune encephalomyelitis and induces a T helper 2 bias in the autoantigen-specific T lymphocyte response. J Immunol 1997;159(1):3–6.

[98] Matejuk A, Hopke C, Vandenbark AA, Hurn PD, Offner H. Middle-age male mice have increased severity of experimental autoimmune encephalomyelitis and are unresponsive to testosterone therapy. J. Immunol 2005;174:2387–2395.

[99] Pike CJ. Testosterone attenuates beta-amyloid toxicity in cultured hippocampal neurons. Brain Res 2001;919:160–165.

[100] Chisu V, Manca P, Lepore G, Gadau S, Zedda M, Farina V. Testosterone induces neuroprotection from oxidative stress. Effects on catalase activity and 3-nitro-l-tyrosine incorporation into alpha-tubulin in a mouse neuroblastoma cell line. Arch Ital Biol 2006;144:63–73.

[101] Chisu V, Manca P, Zedda M, Lepore G, Gadau S, Farina V. Effects of testosterone on differentiation and oxidative stress resistance in C1300 neuroblastoma cells. Neuro Endocrinol Lett 2006;27:807–812.

[102] Rasika S, Alvarez-Buylla A, Nottebohm F. BDNF mediates the effects of testosterone on the survival of new neurons in an adult brain. Neuron 1999;22(1):53–62.

[103] Airas L. Hormonal and gender-related immune changes in multiple sclerosis. Acta Neurol Scand 2015;132(199):62–70.

[104] Confavreux C, Hutchinson M, Hours MM, Cortinovis-Tourniaire P, Moreau T. Rate of pregnancy related relapse in multiple sclerosis. New Engl J Med 1998;339(5):285–291.

[105] Roullet E, Verdier-Taillefer M-H, Amarenco P, Gharbi G, Alperovitch A, Marteau R. Pregnancy and multiple sclerosis: a longitudinal study of 125 remittent patients. J Neurol Neurosurg Psychiatry 1993;56:1062–1965.

[106] Sadovnik AD, Eisen K, Hashimoto SA, Farquhar R, Yee IM, Hooge J, Kastrukoff L, Oger JJ, Paty DW. Pregnancy and multiple sclerosis: a prospective study. Arch Neurol 1994;51:1120–1124.

[107] Worthington J, Jones R, Crawford M, Forti A. Pregnancy and multiple sclerosis: a three year prospective study. J Neurol 1994;241:228–233.

[108] Finkelsztejn A, Brooks JB, Paschoal FM Jr, Fragoso YD. What can we really tell women with multiple sclerosis regarding pregnancy? A systematic review and meta-analysis of the literature. BJOG 2011;118(7):790–797.

[109] van Valdererveen MAA, Tas MW, Barkhof F, Polman CH, Frequin ST, Hommes OR, Valk J. Magnetic resonance evaluation of disease activity during pregnancy in multiple sclerosis. Neurol 1994;44:327–329.

[110] Paavilainen T, Kurki T, Parkkola R, Färkkilä M, Salonen O, Dastidar P, Elovaara I, Airas L. Magnetic resonance imaging of the brain used to detect early post-partum activation of multiple sclerosis. Eur J Neurol 2007;14:1216–1221.

[111] Harbo HF, Gold R, Tintoré M. Sex and gender issues in multiple sclerosis. Ther Adv Neurol Disord 2013;6(4):237–248.

[112] Voskuhl, R Gold, S. Sex-related factors in multiple sclerosis susceptibility and progression. Nat Rev Neurol 2012;8:255–263.

[113] Langer-Gould A, Gupta R, Huang S, Hagan A, Atkuri K, Leimpeter AD, Albers KB, Greenwood E, Van Den Eeden SK, Steinman L, Nelson LM. Interferon-gamma-producing T cells, pregnancy, and postpartum relapses of multiple sclerosis. Arch Neurol 2010;67(1):51–57.

[114] Gilmore W, Arias M, Stroud N, Stek A, Mccarthy Ka, Correale J. Preliminary studies of cytokine secretion patterns associated with pregnancy in MS patients. J Neurol Sci 2004;224:69–76.

[115] Sánchez-Ramón S, Navarro A J, Aristimuño C, Rodríguez-Mahou M, Bellón JM, Fernández-Cruz E, de Andrés C. Pregnancy-induced expansion of regulatory T-lymphocytes may mediate protection to multiple sclerosis activity. Immunol Lett 2005;96:195–201.

[116] Saito S, Nakashima A, Shima T, Ito M. Th1/Th2/Th17 and regulatory T-cell paradigm in pregnancy. Am J Reprod Immunol 2010;63(6):601–610.

[117] Patas K, Engler JB, Friese MA, Gold SM. Pregnancy and multiple sclerosis: feto-maternal immune cross talk and its implications for disease activity. J Reprod Immunol 2013;97:140–146.

[118] Tai P, Wang J, Jin H, Song X, Yan J, Kang Y, Zhao L, An X, Du X, Chen X, Wang S, Xia G, Wang B. Induction of regulatory T cells by physiological level estrogen. J Cell Physiol 2008;214(2):456–464.

[119] Saraste M, Vaisanen S, Alanen A, Airas L. Clinical and immunologic evaluation of women with multiple sclerosis during and after pregnancy. Gend Med 2007;4:45–55.

[120] Neuteboom RF, Verbraak E, Voerman JS, van Meurs M, Steegers EA, de Groot CJ, Laman JD, Hintzen RQ. First trimester interleukin 8 levels are associated with postpartum relapse in multiple sclerosis. Mult Scler 2009;15(11):1356–1358.

[121] Airas L, Nikula T, Huang Yh, Lahesmaa R, Wiendl H. Postpartum-activation of multiple sclerosis is associated with down-regulation of tolerogenic HLA-G. J Neuroimmunol 2007;187:205–211.

[122] Giesser B, Halper J, Cross AH. Multiple sclerosis symptoms fluctuate during menstrual cycle. MS Exchange 1991;3:5.

[123] Zorgdrager A, De Keyser J. Premenstrual exacerbations of multiple sclerosis. J Neurol Neurosurg Psychiatry 1998;65:279–280.

[124] Wilson S, Parrat J, O'Riordan J, Swingler R. Premenstrual worsening of MS symptoms. J Neurol Sci 2001;187(1):336.

[125] Zorgdrager A, De Keyser J. The premenstrual period and exacerbations in multiple sclerosis. Eur Neurol 2002;48(4):204–206.

[126] Jaini R, Altuntas CZ, Loya MG, Tuohy VK. Disruption of estrous cycle homeostasis in mice with experimental autoimmune encephalomyelitis. J Neuroimmunol 2015;279:71–74.

[127] Trenova AG, Slavov GS, Manova MG, Kostadinova II, Vasileva TV. Female sex hormones and cytokine secretion in women with multiple sclerosis. Neurol Res 2013;35(1):95–99.

[128] Zakrzewska-Pniewska B, Gołębiowski M, Zajda M, Szeszkowski W, Podlecka-Piętowska A, Nojszewska M. Sex hormone patterns in women with multiple sclerosis as related to disease activity – a pilot study. Neurol Neurochir Pol 2011;45(6):536–542.

[129] Smith R, Studd JW. A pilot study of the effect upon multiple sclerosis of menopause hormone replacement therapy and menstrual cycle. J R Soc Med 1992;85:612–613.

[130] Holmquist P, Wallberg M, Hamman M, Landtblom AM, Brynhildsen J. Symptoms of multiple sclerosis in women in relation to sex steroid exposure. Maturitas 2006;54(2): 149–153.

[131] Wei T, Lightman SL. The neuroendocrine axis in patients with multiple sclerosis. Brain 1997;120:1067–1076.

[132] de Andrés C, Rodríguez-Sáinz MC, Muñoz-Fernández MA, López-Lazareno N, Rodríguez-Mahou M, Vicente A, Fernández-Cruz E, Sánchez-Ramón S. Short-term sequential analysis of sex hormones and helper T cells type 1 (Th1) and helper T cells type 2 (Th2) cytokines during and after multiple sclerosis relapse. Eur Cytokine Netw 2004;15(3):197–202.

[133] Bove R, Musallam A, Healy BC, Raghavan K, Glanz BI, Bakshi R, Weiner H, De Jager PL, Miller KK, Chitnis T. Low testosterone is associated with disability in men with multiple sclerosis. Mult Scler 2014;20(12):1584–1592.

[134] Pozzilli C, Tomassini V, Marinelli F, Paolillo A, Gasperini C, Bastianello S. 'Gender gap' in multiple sclerosis: magnetic resonance imaging evidence. Eur J Neurol 2003;10(1): 95–97.

[135] Calabrese M, De Stefano N, Atzori M, Bernardi V, Mattisi I, Barachino L, Morra A, Rinaldi L, Romualdi C, Perini P, Battistin L, Gallo P. Detection of cortical inflammatory lesions by double inversion recovery magnetic resonance imaging in patients with multiple sclerosis. Arch Neurol 2007;64(10):1416–1422.

[136] Pozzilli C, Falaschi P,Mainero C, Martocchia A, D'Urso R, Proietti A, Frontoni M, Bastianello S, Filippi M. MRI in multiple sclerosis during the menstrual cycle: relationship with sex hormone patterns. Neurol 1999;53:622–624.

[137] Tomassini V, Giugni E, Mainero C, Onesti E, Giuliani S, Paolillo A, Salvetti M, Pozzilli C. Sex hormones in multiple sclerosis: relationship with disease activity as measured by MRI. J Neurol Sci 2001;187(1):433.

[138] Tomassini V, Onesti E, Mainero C, Giugni E, Paolillo A, Salvetti M, Nicoletti F, Pozzilli C. Sex hormones modulate brain damage in multiple sclerosis: MRI evidence. J Neurol Neurosurg Psychiatry 2005;76:272–275.

[139] Luchetti S, van Eden CG, Schuurman K, van Strien ME, Swaab DF, Huitinga I. Gender differences in multiple sclerosis: induction of estrogen signaling in male and progesterone signaling in female lesions. J Neuropathol Exp Neurol 2014;73(2):123–135.

[140] Sicotte NL, Liva SM, Klutch R, Pfeiffer P, Bouvier S, Odesa S, Wu TC, Voskuhl RR. Treatment of multiple sclerosis with the pregnancy hormone estriol. Ann Neurol 2002;52(4):421–428.

[141] Soldan SS, Retuerto AIA, Sicotte NL, Voskuhl RR. Immune modulation in multiple sclerosis patients treated with pregnancy hormone estriol. J Immunol 2003;171:6267–6274.

[142] Motamed MR, Fereshtehnejad SM. The comparison of sex hormones' and interferon's impacts on the number of relapses and the progression of disability in relapsing-remitting multiple sclerosis. Mult Scler Clin Lab Res 2005;11(1):174.

[143] Vukusic S, Ionescu I, El-Etr M, Schumacher M, Baulieu EE, Cornu C, Confavreux C; Prevention of post-partum relapses with progestin and estradiol in Multiple Sclerosis Study Group. The Prevention of Post-Partum Relapses with Progestin and Estradiol in Multiple Sclerosis (POPART'MUS) trial: rationale, objectives and state of advancement. J Neurol Sci 2009;286(1–2):114–118.

[144] Sicotte NL, Giesser BS, Tandon V, Klutch R, Steiner B, Drain AE, Shattuck DW, Hull L, Wang HJ, Elashoff RM, Swerdloff RS, Voskuhl RR. Testosterone treatment in multiple sclerosis: a pilot study. Arch Neurol 2007;64(5):683–688.

[145] Gold SM, Chalifoux S, Giesser BS, Voskuhl RR. Immune modulation and increased neurotrophic factor production in multiple sclerosis patients treated with testosterone. J Neuroinflammation 2008;5:32.

Chapter 12

Neuroprotection and Recovery in Multiple Sclerosis

Dafin F. Muresanu, Maria Balea, Olivia Rosu,
Anca Buzoianu and Dana Slavoaca

Additional information is available at the end of the chapter

http://dx.doi.org/10.5772/63829

Abstract

Multiple sclerosis is a complex and heterogeneous immune-mediated disease that results in the progressive accumulation of mental and physical symptoms. Currently approved disease-modifying drugs (DMDs) are immunomodulatory or immunosuppressive, but these drugs have little effect on disease progression. In addition to studies that have directly targeted inflammation and immune responses, a large number of studies, most of them experimental, have investigated neuroprotective therapies and remyelination strategies. However, to date, attempts to provide neuroprotection have failed not just in multiple sclerosis but in neurological disorders in general; this situation has emphasized the need to revise the old paradigm of a "magic bullet" with a single mechanism of action. Remyelination strategies involve either promoting endogenous remyelination or replacing lost myelinating cells through exogenous sources. However, several puzzle pieces regarding the physiology of remyelination remain unknown, including feasible treatment monitoring methods, the selection of patients, and the optimal time of treatment initiation. This chapter will describe the direct and indirect neuroprotective effects of DMDs, as suggested by basic research studies and confirmed by clinical studies in some cases. Current knowledge of potential neuroprotective therapies and remyelination strategies is also reviewed.

Keywords: multiple sclerosis, neuroprotection, ion channel modulation, remyelination, systems biology

1. Introduction

Multiple sclerosis (MS) is characterized by complex interactions between pathological pathways and heterogeneity regarding lesions, progression, clinical symptoms, and immune responses.

Recently, significant advances in MS therapy have been made, but these advances have been limited to the prevention of relapse, and long-term results are conflicting.

Understanding of endogenous defense activity (**Figure 1**), including neurotrophicity, neuroprotection, neuroplasticity, neurogenesis, and remyelination, is essential for pharmacological neuroprotection and enhanced neurorecovery. Neurotrophicity includes the processes necessary for the maintenance of a normal phenotype. Neuroprotection is the sum of all processes aimed at counterbalancing the pathophysiological mechanisms that are induced by the alteration of neuro-immune responses. Neuroplasticity represents the sum of the structural and functional changes that must occur for adaptation to new internal or environmental stimuli. Neurogenesis, in a broad sense, refers to the capacity of brain tissue to generate new neurons, astrocytes, and oligodendrocytes [1]. Remyelination is a physiological regenerative process that requires the activation of oligodendrocyte precursor cells (OPCs), their migration, recruitment, and differentiation into remyelinating oligodendrocytes and their interaction with denuded axons. Changes in these steps, which are characteristic of MS, promote neurodegeneration.

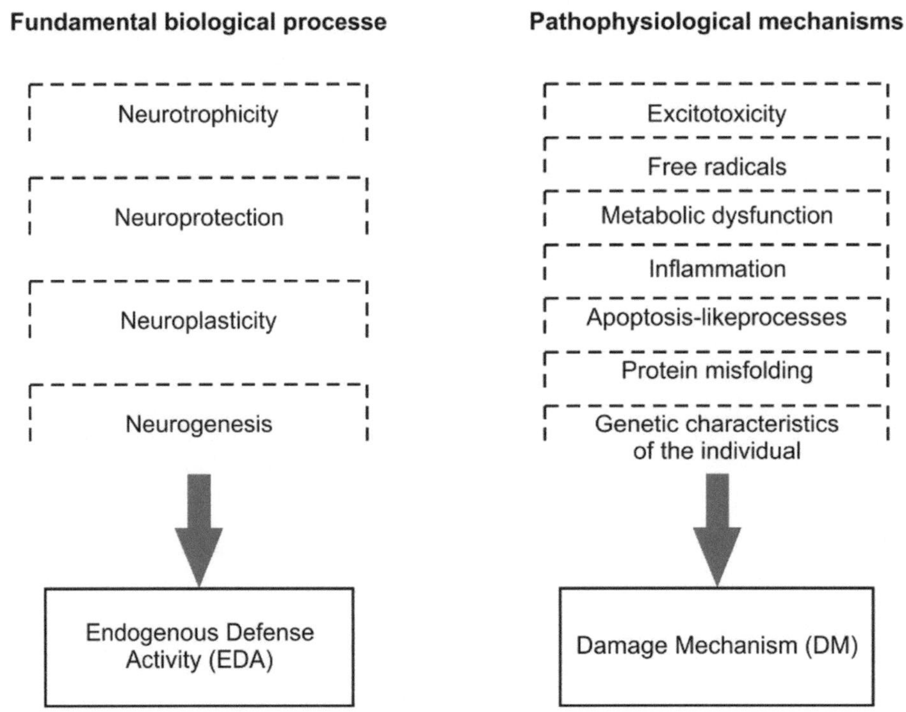

Figure 1. Endogenous defense activity and damage mechanism.

Classical neuroprotection approaches include the use of the already Food and Drug Administration (FDA)-approved disease modifying drugs (DMDs) and a wide spectrum of pharmacological compounds that interact with one or more pathological processes (inflammation,

http://dx.doi.org/10.5772/63829

oxidative damage, mitochondrial damage, and intracellular Ca^{2+} overload), as an attempt to prevent axonal degeneration. Pro-myelination therapies appear to be a promising approach, but several puzzle pieces regarding the physiology of remyelination, feasible treatment monitoring methods, the selection of patients, and the optimal time of treatment initiation remain unknown. However, neurodegeneration is not always related to demyelination, leading to the development of combination therapies that include agents that prevent neurodegeneration, modulate neuroinflammation, and immune responses and promote remyelination [2].

2. Neuroprotective effects of disease modifying drugs (DMDs)

Several DMDs are currently approved by the FDA for MS: interferons (interferon beta 1b or IFNB-1b, interferon beta-1a or IFNB-1a), glatiramer acetate (GA), traditional immunosuppressants (mitoxantrone), fingolimod, and monoclonal antibodies (natalizumab, alemtuzumab, and daclizumab) as well as the recently approved drugs teriflunomide and dimethyl fumarate (DMF). The main target of these molecules is the modulation of immune mechanisms and inflammation, along with a debatable effect on disease progression. **Table 1** summarizes the available information about FDA-approved DMDs, including their mechanisms of action and severe adverse effects [**Table 1**]. The neuroprotective effects of these agents against neurodegeneration and their ability to promote reparative processes are still under investigation.

FDA-approved DMDs	Indication	Primary mechanisms of action	Neuroprotective effects—results from basic research studies	Neuroprotective effects—results from clinical research studies	Severe adverse effects
Interferon beta-1b (Betaseron, Extavia)	First line therapy for RR-MS, SP-MS, and CIS	Suppresses the proliferation of MBP-specific T cells. Inhibits the secretion of pro-inflammatory cytokines	Stabilizes BBB barrier. Protect endothelial cells from apoptosis Decrease the expression of matrix metalloproteinases. Anti-inflammatory effects. Antioxidative and anti-excitotoxic effect. Increase BDNF and NGF levels [3–5]	Higher serum levels of BDNF in patients treated with IFNβ [6–8] Reduces the likelihood of the development of black holes and reduces the size of pre-existing ones [9]	Hepatotoxicity, congestive heart failure, seizures, depression or suicidal thoughts

FDA-approved DMDs	Indication	Primary mechanisms of action	Neuroprotective effects—results from basic research studies	Neuroprotective effects—results from clinical research studies	Severe adverse effects
//5Interferon beta-1a (Avonex; Rebif)	First line therapy for RR-MS, SP-MS, and CIS (only Avonex)	Suppresses the proliferation of MBP-specific T cells. Inhibits the secretion of pro-inflammatory cytokines	–	–	Hepatotoxicity, congestive heart failure, seizures, depression or suicidal thoughts
Peg interferon beta-1a (Plegridy)	First-line therapy for RR-MS	Suppresses the proliferation of MBP-specific T cells. Inhibits the secretion of pro-inflamma-tory cytokines	–	–	Hepatotoxicity, congestive heart failure, seizures, depression or suicidal thoughts
Glatiramer acetate (Copaxone)	First-line therapy for RR-MS and CIS	Suppresses the proliferation of MBP-specific T cells. Shifts the population of T cells from proinflammatory Th1 cells to regulatory Th2 cells	Anti-inflammatory, antioxidative, and anti-apoptotic effects [10, 11]. Increased BDNF and IGF-2 Pro-remyelination and pro-regenerative proprieties [12, 13]	Conflicting results: there found both increased and no effect upon serum BDNF levels [14–16]. Imaging data supports the neuroprotective and pro-myelinating properties of GA by showing that patients treated with GA are less likely to develop "black holes" than non-treated patients and have demonstrated a significant increase in the NAA–Cr ratio compared to pre-treatment values	Injection site lipoatrophy and necrosis, panic disorder, bowel disorder

FDA-approved DMDs	Indication	Primary mechanisms of action	Neuroprotective effects—results from basic research studies	Neuroprotective effects—results from clinical research studies [17]	Severe adverse effects
Mitoxantrone (Novantrone)	Third-line therapy for SP-MS, and worsening RR-MS	Suppresses the proliferation of T cells, B cells, and macrophages. Enhances T-cell suppressor function and inhibits B-cell function and antibody production. Inhibits macrophage-mediated myelin degradation	–	–	Secondary acute myelogenous leukemia, cardiotoxicity
Fingolimod (Gilenya)	First- or second-line therapy for RR-MS and SP-MS	Sequesters lymphocytes in lymph nodes	Promotes oligodentrocyte extension Increases BDNF and GDNF production [18]	–	Macular edema, bradyarrhythmia, PML, hypotension, herpes infection, hepatotoxicity
Natalizumab (Tysabri)	Second- or third line therapy for RR-MS	Inhibits leukocytes migration	–		PML, allergic reactions including anaphylactic shock, infections, hepatotoxicity
Daclizumab (Zinbryta; Zenepax)	Second line therapy for RR-MS	Inhibits the activation of T cells and inhibits survival of already activated T cells; inhibits secretion of pro-inflammatory cytokines. Normalizes the number of circulating LTi cells	–		Infections, cutaneous events, malignancies, auto-immunity

FDA-approved DMDs	Indication	Primary mechanisms of action	Neuroprotective effects—results from basic research studies	Neuroprotective effects—results from clinical research studies	Severe adverse effects
Teriflunomide (Aubagio)	First-line therapy for RR-MS	Inhibits the activation and proliferation of stimulated lymphocytes	–	–	Hepatotoxicity, peripheral neuropathy, hyperkalemia, transient acute renal failure, severe skin reactions
Dimethyl fumarate (Tecfidera)	First line therapy for RR-MS	Reduce transendothelial migration of activated leukocytes	Antioxidative effects by activation of Nrf2 [19, 20]	–	Lymphopenia
Alemtuzumab (Lemtrada)	Second line therapy for RR-MS	Lymphocyte B and T depletion; decrease of pro-inflammatory cytokines	Anti-inflammatory effects Induction of neurotrophin producing lymphocytes Preservation of axonal conductance Stabilizes blood–brain barrier [21]	It significantly decreases the T2-weighted lesion burden compared to IFNβ [22]	Infusion-associated reactions, infections, auto-immunity

Abbreviations: LTi—lymphoid tissue inducer; IGF-2—insulin growth factor; MPB—myelin-basic protein; BDNF—brain-derived neurotrophic factor; GDNF—glial cell-derived nerve factor; Nrf2—nuclear factor erythroid 2-related factor; BBB—blood–brain barrier, RR-MS—relapse remitting MS; SP-MM—secondary progressive MS, CIS—clinical-isolated syndrome; PML—progressive multifocal leukoencephalopathy; LTi—lymphoid tissue inducer.

Table 1. The neuroprotective effects of FDA-approved DMD.

In addition to the currently FDA-approved DMDs, some promising new agents are already in ongoing late-phase clinical trials, such as laquinomid, ozanimod, ponesimod, siponimod, ocrelizumab, ofatumumab, masitinib, and cladribine. Few data related to the mechanisms of action of these drugs are currently available. Of these compounds, laquinimod is the only one that appears to have neuroprotective properties, and laquinimod is currently being tested in patients with RR-MS in a third phase III trial, CONCERTO [23]. Basic research studies suggest that in addition to its neuromodulatory and anti-inflammatory effects, laquinimod also displays neuroprotective effects through several mechanisms, including reducing excitotox-

http://dx.doi.org/10.5772/63829

icity, increasing serum levels of BDNF, downregulating the astrocytic pro-inflammatory response, reducing astrocytic nuclear factor κB (NFκB) activity, and preserving cannabinoid receptor type 1 expression [24]. However, to date, the results of phase II and III clinical trials have failed to show a clear effect of laquinimod in RR-MS patients [25, 26].

3. Other neuroprotective strategies

In addition to DMDs, there are many additional potential neuroprotective agents, including ion channel modulators, glutamate antagonists, growth factors, sex hormones, statins, and immunophilin ligands. Most of these were tested only in experimental studies as a means to target molecular pathways involved in neurodegeneration or, in contrast, to stimulate endogenous defense mechanisms. There is increasing interest in pleiotropic molecules such as 5-HTR3 antagonists [27], polymerized nano-curcumin [28], and tyrphostin AG 126 [29]; in molecules that can modulate the kynurenine pathway [30]; in cannabinoid compounds [31–33]; and in combination therapies of DMDs with pleiotropic molecules.

One of the factors that contributes to the persistence of inflammation in MS is sustained activation of the transcription of nuclear factor kappa B (NFκB), which is an important hub for several molecular mechanisms involved in apoptosis and in immune and inflammatory responses. Glucocorticoid-induced leucine zipper (GILZ) is a glucocorticoid-responsive protein that binds the p65 unit of NFκB and thus can reduce the immuno-inflammatory response. In cell cultures, a synthetic peptide (GILZ-P) derived from the proline-rich region of GILZ suppressed NFκB activation and prevented glutamate neurotoxicity [34]. Additionally, in an in vitro study, intraperitoneal administration of GILZ-P modulated the Th1/Th2 balance and ameliorated the symptomatology of experimental autoimmune encephalomyelitis (EAE) [35]. The paracaspase mucosa-associated lymphoid tissue lymphoma translocation protein 1 (MALT1) is another signaling molecule that triggers lymphocyte activation through NFκB signaling and also acts as a cysteine protease. To test the hypothesis that MALT1 inhibitors could be used to treat lymphocyte-mediated pathologies, the therapeutic potential of mepazine (a recently identified MALT1 inhibitor) was studied in mice with EAE. When mepazine was prophylactically administered, it significantly reduced clinical disease symptoms and histopathological parameters. Moreover, its therapeutic administration clearly promotes disease remission [36].

The nuclear receptor-related 1 protein (Nurr1) is a member of the class of steroid nuclear hormone receptors, and its activity is significantly downregulated in neurodegenerative disorders such as MS; its levels are also negatively correlated with EDSS progression. In mice with EAE, the administration of isoxazolo-pyridinone, an activator of the Nurr1 signaling pathway, delays EAE onset and reduces its severity. Therapeutic administration of isoxazolo-pyridinone also reduced neuro-inflammatory and histopathological alterations in the spinal cord but not the course of EAE [37].

KV1.3, the third member of the shaker-related subfamily of voltage-gated potassium channels, is known to modulate calcium signaling to induce T cell proliferation (effector memory T cells

—TEM), immune system activation and cytokine production. Toxins derived from animal venoms can target ion channels, including KV1.3, and offer a means to diminish the activation and proliferation of TEM cells and to improve of the pathology underlying autoimmune diseases. For example, in a rat acute EAE model, ADWX-1, an analog of scorpion toxin, reduced the number of T cells and the secretion of inflammatory factors. These toxic peptides could be used to obtain better clinical results without neurological impairment [38]. There is increasing interest in bee venom therapy, which experimental studies have shown can ameliorate the symptomatology of EAE by decreasing inflammation and demyelination [39]. However, additional clinical evidence is needed.

The mitochondrial permeability transition pore (PT pore) is a drug target for neurodegenerative conditions and for ischemia-reperfusion injury. Cyclophilin D (CypD) is a positive regulator of the pore, and its downregulation improves outcomes in animal models of stroke. However, this isomerase is not selective and may have toxic effects. A new synthesized mitochondria-targeting CypD inhibitor, JW47, displayed selective cellular inhibition and reduced cellular toxicity. In an EAE model, JW47 significantly protected axons and improved motor assessments with minimal immunosuppression. These findings suggest that selective CypD inhibition could become a viable therapeutic strategy for MS [40].

Granzyme B (GrB) is a serine protease released from the granules of cytotoxic T cells, which can induce cell death by disrupting a variety of intra/extracellular protein substrates. GrB-expressing T cells were identified in close proximity to oligodendrocytes and demyelinating axons in acute MS lesions and were thus associated with neuronal loss. The GrB inhibitor serpina3n, which was isolated from mouse Sertoli cells, can inhibit the enzymatic activity of this protease. The administration of serpina3n attenuated disease severity in an animal model of MS by reducing T cell-mediated neuronal death and axonal injury. These observations suggest that serpina3n could be used to decrease inflammation-mediated neurodegeneration [41].

Experimental studies have shown that fasudil—an inhibitor of Rho kinase (ROCK)—can suppress experimental EAE when administered via multiple, short-term injections. Later, a novel ROCK inhibitor that can be delivered intranasally was developed. This inhibitor, FSD-C10, reaches the CNS faster and in a much lower dose. FSD-C10 reduced EAE severity and CNS inflammatory infiltration and promoted neuroprotection by inducing CNS production of IL-10, NGF, and BDNF and by inhibiting the production of multiple pro-inflammatory cytokines [42].

Eriocalyxin B (EriB) is a diterpenoid extracted from Isodon eriocalyx, a perennial herb from southwest China that is used as an anti-inflammatory remedy in traditional Chinese medicine. EriB has been reported to induce apoptosis in leukemia and lymphoma by elevating the intracellular levels of reactive oxygen species and by suppressing the NFκB pathway. In an EAE model, EriB alleviated symptoms, delayed disease onset, decreased T cell populations, inhibited the NFκB pathway and reduced CNS inflammation and demyelination, improving the course of the disease [43]. Adenanthin, which is also a diterpenoid isolated from the leaves of Isodon adenanthus, displays preventive and therapeutic effects in EAE, as demonstrated by improved clinical scores as well as by reduced infiltration of inflammatory cells and demyelination in the CNS [44, 45].

Regarding sex hormones, 2-methoxyestradiol (2ME2)—the endogenous metabolite of estradiol and an antimitotic and antiangiogenic cancer drug—was found to suppress the development of mouse EAE, as it inhibited lymphocyte activation, cytokine production, and proliferation in a dose-dependent manner [46]. Other studies have shown that estrogen and estrogen receptor agonists reduce the severity of EAE in animals when they are administered after disease onset; these agents inhibit several inflammatory cytokines, induce apoptosis in T cells, and also regulate the expression of adhesion and accessory molecules by endothelial cells, altering leukocyte migration [47]. In addition, the β estrogen receptor has been demonstrated to modulate microglial activity. The β estrogen receptor agonist LY3201 can suppress activated microglia and NFκB activation in both microglia and T cells. All of these outcomes can be achieved without negative effects on the pituitary gland, mammary glands, or uterus [48].

Nevertheless, in animal models of demyelination, progesterone and synthetic progestins have been observed to attenuate myelin loss and to reduce clinical symptom severity. One study showed that progesterone and Nosterone (a synthetic 19-nor-progesterone derivative) promoted remyelination and attenuated inflammatory responses in female mice with severe chronic demyelinating lesions. The remyelinating effect of progesterone was receptor-dependent and began in the corpus callosum. Moreover, it enhanced the number of mature oligodendrocytes and their progenitors as well, indicating that these hormones could represent promising therapeutic agents for demyelinating diseases [49].

Statins are widely used to treat vascular diseases, but they also have immunomodulatory and neuroprotective properties that could make them possible treatment candidates for neurodegenerative disorders. Lovastatin has been found to improve clinical symptoms associated with EAE as well as to reduce neuroinflammatory mediators such as iNOS, TNF-α and interferon gamma (IFNγ). Similarly, atorvastatin has also been shown to ameliorate EAE symptomatology by modulating T cell immunity [50]. One double-blind, controlled trial used simvastatin in patients with secondary progressive MS. High-dose simvastatin reduced the rate of whole-brain atrophy by 43% compared with placebo and was safe and well tolerated. Furthermore, differences between the simvastatin-treated and control groups were consistently observed over 12 and 25 months. A small but significant improvement in disability outcomes and a non-significant reduction in T2 lesion accumulation were also observed [51].

SWABIMS was a multi-center, randomized, parallel-group, rater-blinded study conducted in 8 Swiss hospitals that evaluated the efficacy, safety, and tolerability of daily administration of 40 mg atorvastatin and subcutaneous IFNB-1b compared to monotherapy with IFNB-1b. At the end of the study, both groups had an equivalent number of patients with new lesions on T2-weighted MRI images. Additionally, none of the secondary endpoints, including the number of new lesions and total lesion volume on T2-weighted images, the total number of new Gd-enhancing lesions on T1-weighted images, total brain volume, grey matter volume, white matter volume, EDSS, relapse rate and number of relapse-free patients, did showed any significant differences, suggesting that atorvastatin did not have a beneficial effect on relapsing-remitting MS [52].

Recent data from an established rat model of MS suggest that inhibiting excitatory glutamatergic neurotransmission may have neuroprotective effects. One of these studies investigated whether drugs such as amantadine and memantine (antagonists of NMDA glutamate receptors), LY 367385 (a selective mGluR1 antagonist) or MPEP (an mGluR5 antagonist) could improve the condition of rats with EAE. On the one hand, amantadine and memantine reduced the development and duration of neurological deficits and modified all of the assessed parameters. On the other hand, LY 367385 and MPEP did not influence the condition of treated animals when they were administered alone or in conjunction with NMDA antagonists [53]. Another study evaluated if selective antagonism of the NR2B subtype of NMDA receptors (which are considered to play a more pivotal role in neurodegeneration) could be more effective than memantine in EAE mice. Therapeutic administration of RO25-6981 (a selective inhibitor of NR2B) caused a more significant decrease in neurological deficits, inflammation, myelin degradation, and degeneration of axons from the spinal cord, suggesting that this drug may be an effective treatment strategy to slow down the clinical deterioration that causes disability in MS [54].

The metabotropic glutamate receptor 4 (mGluR4) has immunomodulatory properties, such that a positive allosteric modulator of the receptor, ADX88178, protects mice with relapsing-remitting EAE. ADX88178 is a newly developed drug with high selectivity and potency, optimal pharmacokinetics, good brain penetrance, and almost no toxicity. Its administration in EAE converted the disease into a form of mild chronic neuroinflammation that remained stable for two months after the drug treatment was discontinued [55].

Recent studies have demonstrated that atypical antipsychotic agents (antagonists of dopamine D2 and serotonin 5-HT2a receptors) have immunomodulatory properties, both peripherally and within the CNS. In an EAE animal model, chronic oral administration of risperidone improved disease severity, decreased both the size and the number of spinal cord lesions and substantially reduced antigen-specific interleukins such as IL-17a, IL-2, and IL-4 and the activation of microglia and macrophages in the CNS. In addition, another antipsychotic agent, clozapine, showed a similar ability to modify macrophages and to reduce disease severity. Together, these studies indicate that atypical agents could treat immune-mediated diseases such as MS [56].

Polyphenolic flavonoids and non-flavonoids have potent antioxidant abilities, but they can also target different molecules and affect multiple signaling pathways. Resveratrol, a phenol found in grapes and red wines, is considered to have neuroprotective effects. In EAE, it induces the apoptosis of activated T cells in the periphery and suppresses pro-inflammatory responses. Another plant-derived substance, oleanolic acid (a triterpenoid), is known to have potent anti-inflammatory properties. Treatment with oleanolic acid has been reported to prevent EAE by suppressing peripheral inflammation and preventing CNS infiltration of inflammatory cells (due to blockade of the NF-κB pathway [45]. Other studies have shown that flavonoids are naturally immunomodulatory compounds that can limit demyelination, reduce neuroinflammation, and downregulate immune functions. For example, luteolin provides neuroprotection by reducing axonal damage and, together with quercetin and fisetin, is able to decrease the amount of myelin phagocytosed by macrophages; thus, luteolin may help prevent MS [57].

Polyphenolic curcuminoids are the mixtures of curcumin, desmethoxycurcumin, and bisdemethoxycurcumin, which are derived from turmeric (*Curcuma longa*). Both the mixtures and the individual components have been suggested to influence inflammatory and apoptotic genes and the regulation of signal transduction pathways that lead to the activation of transcription factors. In EAE, treatment with curcumin modulates pro- and anti-inflammatory responses, prevents the differentiation of neural antigen-specific T cells, decreases oxidative stress, improves remyelination and promotes neurogenesis [28]. However, despite the promising therapeutic potential of curcumin, its poor water solubility, fast degradation profile and poor bioavailability are significant hurdles for its clinical use.

The kynurenine pathway is known to have a regulatory function in the immune system. Alterations of this pathway have been described in preclinical and clinical investigations of MS. These data led to the identification of potential therapeutic targets, such as synthetic tryptophan analogs, endogenous tryptophan metabolites, structural analogs, indoleamine-2, 3-dioxygenase inhibitors, and kynurenine-3-monooxygenase inhibitors [30]. Additionally, high levels of a by-product of the kynurenine pathway, quinolinic acid, were found in EAE mice and MS patients. Sundaram et al. demonstrated two possible strategies to limit quinolinic acid gliotoxicity: by neutralizing quinolinic acid's effects with monoclonal antibodies or by inhibiting quinolinic acid production using specific KP enzyme inhibitors. These observations could represent a novel therapeutic approach in MS [58].

Cannabidiol (CBD) is a non-psychotropic cannabinoid constituent of *Cannabis sativa* that is known to possess anti-inflammatory and immunosuppressive properties. In a viral model of MS, CBD decreased the transmigration of blood leukocytes by downregulating the expression of VCAM-1, chemokines and the cytokine IL-1β and by attenuating the activation of microglia. Its administration had long-lasting effects and ameliorated motor deficits during the chronic phase of the disease, demonstrating the significant therapeutic potential of this compound [59]. Another study of CBD as a topical 1% cream also had surprisingly good results too. The daily treatment, initiated at the time of symptomatic disease onset, displayed neuroprotective effects against EAE, diminishing clinical disease scores (EDSS) by recovering hind limb paralysis and by ameliorating lymphocytic infiltration and demyelination in spinal cord tissues [60]. However, when the CUPID trial investigated if oral dronabinol (Δ^9-tetrahydrocannabinol) might slow the course of progressive MS, it had no overall effect on disease progression, although there were no serious safety concerns [61].

Epigallocatechin-3-gallate (EGCG), one of the major polyphenolic extracts of green tea, has been shown to exhibit neuroprotective effects against toxic insults and neuronal injury. In an EAE animal model, the administration of EGCG attenuated clinical symptoms and leukocyte infiltration and demyelination in the CNS. Moreover, EGCG inhibited the NF-κB-mediated transactivation of inflammatory mediators, reducing the production of interferons, IL-17, IL-6, IL-1, and tumor necrosis factors [62]. These results were corroborated by other studies, which demonstrated that EGCG, due to its antioxidative properties, could reduce the clinical severity of EAE by limiting brain inflammation and reducing neuronal damage [63]. In addition, GA and EGCG combination therapy had synergistic protective effects in vitro and in vivo, with good results and no unexpected adverse events [64].

Ginseng has been used in traditional medicine for over 2000 years due to its antianxiety, antidepressant, and cognition-enhancing properties. Moreover, its effects on the brain are related to glutamatergic and monoaminergic transmission, estrogen signaling, nitric oxide production, neuronal survival, apoptosis, neural stem cells, and neuroregeneration. The efficacy of ginsenoside Rd has been studied in mice with EAE. The results were promising because the ginsenoside reduced the permeability of the blood–brain barrier, regulated the secretion of INF-gamma and IL-4 and decreased disease severity [65].

Based on the observational studies that showed that low levels of vitamin D represent a risk factor for the development of MS [66, 67], treatment with vitamin D has become increasingly attractive and has been tested in both experimental and clinical trials. Vitamin D appeared to modulate upon immune responses and inflammation, but clinical studies have not yet shown a clear benefit [68, 69].

In addition to pharmaceutical compounds, clinical and basic research studies have also highlighted that voluntary exercise can promote both neuroprotection and neuroregeneration [70, 71]. An experiment conducted in mice with EAE showed that the exercising mice (on a running wheel) presented a less severe neurological disease score, later disease onset and a significant reduction of inflammatory cell infiltration and demyelination in the ventral white matter tracts of the lumbar spinal cord [71]. Studies of patients with MS also support these observations, physical excesses determining not only improvement of muscle function and walking endurance, but also of cognitive abilities [72–75].

4. Ion channel modulation

Among the molecules that make up neurons, ion channels are especially important, because they provide them their signaling abilities. In multiple sclerosis, there were described several types of ion channels dysfunctioning:

- Ectopic distribution of calcium channels, up-regulated within the axon membrane, during the demyelinating process. Increased intracellular calcium levels activate calcium-dependent proteases (calpains) that can degrade axonal proteins, contributing to the axonal injury. Blocking the calcium channels can protect myelinated axons from axotomy-induced and anoxia-induced degeneration (see **Figure 2**) [76].
- Transcriptional channelopathy that described in cerebellar Purkinje neurons. Studies showed that Nav1.8 gene (normally inactivated in the cerebellum) is aberrantly activated in Purkinje neurons, producing the Nav1.8 protein, possibly responsible for cerebellar deficits [77].
- Ion channel dysfunctioning during remyelination—redistribution and clustering of ion channels [78–81].

In MS, excessive accumulation of Ca^{2+} ions is known to contribute to axonal degeneration in the central nervous system (CNS) through the activation of acid-sensing ion channel type 1a

http://dx.doi.org/10.5772/63829

(ASIC1). ASIC1 is considered a mediator of neuronal injury in stroke and CNS inflammation due to its ability to modulate Na^+ and Ca^{2+} flux. So, it could be possible to attenuate axonal loss by disrupting the ASIC1a gene or by using a nonspecific blocker of these channels, such as amiloride (a diuretic with a proven safety record) [82]. Recently, a single-arm, longitudinal trial of amiloride showed an important reduction of brain atrophy in the primary progressive form of MS. The aim of Amiloride Clinical Trial in Optic Neuritis (ACTION), an ongoing phase II clinical trial, is to demonstrate the neuroprotective effect of amiloride in acute optic neuritis (a common manifestation of MS) using a multimodal approach that combines structural and functional outcomes with clinical measures [83].

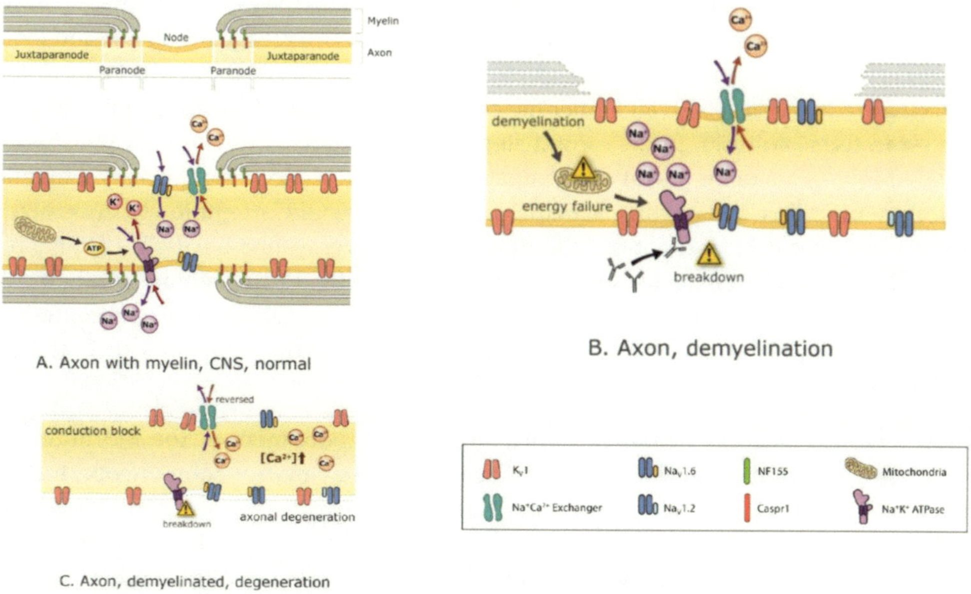

Figure 2. Mechanisms of demyelination-related neurodegeneration. Demyelination can result progressively in ionic disequilibria, energy crisis, conduction block, and eventually neurodegeneration. (A) a normal node of Ranvier with juxtaparanodal, paranodal, and nodal regions intact, depicting Na^+, K^+, and Ca^{2+} ions flowing through their respective channels with mitochondria supplying the ATP for energy-dependent Na^+K^+ ATPases that re-establish the ion gradients depleted by ion flux through channels. Numerous different ion channels are present in the axon but only a small subset is depicted here; (B) partial demyelination results in dispersal of nodal ion channels, energy insufficiency, and disequilibria of ion gradients; (C) complete demyelination can result in conduction block and axonal degeneration due to the accumulation of intracellular Ca^{2+} that results from energy crisis and disruption of ionic balances. Abbreviations: Kv1—potassium channel type 1; Nav1.6 and Nav1.2—sodium channel types 1.6 and 1.2; Na^+ Ca^+ Exchanger—Na-Ca exchange pump; Na^+K^+ ATPase—ATP (energy)-dependent Na-K exchange pump; CASPR1—contactin-associated protein 1 (interaction molecule between myelinating cell with axon); NF155—neurofascin 155 (predominant interaction molecule between myelin and axon at paranodal axo-glial junction) http://www.mdpi.com/1422-0067/16/9/21215.

4-Aminopyridine (Fampridine) is a potassium channel blocker that improves axonal conductivity in demyelinated lesions by targeting the potassium channel subtypes Kv1.1, Kv1.2, and Kv1.4 and thus correcting the leakage of potassium ions. Even if it has no impact upon disease incidence and severity, it has been already approved for improvement of fatigue, walking speed, and strength in MS patients [84].

Other potential agents that can target ion channels are lamotrigine, phenytoin, flecainide, topiramate, carbamazepine, and glibenclamide, but even if some of them have some positive results in animal studies, there is lack of clinical data regarding their efficacy in MS [85].

5. Remyelinating strategies in MS

For successful remyelination to take place, OPCs must undergo several necessary and sequential steps. This very intricate process can fail if not regulated effectively. In the first step —the activation phase—OPCs must proliferate, which involves the expression of several genes and transcription factors by either activated microglia or astrocytes within the lesion [86, 87]. Mediators such as the proteins Cdk2 and p27Kip-1, platelet-derived growth factor (PDGF), fibroblast growth factor (FGF), and other factors have been demonstrated to have a proliferative effect in tissue cultures. In the second step—the migration or recruitment phase—OPCs are guided to migrate to the site of demyelination by chemotactic factors such as semaphorin receptors, neuropilins, and plexins. Semaphorin 3A impairs OPC migration to the lesion site, whereas semaphorin 3F promotes OPC migration and remyelination [88]. PDGFα is the archetypal chemotactic factor for OPCs, although it is difficult to separate its chemotactic effects from its effect on OPC proliferation. In the third step, OPCs must differentiate into remyelinating oligodendrocytes in a process driven by transcription factors such as Nkx2.2 and Olig2 [89].

Many changes in both the cytoarchitecture and microenvironment of the MS brain could prevent remyelination by endogenous OPCs. Extracellular matrix components, including fibronectin, hyaluronic acid (HA), and chondroitin sulfate proteoglycans (CSPGs), can block the differentiation of OPCs and premyelinating oligodendrocytes [90]. Components of damaged myelin, such as myelin-associated glycoprotein (MAG), oligodendrocyte myelin glycoprotein (OMgp), and NOGO-A, which signal through the Nogo 1 receptor and its co-receptors p75, TROY and LINGO-1 (leucine-rich repeat- and Ig domain-containing Nogo receptor-interacting protein 1) inhibit both axonal regeneration and oligodendrocyte differentiation and remyelination [91, 92]. The differentiation phase can also be influenced by intrinsic signaling pathways (Notch signaling, Wnt signaling, and Retinoid X receptor (RXR) signaling) and extrinsic competitors (LINGO-1, semaphorin 3A, sonic hedgehog (Shh), fibroblast growth factor, insulin-like growth factor 1 (IGF-1), BDNF, chemokine CXCL 12, and bone morphogenic proteins (BMPs). The Notch signaling pathway is an important regulator of the balance between OPC proliferation and differentiation in the developing CNS as well as PNS. Notch 1 is a surface receptor expressed by both developing and mature oligodendrocytes. The ligand engaged with the Notch receptor determines whether the canonical or non-canonical signaling pathway is activated. The canonical Notch 1 signaling pathway, which is mediated through Jagged 1, prevents OPC differentiation, whereas the non-canonical signaling pathway mediated through contactin promotes differentiation [93]. The canonical Wnt-β-catenin signaling pathways negatively regulate the production and differentiation of oligodendrocytes during both developmental myelination and remyelination. Some data suggest that the inhibition of Wnt via Axin2 promotes oligodendrocyte differentiation and remyelination [94].

Remyelination is not regulated by a single molecule or mediator but through a combination of signaling pathways that act on OPCs and oligodendrocytes as well as on other cellular players such as microglia, astrocytes, and even blood vessels. The discovery of new molecular players and of pharmacological strategies to act on them is currently a priority of the field so that new therapeutic agents that can change the natural history of MS can be developed.

Currently, from all potential remyelinating strategies for MS that stimulate OPC differentiation and enhance remyelination that include all the pathways and the signaling molecules described above [95–100], only anti-LINGO-1 antibodies have been tested in clinical trials. A phase II trial is ongoing and will provide additional information about safety, tolerability, and efficacy (NCT01864148).

The transplantation of exogenous OPCs into the CNS appears to be an attractive solution for MS, but unanswered questions render this procedure unfeasible in MS; these open questions include how to overcome the limited migration potential of transplanted OPCs, how to control the proliferation and differentiation process, and how to avoid immunosuppression treatment [101].

6. Concluding remarks from a systems biology perspective

The dynamic interactions between environmental factors and epigenetic mechanisms that involve multiple pathways and processes suggest the need for a system-based approach to understand MS physiopathology and to implement new pharmacological therapies.

Targeting neuroprotection is always ambitious, not only in MS, but in neurology in general, mostly because of a poor understanding of the complexity of interconnections between different cellular and molecular processes. In complex diseases such as MS there is a milieu of dynamical interplay between networks of genes and signaling proteins, lipids, carbohydrate molecules that can have concomitant roles in inflammation, immune systems reactivity, demyelination, neurodegeneration, neuroprotection, remyelination. For example, the network of p38 mitogen-activated protein kinase (MAPK) signaling pathway can trigger both inflammation and neuroprotection. MAPK is activated by cell stress, playing a key role in immune responses and has been intensively investigated in relation with EAE pathogenesis [102]. Taking in account this multitude of interactions, the currently trend is to inhibit/potentiate selectively a single molecular pathway, for example, acting only on p38α MAPK and not also on p38β MAPK [103].

However, over-selective interventions have an important disadvantage. Imbalances in complex systems always affect concomitant different subsystems between which there is a significant cross-talk. This leads to several pathological outcomes, for example, to inflammation, demyelination, and neurodegeneration which potentiate each other, so targeting a single pathway seems senseless. Additionally, some of these processes occur as compensatory mechanisms and become maladaptive and trigger the emergence and expansion of vicious circles due to the alteration of modulatory mechanisms. For example, in a demyelinated axon, homeostatic plasticity that involves the redistribution of ion channels occurs, and this redistribution contributes to the failure of AP conduction and finally generates a metabolic crisis. Intercorrelation between the molecular mechanisms that underlie inflammation, apoptosis, oxidative stress, increased Ca^{2+} load, mitochondrial dysfunction, microglial activation, and blood–brain barrier dysfunction is responsible for the expansion of vicious circles that generate a nonlinear pattern of clinical evolution. From this perspective, the traditional idea of a "magic bullet" seems too simplistic to achieve sufficient neuroprotection.

An interesting explanation of these mechanisms derives from the theory of complex biological systems, which are characterized by criticality and degeneracy. Degeneracy describes the ability of structurally and functionally distinct pathways to produce the same output. This characteristic supports the existence of multifunctional components that can perform similar functions under certain conditions. A direct consequence of degeneracy is the assurance of quick compensation if one of these mechanisms fails. However, in pathological conditions, degeneracy can lead to a chronic, robust state in which a unimodal therapeutic approach that targets a single pathway will fail to ensure the sustainable irreversibility of the pathological process. According to this idea, the combination of therapies that utilize pharmacological compounds with synergic effects but different mechanisms of action or individual multimodal, pleiotropic therapies, with modulatory properties that can target as many pathways as possible offer a feasible therapeutic approach.

Last, but not least, it is very important to take in account that everyone has a different genetic polymorphism that leads to different phenotypes which can have an important influence upon the reactivity of molecular networks. This patient inter-variability may be responsible for both heterogeneity in disease progression and treatment response, leading to an open door to metabolomics [104].

Author details

Dafin F. Muresanu[1,2*], Maria Balea[1,2], Olivia Rosu[1], Anca Buzoianu[3] and Dana Slavoaca[1,2]

*Address all correspondence to: dafinm@ssnn.ro

1 Department of Clinical Neurosciences, "Iuliu Hatieganu" University of Medicine and Pharmacy, Cluj-Napoca, Romania

2 "RoNeuro" Institute for Neurological Research and Diagnostic, Cluj-Napoca, Romania

3 Department of Clinical Pharmacology and Toxicology, "Iuliu Hatieganu" University of Medicine and Pharmacy, Cluj-Napoca, Romania

References

[1] Muresanu DF, Buzoianu A, Florian SI, von Wild T. Towards a roadmap in brain protection and recovery. J Cell Mol Med. 2012;16(12):2861–71. doi:10.1111/j.1582-4934.2012.01605.x.

[2] Salvetti M, Landsman D, Schwarz-Lam P, Comi G, Thompson AJ, Fox RJ. Progressive MS: from pathophysiology to drug discovery. Mult Scler. 2015 Oct;21(11):1376–84. doi:10.1177/1352458515603802.

[3] Jin S, Kawanokuchi J, Mizuno T, Wang J, Sonobe Y, Takeuchi H, Suzumura A. Interferon-beta is neuroprotective against the toxicity induced by activated microglia. Brain Res. 2007;1179:140–6.

[4] Kieseier BC. The mechanism of action of interferon-β in relapsing multiple sclerosis. CNS Drugs. 2011 Jun 1;25(6):491–502. doi:10.2165/11591110-000000000-00000

[5] Lindquist S, Hassinger S, Lindquist JA, Sailer M. The balance of pro-inflammatory and trophic factors in multiple sclerosis patients: effects of acute relapse and immunomodulatory treatment. Mult Scler. 2011;17(7):851–66. doi:10.1177/1352458511399797.

[6] Caggiula M, Batocchi AP, Frisullo G, Angelucci F, Patanella AK, Sancricca C, Nociti V, Tonali PA, Mirabella M. Neurotrophic factors in relapsing remitting and secondary progressive multiple sclerosis patients during interferon beta therapy. Clin Immunol. 2006;118(1):77–82.

[7] Lalive PH, Kantengwa S, Benkhoucha M, Juillard C, Chofflon M. Interferon-beta induces brain-derived neurotrophic factor in peripheral blood mononuclear cells of multiple sclerosis patients. J Neuroimmunol. 2008;197(2):147–51. doi:10.1016/j.jneuroim.2008.04.033.

[8] Mehrpour M, Akhoundi FH, Delgosha M, Keyvani H, Motamed MR, Sheibani B, Meysamie A. Increased serum brain-derived neurotrophic factor in multiple sclerosis patients on interferon-β and its impact on functional abilities. Neurologist. 2015 Oct;20(4):57–60. doi:10.1097/NRL.0000000000000053.

[9] Cadavid D, Wolansky LJ, Skurnick J, et al. Efficacy of treatment of MS with IFN-1b or glatiramer acetate by monthly brain MRI in the BECOME study. Neurology 2009;72:1976 –83. doi:10.1212/01.wnl.0000345970.73354.17.

[10] Aharoni R. Immunomodulation neuroprotection and remyelination—the fundamental therapeutic effects of glatiramer acetate: a critical review. J Autoimmun. 2014;54:81–92. doi:10.1016/j.jaut.2014.05.005.

[11] Gentile A, Rossi S, Studer V, et al. Glatiramer acetate protects against inflammatory synaptopathy in experimental autoimmune encephalomyelitis. J Neuroimmune Pharmacol.2013;8:651–63.doi:10.1007/s11481-013-9436-x.

[12] Liblau R. Glatiramer acetate for the treatment of multiple sclerosis: evidence for a dual anti-inflammatory and neuroprotective role. J Neurol Sci. 2009;287 Suppl 1:S17–23. doi: 10.1016/S0022-510X(09)71296-1.

[13] Aharoni R. Immunomodulation neuroprotection and remyelination—the fundamental therapeutic effects of glatiramer acetate: a critical review. J Autoimmun. 2014 Nov; 54:81–92. doi:10.1016/j.jaut.2014.05.005.

[14] Azoulay D, Vachapova V, Shihman B, Miler A, Karni A. Lower brain-derived neurotrophic factor in serum of relapsing remitting MS: reversal by glatiramer acetate. J Neuroimmunol. 2005 Oct;167(1–2):215–8.

[15] Vacaras V, Major ZZ, Muresanu DF, Krausz TL, Marginean I, Buzoianu DA. Effect of glatiramer acetate on peripheral blood brain-derived neurotrophic factor and phosphorylated TrκB levels in relapsing-remitting multiple sclerosis. CNS Neurol Disord Drug Targets. 2014;13(4):647–51.

[16] Ehling R, Di Pauli F, Lackner P, Rainer C, Kraus V, Hegen H, et al. Impact of glatiramer acetate on paraclinical markers of neuroprotection in multiple sclerosis: a prospective observational clinical trial. J Neuroimmunol. 2015;287:98–105. doi:10.1016/j.jneuroim.2015.08.004.

[17] Aharoni R, Arnon R, Eilam R. Neurogenesis and neuroprotection induced by peripheral immunomodulatory treatment of experimental autoimmune encephalomyelitis. J Neurosci 2005;25:8217e28.

[18] Giunti D, Parodi B, Cordano C, Uccelli A, Kerlero de Rosbo N. Can we switch microglia's phenotype to foster neuroprotection? Focus on multiple sclerosis. Immunology. 2014 Mar;141(3):328–39. doi:10.1111/imm.12177.

[19] di Nuzzo L, Orlando R, Nasca C, Nicoletti F. Molecular pharmacodynamics of new oral drugs used in the treatment of multiple sclerosis. Drug Des Devel Ther. 2014;8:555–68. doi:10.2147/DDDT.

[20] Wilms H, Sievers J, Rickert U, Rostami-Yazdi M, Mrowietz U, Lucius R. Dimethylfumarate inhibits microglial and astrocytic inflammation by suppressing the synthesis of nitric oxide, IL-1β, TNF-α and IL-6 in an in-vitro model of brain inflammation. J Neuroinflamm. 2010;7:30. doi:10.1186/1742-2094-7-30.

[21] Jones JL, Anderson JM, Phuah CL, Fox EJ, Selmaj K, Margolin D, et al. Improvement in disability after alemtuzumab treatment of multiple sclerosis is associated with neuroprotective autoimmunity. Brain. 2010 Aug;133(Pt 8):2232–47. doi:10.1093/brain/awq176.

[22] Cohen JA, Coles AJ, Arnold DL, et al. Alemtuzumab versus interferon β 1a as first-line treatment for patients with relapsing remitting multiple sclerosis: a randomized controlled phase 3 trial. Lancet. 2012;380:1819–28. doi:10.1155/2013/249101

[23] ClinicalTrials.gov [Internet]. Bethesda (MD): National Library of Medicine (US). 2016 May 10 – Identifier NCT01707992, The Efficacy and Safety and Tolerability of Laqui-

nimod in Subjects With Relapsing Remitting Multiple Sclerosis (RRMS) (CONCERTO) 2016 Feb 18 [cited 2016 Feb 18]. Available from: https://clinicaltrials.gov/ct2/show/NCT01707992?term=NCT01707992&rank=1

[24] Kieseier BC. Defining a role for laquinimod in multiple sclerosis. Ther Adv Neurol Disord. 2014;7(4):195–205. doi:10.1177/1756285614529615.

[25] Comi G, Jeffery D, Kappos L, et al. Placebo-controlled trial of oral laquinimod for multiple sclerosis. N Engl J Med. 2012;366:1000–9. doi:10.1056/NEJMoa1104318.

[26] Vollmer TL, Sorensen PS, Selmaj K, et al. BRAVO Study Group. A randomized placebo-controlled phase III trial of oral laquinimod for multiple sclerosis. J Neurol. 2014;261:773–83. doi:10.1007/s00415-014-7264-4.

[27] Fakhfouri G, Mousavizadeh K, Mehr SE, Dehpour AR, Zirak MR, et al. From chemotherapy-induced emesis to neuroprotection: therapeutic opportunities for 5-HT3 receptor antagonists. Mol Neurobiol. 2015 Dec;52(3):1670–9. doi:10.1007/s12035-014-8957-5.

[28] Mohajeri M, Sadeghizadeh M, Najafi F, Javan M. Polymerized nano-curcumin attenuates neurological symptoms in EAE model of multiple sclerosis through down regulation of inflammatory and oxidative processes and enhancing neuroprotection and myelin repair. Neuropharmacology. 2015 Jul 23;99:156–67. doi:10.1016/j.neuropharm.2015.07.013.

[29] Menzfeld C, John M, van Rossum D, Regen T, Scheffel J, Janova H, et al. Tyrphostin AG126 exerts neuroprotection in CNS inflammation by a dual mechanism. Glia. 2015;63:1083–99. doi:10.1002/glia.22803.

[30] Rajda C, Majláth Z, Pukoli D, Vécsei L. Kynurenines and multiple sclerosis: the dialogue between the immune system and the central nervous system. Int J Mol Sci. 2015;16(8):18270–82. doi:10.3390/ijms160818270.

[31] Fernández-Ruiz J, Moro MA, Martínez-Orgado J. Cannabinoids in neurodegenerative disorders and stroke/brain trauma: from preclinical models to clinical applications. Neurotherapeutics. 2015;12(4):793–806. doi:10.1007/s13311-015-0381-7.

[32] Romero K, Pavisian B, Staines WR, Feinstein A. Multiple sclerosis, cannabis, and cognition: a structural MRI study. Neuroimage Clin. 2015;8:140–7. doi:10.1016/j.nicl.2015.04.006.

[33] Pryce G, Riddall DR, Selwood DL, Giovannoni G, Baker D. Neuroprotection in experimental autoimmune encephalomyelitis and progressive multiple sclerosis by cannabis-based cannabinoids. J Neuroimmune Pharmacol. 2015;10(2):281–92. doi:10.1007/s11481-014-9575-8.

[34] Srinivasan M, Blackburn C, Lahiri DK. Functional characterization of a competitive peptide antagonist of p65 in human macrophage-like cells suggests therapeutic

potential for chronic inflammation. Drug Des Dev Ther 2014;8:2409–21. doi:10.2147/DDDT.S59722.

[35] Srinivasan M, Janardhanam S. Novel p65 binding glucocorticoid-induced leucine zipper peptide suppresses experimental autoimmune encephalomyelitis. J Biol Chem. 2011;286(52):44799–810. doi:10.1074/jbc.M111.279257.

[36] McGuire C, Elton L, Wieghofer P, Staal J, Voet S, Demeyer A, et al. Pharmacological inhibition of MALT1 protease activity protects mice in a mouse model of multiple sclerosis. J Neuroinflamm. 2014;11:124. doi:10.1186/1742-2094-11-124.

[37] Montarolo F, Raffaele C, Perga S, Martire S, Finardi A, et al. Effects of Isoxazolo-Pyridinone 7e, a potent activator of the Nurr1 signaling pathway, on experimental autoimmune encephalomyelitis in mice. PLoS ONE. 2014;9(9): e108791. doi:10.1371/journal.pone.0108791

[38] Zhao Y, Huang J, Yuan X, Peng B, Liu W, Han S, et al. Toxins targeting the KV1.3 channel: potential immunomodulators for autoimmune diseases. Toxins. 2015;7:1749–64. doi:10.3390/toxins7051749.

[39] Silva J, Monge-Fuentes V, Gomes F, Lopes K, dos Anjos L, Campos G, et al. Pharmacological alternatives for the treatment of neurodegenerative disorders: wasp and bee venoms and their components as new neuroactive tools. Toxins (Basel). 2015 Aug 18;7(8):3179–209. doi:10.3390/toxins7083179.

[40] Warne J, Pryce G, Hill JM, Shi X, Lennerås F, Puentes F, et al. Selective Inhibition of the Mitochondrial Permeability Transition Pore Protects against Neurodegeneration in Experimental Multiple Sclerosis. J Biol Chem. 2016; 291(9):4356-73. doi: 10.1074/jbc.M115.700385.

[41] Haile Y, Carmine-Simmen K, Olechowski C, Kerr B, Bleackley RC, Giuliani F. Granzyme B-inhibitor serpina3n induces neuroprotection in vitro and in vivo. J Neuroinflamm. 2015;12:157. doi:10.1186/s12974-015-0376-7.

[42] Li YH, Yu JZ, Liu CY, Zhang H, Zhang HF, Yang WF, et al. Intranasal delivery of FSD-C10, a novel Rho kinase inhibitor, exhibits therapeutic potential in experimental autoimmune encephalomyelitis. Immunology. 2014;143:219–29. doi:10.1111/imm.12303.

[43] Lu Y, Chen B, Song J-H, Zhen T, Wang B-Y, Li x, et al. Eriocalyxin B ameliorates experimental autoimmune encephalomyelitis by suppressing Th1 and Th17 cells. Proc Natl Acad Sci U S A. 2013 Feb 5;110(6):2258–63. doi:10.1073/pnas.1222426110.

[44] Yin Q-Q, Liu C-H, Wu Y-L, Wu S-F, Wang Y, Zhang X, et al. Preventive and therapeutic effects of Adenanthin on experimental autoimmune encephalomyelitis by inhibiting NF-κB signaling. J Immunol. 2013;191:2115–25. doi:10.4049/jimmunol.1203546.

[45] Srinivasan M, Lahiri DK. Significance of NF-κB as a pivotal therapeutic target in the neurodegenerative pathologies of Alzheimer's disease and multiple sclerosis. Expert Opin Ther Targets. 2014; 19(4):1–17.

[46] Duncan GS, Brenner D, Tusche MW, Brustle A, Knobbe CB, Elia AJ, et al. 2-Methoxyestradiol inhibits experimental autoimmune encephalomyelitis through suppression of immune cell activation. Proc Natl Acad Sci U S A. 2012 Dec 18;109(51):21034–9. doi: 10.1073/pnas.1215558110.

[47] Chakrabarti M, Haque A, Banik N, Nagarkatti P, Nagarkatti M, Ray SK. Estrogen receptor agonists for attenuation of neuroinflammation and neurodegeneration. Brain Res Bull. 2014 October;109:22–31. doi:10.1016/j.brainresbull.2014.09.004.

[48] Wu W-F, Tan X-J, Dai Y-B, Krishnan V, Warner M, Gustafsson J-A. Targeting estrogen receptor β in microglia and T cells to treat experimental autoimmune encephalomyelitis. Proc Natl Acad Sci U S A. 2013 Feb 26;110(9):3543–8. doi:10.1073/pnas.1300313110.

[49] El-Etr M, Rame M, Boucher C, Ghoumari A, Kumar N, Liere P, et al. Progesterone and Nestorone promote myelin regeneration in chronic demyelinating lesions of corpus callosum and cerebral cortex. Glia. 2015 January;63(1):104–17. doi:10.1002/glia.22736.

[50] McFarland AJ, Anoopkumar-Dukie S, Arora DS, Grant GD, McDermott CM, Perkins AV, et al. Molecular mechanisms underlying the effects of statins in the central nervous system. Int J Mol Sci. 2014;15:20607–37. doi:10.3390/ijms151120607.

[51] Chataway J, Schuerer N, Alsanousi A, Chan D, MacManus D, Hunter K, et al. Effect of high-dose simvastatin on brain atrophy and disability in progressive multiple sclerosis (MS-STAT): a randomized, placebo-controlled, phase 2 trial. Lancet. 2014 Jun 28;383(9936):2213–21. doi:10.1016/S0140-6736(13)62242-4.

[52] Kamm CP, El-Koussy M, Humpert S, Findling O, von Bredow F, Burren Y, et al. Atorvastatin added to interferon beta for relapsing multiple sclerosis: a randomized controlled trial. J Neurol. 2012;259:2401–13. doi:10.1007/s00415-012-6513-7.

[53] Sulkowski G, Dabrowska-Bouta B, Struzynska L. Modulation of neurological deficits and expression of glutamate receptors during experimental autoimmune encephalomyelitis after treatment with selected antagonists of glutamate receptors. Biomed Res Int. 2013;2013:186068. doi:10.1155/2013/186068.

[54] Farjam M, Beigi Zarandi FB, Farjadian S, Geramizadeh B, Nikseresht R, Panjehshahin MR. Inhibition of NR2B-containing N-methyl-D-aspartate receptors (NMDARs) in experimental autoimmune encephalomyelitis, a model of multiple sclerosis. Iran J Pharm Res. 2014;13(2):695–705.

[55] Volpi C, Mondanelli G, Pallotta MT, Vacca C, Iacono A, Gargaro M. Allosteric modulation of metabotropic glutamate receptor 4 activates IDO1-dependent, immunoregu-

latory signaling in dendritic cells. Neuropharmacology. 2016;102:59–71. doi:10.1016/j.neuropharm.2015.10.036

[56] O'Sullivan D, Green L, Stone S, Zareie P, Kharkrang M, Fong D, et al. Treatment with the antipsychotic agent, risperidone, reduces disease severity in experimental autoimmune encephalomyelitis. PLoS ONE. 2014;9(8):e104430. doi:10.1371/journal.pone.0104430.

[57] Solanki I, Parihar P, Mansuri MK, Parihar MS. Flavonoid-based therapies in the early management of neurodegenerative diseases. American society for nutrition. Adv Nutr. 2015;6:64–72. doi:10.3945/an.114.007500.

[58] Sundaram G, Brew BJ, Jones SP, Adams S, Lim CK, Guillemin GJ. Quinolinic acid toxicity on oligodendroglial cells: relevance for multiple sclerosis and therapeutic strategies. J Neuroinflamm. 2014;11:204. doi:10.1186/s12974-014-0204-5.

[59] Mecha M, Feliu A, Inigo PM, Mestre L, Carrillo-Salinas FJ, Guaza C. Cannabidiol provides long-lasting protection against the deleterious effects of inflammation in a viral model of multiple sclerosis: A role for A2A receptors. Neurobiol Dis. 2013;59:141–50. doi:10.1016/j.nbd.2013.06.016.

[60] Giacoppo S, Galuppo M, Pollastro F, Grassi G, Bramanti P, Mazzon E. A new formulation of cannabidiol in cream shows therapeutic effects in a mouse model of experimental autoimmune encephalomyelitis. DARU J Pharm Sci. 2015;2:48. doi:10.1186/s40199-015-0131-8.

[61] Zajicek J, Ball S, Wright D, Vickery J, Nunn A, Miller D, et al. Effect of dronabinol on progression in progressive multiple sclerosis (CUPID): a randomized, placebo-controlled trial. Lancet. 2013;12:857–65. doi:10.1016/S1474-4422(13)70159-5.

[62] Wang J, Ren Z, Xu Y, Xiao S, Meydani SN, Wu D. Epigallocatechin-3-gallate ameliorates experimental autoimmune encephalomyelitis by altering balance among CD4-T-cell subsets. Am J Pathol. 2012;180:1. doi:10.1016/j.ajpath.2011.09.007.

[63] Aktas O, Prozorovski T, Smorodchenko A, Savaskan NE, Lauster R, Kloetzel PM, et al. Green tea epigallocatechin-3-gallate mediates T cellular NF-κB inhibition and exerts neuroprotection in autoimmune encephalomyelitis. J Immunol. 2014;173:5794–800. doi:10.1523/JNEUROSCI.1521-05.2005.

[64] Herges K, Millward JM, Hentschel N, Infante-Duarte C, Aktas O, Zipp F. Neuroprotective effect of combination therapy of glatiramer acetate and epigallocatechin-3-gallate in neuroinflammation. PLoS ONE. 2011;6(10):e25456. doi:10.1371/journal.pone.0025456.

[65] Ong W-Y, Faroqui T, Koh H-L, Faroqui AA, Ling E-A. Protective effects of ginseng in neurological disorders. Front Aging Neurosci. 2015;7:129. doi:10.3389/fnagi.2015.00129.

[66] Mowry EM, Waubant E, McCulloch CE, Okuda DT, Evangelista AA, Lincoln RR, et al. Vitamin D status predicts new brain magnetic resonance imaging activity in multiple sclerosis. Ann Neurol. 2012 Aug;72(2):234–40. doi:10.1002/ana.23591.

[67] Mowry EM, Pelletier D, Gao Z, Howell MD, Zamvil SS, Waubant E. Vitamin D in clinically isolated syndrome: evidence for possible neuroprotection. Eur J Neurol. 2016;23(2):327–32. doi:10.1111/ene.12844.

[68] Burton JM, Kimball S, Vieth R, Bar-Or A, Dosch HM, Cheung R, et al. A phase I/II dose-escalation trial of vitamin D3 and calcium in multiple sclerosis. Neurology. 2010;74(23): 1852–9. doi:10.1212/WNL.0b013e3181e1cec2.

[69] Fitzgerald KC, Munger KL, Köchert K, Arnason BG, Comi G, Cook S, et al. Association of vitamin D levels with multiple sclerosis activity and progression in patients receiving interferon beta-1b. JAMA Neurol. 2015 Dec 1;72(12):1458–65. doi:10.1001/jamaneurol. 2015.2742

[70] Giesser BS. Exercise in the management of persons with multiple sclerosis. Ther Adv Neurol Disord. 2015;8(3):123–30. doi:10.1177/1756285615576663.

[71] Pryor WM, Freeman KG, Larson RD, Edwards GL, White LJ. Chronic exercise confers neuroprotection in experimental autoimmune encephalomyelitis. J Neurosci Res. 2015;93(5):697–706. doi:10.1002/jnr.23528.

[72] Moradi M, Ali Sahrain M, Aghsaie A, Kordi MR, Meysamie A, Abolhasani M, et al. Effects of eight-week resistance training program in men with multiple sclerosis. Asian J Sports Med. 2015 June;6(2):e22838. doi:10.5812/asjsm.6(2)2015.22838.

[73] Wens I, Dalgas U, Vandenabeele F, Grevendonk L, Verboven K, Hansen D, et al. High intensity exercise in multiple sclerosis: effects on muscle contractile characteristics and exercise capacity, a randomized controlled trial. PLoS ONE. 2015;10(9):e0133697. doi: 10.1371/journal/pone.0133697.

[74] Ebrahimi A, Eftekhari E, Etemadifar M. Effects of whole body vibration on hormonal & functional indices in patients with multiple sclerosis. Indian J Med Res. 2015;142:450–8. doi:10.4103/0971-5916.169210

[75] Sangelaji B, Estebsari F, Nabavi SM, Jamshidi E, Morsalis D, Dastoorpoor M. The effect of exercise therapy on cognitive functions in multiple sclerosis patients: a pilot study. Med J Islam Repub Iran. 2015;29:205.

[76] Coggan JS, Bittner S, Stiefel KM, Meuth SG, Prescott SA. Physiological dynamics in demyelinating diseases: unraveling complex relationships through computer modeling. Int J Mol Sci. 2015;16(9):21215–36.

[77] Waxman SG. Ion channels and neuronal dysfunction in multiple sclerosis. Arch Neurol. 2002 Sep;59:1377–80.

[78] Shrager P. Ionic channels and signal conduction in single remyelinating frog nerve fibers. J Physiol. 1988;404:695–712.

[79] Rasband MN, Trimmer JS, Schwarz TL, Levinson SR, Ellisman MH, Schachner M, et al. Potassium channel distribution, clustering and function in remyelinating rat axons. J Neurosci. 1998;18:36–47.

[80] Black JA, Waxman SG, Smith KJ. Remyelination of dorsal column axons by endogenous Schwann cells restores the normal pattern of Nav1.6 and Kv1.2 at nodes of Ranvier. Brain. 2006;129(Pt 5): 1319–29. doi:10.1093/brain/awl057.

[81] Rasband MN, Trimmer J. Developmental clustering of ion channels at and near the node of Ranvier. Dev Biol. 2001;236:5–16. doi:10.1006/dbio.2001.0326.105.

[82] Kweon HJ, Suh BC. Acid-sensing ion channels (ASICs): therapeutic targets for neurological diseases and their regulation. BMB Rep. 2013;46(6):295–304.

[83] Arnold R, Huynh W, Kiernan MC, Krishnan AV. Ion channel modulation as a therapeutic approach in multiple sclerosis. Curr Med Chem. 2015;22(38):4366–78.

[84] McKee JB, Elston J, Evangelou N, et al. Amiloride Clinical Trial In Optic Neuritis (ACTION) protocol: a randomized, double blind, placebo controlled trial. BMJ Open. 2015;5:e009200. doi:10.1136/bmjopen-2015-009200.

[85] Bittner S, Meuth SG. Targeting ion channels for the treatment of autoimmune neuroinflammation. Ther Adv Neurol Disord. 2013;6(5):322–36. doi: 10.1177/1756285613487782.

[86] Rhodes KE, Raivich G, Fawcett JW. The injury response of oligodendrocyte precursor cells is induced by platelets, macrophages and inflammation-associated cytokines. Neuroscience. 2006;140:87–100.

[87] Murtie JC, Zhou YX, Le TQ, Vana AC, Armstrong RC. PDGF and FGF2 pathways regulate distinct oligodendrocyte lineage responses in experimental demyelination with spontaneous remyelination. Neurobiol Dis. 2005;19(1–2):171–82.

[88] Piaton G, Aigrot MS, Williams A, Moyon S, Tepavcevic V, Moutkine I, et al. Class 3 semaphorins influence oligodendrocyte precursor recruitment and remyelination in adult central nervous system. Brain. 2011;134(Pt 4):1156–67. doi:10.1093/brain/awr022

[89] Fancy SP, Chan JR, Baranzini SE, Franklin RJ, Rowitch DH. Myelin regeneration: a recapitulation of development? Annu Rev Neurosci. 2011;34:21–43. doi:10.1146/annurev-neuro-061010-113629.

[90] Mohan H, Krumbholz M, Sharma R, Eisele S, Junker A, Sixt M, et al. Extracellular matrix in multiple sclerosis lesions: fibrillar collagens, biglycan and decorin are upregulated and associated with infiltrating immune cells. Brain Pathol. 2010;20(5):966–75. doi: 10.1111/j.1750-3639.2010.00399.x.

[91] Yang Y, Liu Y, Wei P, Peng H, Winger R, Hussain RZ, et al. Silencing Nogo-A promotes functional recovery in demyelinating disease. Annals of neurology. 2010;67(4), 498–507. doi:10.1002/ana.21935

[92] Pepinsky RB, Walus L, Shao Z, et al. Production of a PEGylated Fab' of the anti-LINGO-1 Li33 antibody and assessment of its biochemical and functional properties in vitro and in a rat model of remyelination. Bioconjug Chem. 2011;22(2):200–10. doi: 10.1021/bc1002746

[93] Aparicio E, Mathieu P, Pereira Luppi M, Almeira Gubiani MF, Adamo AM. The notch signaling pathway: its role in focal CNS demyelination and apotransferrin-induced remyelination. J Neurochem. 2013;127(6):819–36. doi:10.1111/jnc.12440.

[94] Taveggia C, Feltri ML, Wrabetz L. Signals to promote myelin formation and repair. Nat Rev Neurol. 2010;6:276–87. doi:10.1038/nrneurol.2010.37

[95] Warrington AE, Bieber AJ, Ciric B, Pease LR, Van Keulen V, Rodriguez M. A recombinant human IgM promotes myelin repair after a single, very low dose. J Neurosci Res. 2007;85(5):967–76.

[96] Magalon K, Zimmer C, Cayre M, Khaldi J, Bourbon C, Robles I, et al. Olesoxime accelerates myelination and promotes repair in models of demyelination. Ann Neurol. 2012;71(2):213–26. doi:10.1002/ana.22593.

[97] Fancy SP, Harrington EP, Yuen TJ, Silbereis JC, Zhao C, et al. Axin2 as regulatory and therapeutic target in newborn brain injury and remyelination. Nat Neurosci. 2011;14: 1009–16. doi:10.1038/nn.2855.

[98] Huang JK, Jarjour AA, Nait Oumesmar B, Kerninon C, Williams A, Krezel W, et al. Retinoid X receptor gamma signaling accelerates CNS remyelination. Nat Neurosci. 2011;14(1):45–53. doi:10.1038/nn.2702

[99] Patel JR, McCandless EE, Dorsey D, Klein RS. CXCR4 promotes differentiation of oligodendrocyte progenitors and remyelination. Proc Natl Acad Sci U S A. 2010; 15; 107(24): 11062–7. doi:10.1073/pnas.1006301107.

[100] Ara J, See J, Mamontov P, Hahn A, Bannerman P, Pleasure D, Grinspan JB. Bone morphogenetic proteins 4, 6, and 7 are up-regulated in mouse spinal cord during experimental autoimmune encephalomyelitis. J Neurosci Res. 2008;86(1):125–35.

[101] Harlow DE, Honce JM, Miravalle AA. Remyelination therapy in multiple sclerosis. Front Neurol. 2015 Dec 10;6:257. doi:10.3389/fneur.2015.00257.

[102] Krementsov DN, Thornton TM, Teuscher C, Rincon M. The emerging role of p38 mitogen-activated protein kinase in multiple sclerosis and its models. Mol Cell Biol. 2013;33(19):3728–34. doi:10.1128/MCB.00688-13.

[103] Xing B, 2015; Xing B, Bachstetter AD, Van Eldik LJ. Inhibition of neuronal p38α, but not p38β MAPK, provides neuroprotection against three different neurotoxic insults. J Mol Neurosci. 2015;55(2):509–18. doi:10.1007/s12031-014-0372-x.

[104] Kotelnikova E, Bernardo-Faura M, Silberberg G, Kiani NA, Messinis D, et al. Signaling networks in MS: a systems-based approach to developing new pharmacological therapies. Mult Scler. 2015 Feb;21(2):138–46. doi:10.1177/1352458514543339

Chapter 13

Neuroprotection: A New Therapeutic Approach of Relapsing Remitting Multiple Sclerosis

Juan Espinosa-Parrilla, Marco Pugliese,
Nicole Mahy and Manuel J Rodríguez

Additional information is available at the end of the chapter

http://dx.doi.org/10.5772/63730

Abstract

Neurodegenerative changes occurring early from primary acute immune-mediated inflammation support the hypothesis that multiple sclerosis (MS) is a complex disease. Axonal loss progresses with the disease course and represents the principal driver of disability. In this context, the pursuit of neuroprotective therapies in multiple sclerosis provides new valid alternatives that could significantly impact on disease progression and neurodegenerative changes, including the promotion of restoration of myelin sheaths through the remyelination process. This chapter reviews promising drugs with proposed neuroprotective or neuroregenerative effects that are currently approved or in clinical trials for the treatment of multiple sclerosis. Although the chapter highlights the diazoxide action on neuroinflammation and the results of a clinical trial with this drug, the review also includes other molecules with oral or parenteral administration.

Keywords: relapsing-remitting multiple sclerosis, disease-modifying drugs, neuroprotection, neuroregeneration, neuroinflammation, central nervous system

1. Introduction

Immunosuppressive and immunomodulatory drugs have been designed for years to treat multiple sclerosis (MS), as it was considered the most appropriate approach to balance the effects of the patients' immune reaction. However, the new data recently offered by basic and clinical research increase our understanding of this complex disease, allowing changes in its therapeutic approach. As a consequence, the first disease-modifying drug with a suggested neuroprotective mechanism of action has been recently approved, broadening and improving the therapeutic landscape against MS.

In this chapter, we review new drugs with proposed neuroprotective or neuroregenerative effects that are currently approved or in clinical trials for MS treatment. Although we highlight the diazoxide action on neuroinflammation and the results of a clinical trial with this drug, the review also includes other molecules with oral or parenteral administration.

The articles analysed for this review were selected using PubMed database filtered by English language. Clinical trials were selected at the ClinicalTrials.gov database. Studies in the database labelled as "unknown status" were excluded. The initial search was done in December 2015.

2. Treating neurodegeneration in multiple sclerosis

MS is an autoimmune disease in which elements of the neuronal myelin sheath are recognized as antigens by the immune system. Focal inflammatory and immune actions against neuronal cover cause a neurodegenerative process that leads to neurological impairment. The difficulty to characterize the neurodegenerative process supports the hypothesis that MS is a complex disease, with high variations among individuals. In any case, as a consequence of the immune aggression, an axonal loss progresses with the disease and represents the principal driver of disability in the chronic course of MS [1]. In this context, multiple mechanisms could contribute to demyelination and axonal injury including energy imbalance, ion accumulation, neuroinflammation and astroglial response to oxidative and metabolic stress.

2.1. Chronic neurodegenerative processes in multiple sclerosis

About 85% of MS patients present the so-called relapsing-remitting (RR) form, characterized by unpredictable relapses related to inflammatory activity, followed by periods of months to years of relative quietness. During the remitting period, patients present no new signs of disease activity and, occasionally, partial remissions of symptoms associated with reparative processes are observed [2]. Progressive forms are less frequent forms of initial MS, but about 55–65% of relapsing-remitting multiple sclerosis (RRMS) patients develop a secondary progressive course [1].

At the pathophysiological level, the neurological impairment develops due to focal inflammatory and immune attacks against the neuronal cover, which cause a chronic neurodegenerative process. The reason why and where these focal demyelinating inflammatory lesions appear within the central nervous system (CNS) remains unknown. Current hypothesis establish that CD4-positive T lymphocytes are mainly responsible for the initial autoimmune attack, but with a secondary role in chronic neuronal damage [3]. Resident microglia and astrocytes, and infiltrated macrophages, B lymphocytes, natural killer (NK)-positive and CD8-positive T cells would be the major players in the neurodegenerative process [4, 5].

At the subcellular level, a plethora of inflammatory effectors mediating myelin and neuronal damage have been described. These effectors include molecules such as nitric oxide (NO), reactive oxygen species (ROS), tumour necrosis factor α (TNF-α), interferon γ (IFNγ), granzymes, perforin and matrix metalloproteinases, and also molecular processes such as activation of the complement, antibody secretion and phagocytosis [4, 6, 7]. Furthermore, as a concomitant event, glutamate release from damaged axons will trigger excitotoxicity, which leads to ion imbalance and mitochondrial metabolic stress, feeding neuronal damage and neuroinflammation [8, 9]. Thus, inflammatory damage leads to oligodendrocyte death, axon demyelination, axonal damage, neuronal death and the formation of glial scars. Progressive axonal injury and neuronal loss increase with the course of MS and represent the principal driver of disability.

Key elements that mediate inflammation in MS are microglial cells. Microglia are often considered to be macrophages of the CNS, but a series of recent findings in the mouse have established that they are a unique cell population distinct from macrophages [10]. In normal conditions, microglia present a surveillance state and important roles in normal development, connectivity and plasticity of the CNS. However, they are transformed and activated by a range of signals, such as neuronal death, mechanical injury and toxins [11]. Once activated, they form the first line of defense against infection or injury to the CNS [12]. As a consequence, microglia mediate and trigger a neuroinflammatory response to injury. In MS, this microglial reaction is an early event that often precedes and triggers demyelination and neurodegeneration [13].

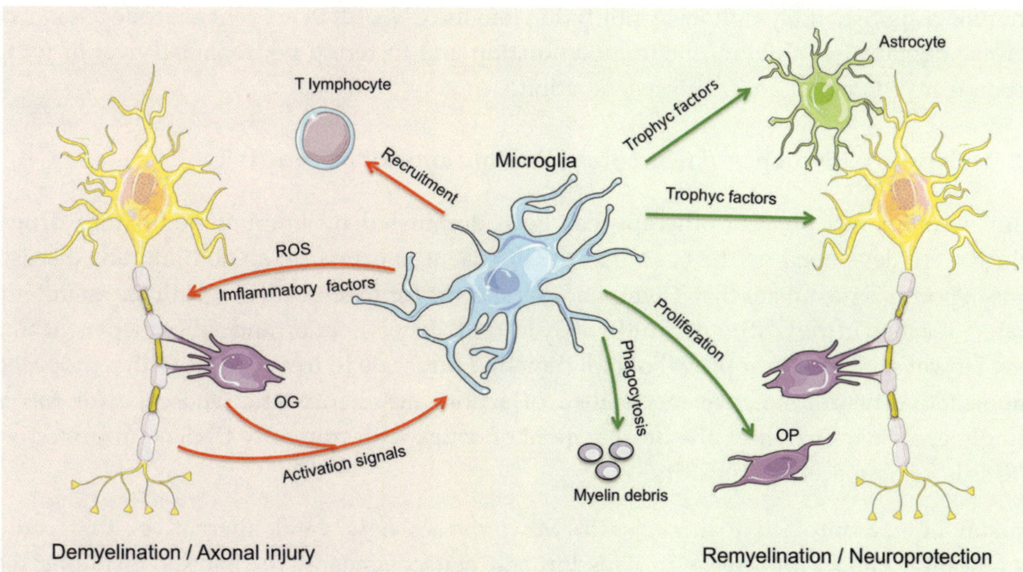

Figure 1. Dual role of microglia in MS. Reactive microglia mediate different pro-inflammatory (red arrows) and neuroprotective processes (green arrows) according to the diversity of signals from the lesioned axons and oligodendrocytes. OG, oligodendrocytes; OP, oligodendrocyte precursors; ROS, reactive oxygen species. (Cell drawings are from SERVIER Medical Art.)

Perivascular microglia are the antigen-presenting cells that recruit myelin-specific T cells and promote the inflammatory process inside the CNS. This process then activates parenchymal microglia by secreting pro-inflammatory and neurotoxic factors such as TNF-α, prostaglandins, interleukin-6 (IL-6), NO or ROS, which elicit myelin damage and neurodegeneration [11, 14]. Whether microglia adopt a phenotype that mostly exacerbates tissue injury or one that promotes brain repair is likely to depend on the diversity of signals from the lesion environment and the response capacity of the cell (**Figure 1**).

As a response to the inflammatory aggression, reparative and regenerative processes are activated and originate MS remissions. This neuroprotective response is led by the activation of microglia and TH2-IL-10 lymphocyte pathways, and results in inhibition of the inflammatory process, up-regulation of antioxidant mechanisms, and secretion of neurotrophic factors. These processes promote remyelination by surviving oligodendrocytes and precursors [15–17]. According to this, the progression of MS symptoms depends on a delicate balance between neuroinflammation and the regenerative process. However, neuronal regeneration is not an easy and common process within the CNS, especially for large myelinated neurons. Although myelin sheath can be partially restored, oligodendrocytes regenerated and axons repaired, and if the inflammatory insult persists, the degenerative damage becomes chronic and cannot be counteracted.

According to these processes, the therapeutic approaches for MS should follow three different but not exclusive strategies: (a) to suppress the autoimmune reaction by inhibiting the initial immune response and lymphocyte infiltration into the CNS, (b) to prevent neurodegenerative chronic damage by inhibiting neuroinflammation and fostering neuronal survival or (c) to promote myelin repair and neuroregeneration.

2.2. Molecules with proposed neuroprotective and antioxidative activity

Until recently, MS pharmacotherapy has been dominated by immunomodulatory drugs, which were developed on the basis that the disease was primarily an autoimmune disease. This hypothesis postulates that T lymphocytes specific for myelin antigens initiate an inflammatory reaction in the CNS, which ultimately leads to demyelination and subsequent neuronal loss. However, since the approval of oral dimethyl fumarate to treat RRMS, with a proposed antioxidative neuroprotective mechanism of action, the therapeutic landscape for MS is rapidly evolving. Currently, the development of drugs with primarily CNS neuroprotective effects is a pharmaceutical priority.

Pursuit of neuroprotective therapies in MS provides new valid alternatives that could significantly impact on disease progression and neurodegenerative changes, including the promotion of myelin sheath restoration through the remyelination process [18]. Thus, fingolimod, laquinimod, Anti-LINGO antibody, (-)-epigallotechin-3-gallate (EGCG) and diazoxide emerge as neuroprotective drugs for the treatment of MS (**Table 1**). Nevertheless, the neuroprotective effect of these compounds has not been fully established and requires further investigation.

http://dx.doi.org/10.5772/63730

Compound	Proposed mechanism of action	Effects	Clinical phase	Key adverse effects
Dimethyl fumarate	Nrf2 up-regulation Induction of IL-4-Th2 response	Anti-inflammatory activity Decreased lymphocyte entry into CNSProtective effects on oligodendrocytes, myelin, axons and neurons	Phase III: DEFINE and CONFIRM Approved	Moderate infections Elevated liver enzymes Leucopenia
Fingolimod	Decreased expression of S1p1 on lymphocytes and other cells	Decrease of T lymphocytes infiltrated in the CNS Anti-inflammatory and neuroprotective microglia phenotypes	Phase III: TRANSFORMS and FREEDOMS Approved	Bradycardia and AV block Severe viral infections Macular oedema
Laquinimod	Unknown Inhibition of NF-kB activation? Inhibition of IL-17expression?	Decreased lymphocyte entry into CNS Axon protection Decrease of pro-inflammatory cytokines Increased BDNF levels	Phase III studies CONCERTO Results expected by 2017	Elevated liver enzymes Infections
Anti-LINGO antibody BIIB033	Blockade of Nogo signaling	promotes axonal integrity/remyelination functional recovery	Phase I NCT01052506 NCT01244139 Phase II: SYNERGY Results expected by 2016	Hypersensitivity reactions Elevated liver enzymes
(–)-Epigallotechin-3-galeate	Inhibition of NF-kB activation Free radical scavenger.	Improves muscle metabolism during moderate exercise in MS patients	Phase II SuniMS completed. No results available NCT01417312 completes	Elevated liver enzymes (1 case)
Diazoxide	Activation of K_{ATP} channels Maintenance of mitochondrial homeostasis and function	Anti-inflammatory activity Neuronal, axonal and myelin protection Modulation of antigen presentation	Phase II: NEUROADVAN completed	Autoimmune hypothyroidism (1 case)

Table 1. Neuroprotective drugs for the treatment of RRMS.

2.2.1. Dimethyl fumarate

Fumaric acid esters (FAEs) are a group of simple low-molecular structured compounds that has been used for long time in the treatment of moderate to severe psoriasis [19]. Due to their immunomodulatory potential, FAEs were also evaluated as a potential treatment for RRMS. At preclinical stages, FAEs showed promising results in myelin oligodendrocyte glycoprotein (MOG)-induced experimental autoimmune encephalomyelitis (MOG-EAE) mice, ameliorating the disease course [20]. In vivo, the mechanism of action of dimethyl fumarate is not completely understood. For some authors, fumarate treatment induces IL-4-producing Th2 dendritic cells [21]. In the human and mice, type II dendritic cells subsequently produce the anti-inflammatory cytokines IL-10 and IL-4 instead of pro-inflammatory IL-12 and IL-23 [21]. This anti-inflammatory activity also causes apoptosis of activated T cells preserving the CNS from influx of activated lymphocytes.

Regarding the neuroprotective role of fumarate, other authors found in vitro and in vivo effects, potentially via up-regulation of the nuclear factor (erythroid-derived 2)-like 2 (Nrf2). Dimethyl fumarate also exerts protective effects on oligodendrocytes, myelin, axons and neurons, and reduces oxidative stress as measured by protein nitrosylation [22]. Nonetheless, as recently shown, the protective effect of dimethyl fumarate could depend on pre-existing tissue expression of Nrf2. Actually, Nrf2 is intrinsically higher in astrocytes and macrophages from active MS lesions and increased Nrf2 levels have been recently reported in oligodendrocytes from active MS lesions [23].

Two randomized, placebo- and active-controlled, double-blind, parallel-group Phase III studies (DEFINE and CONFIRM) of dimethyl fumarate (Code name BG-12) have been conducted (funded by Biogen Idec). The primary end point of these studies was the proportion of patients who had a 2-year relapse. Secondary end points included the annualized relapse rate (ARR), the time to confirmed progression of disability as measured by Expanded Disability Status Scale (EDSS), and findings on brain magnetic resonance imaging scan (MRI) such as the number of gadolinium-enhancing lesions. Both studies described highly significant superiority of BG-12 to placebo on almost all end points in patients with RRMS [24]. In the DEFINE and CONFIRM extension study (ENDORSE), a minimum of 5 years of treatment with the drug was associated with continued benefit and no new/worsening tolerability signals. Thus, in March 2013, the Food and Drug Administration (FDA) approved dimethyl fumarate as a new first-line oral treatment for patients with RRMS. In September 2013, it was also approved in Canada and Australia and, in 2014, the European Commission has approved the use of the drug for the treatment of RRMS in Europe.

2.2.2. Fingolimod

Fingolimod became the first drug approved for relapsing forms of MS in the USA in 2010. However, some safety issues were identified during the drug development process, after completion of trials and in the first months of clinical use in the United States. These issues led to the approval of fingolimod as a second-line drug by the European Medicines Agency (EMA) after the FDA had licensed it as a first-line agent. In addition, contradictory results regarding efficacy on progression of disability in MS patients were found in the two pivotal Phase III trials that allowed fingolimod marketing in most countries [18].

Although fingolimod was primarily believed to be a pure immunosuppressive compound, recent findings revealed direct effects on the CNS [25]. When incorporated to the organism, fingolimod is rapidly phosphorylated by sphingosine kinases [26] and the product of this phosphorylation, phosphofingolimod, is a potent modulator of S1P receptors. Administration of fingolimod and similar S1P1 modulators produce marked beneficial effects on different animal models of MS, especially when administered preventively. The proposed mechanism of action for fingolimod is the inhibition of encephalitogenic T-cell responses and/or their migration into the CNS [27, 28]. According to this, EAE animals treated with fingolimod showed a dramatic decrease of T lymphocytes infiltrated in the CNS and even a reversible peripheral lymphocytopaenia. These animals also showed better myelin preservation and decrease of pro-inflammatory cytokine production [29].

In the CNS, both neurons and glia profusely express S1P receptors. Some of the beneficial effects of fingolimod in EAE and MS could be attributed to SP1 receptor modulation in these cells and result in neuroprotection. Activation of neuronal S1P1 and S1P3 receptors promotes neurogenesis and increases neurite outgrowth, although high and continuous activation of neuronal S1P receptors could lead to overactivation of the glutamatergic system with deleterious effects [30]. In microglia, fingolimod promotes anti-inflammatory and neuroprotective phenotypes, but the exact mechanism of action involved remains unclear [31]. Furthermore, one of the most discussed direct effects of fingolimod on the CNS is on myelin repair and oligodendrocyte regeneration [32, 33].

One Phase II study, followed by an active extension, and two clinical Phase III placebo-controlled and active comparator-controlled clinical trials (named TRANSFORMS and FREEDOMS, sponsored by Novartis) have been performed with fingolimod in patients with RRMS. These studies have demonstrated the efficacy of fingolimod in treating RRMS [34, 35]. More recently, FREEDOMS II, a third Phase III trial of fingolimod, was conducted predominantly in USA and Canada. The trial replicated the findings of FREEDOMS regarding the ARR and MRI outcomes, but the significant effect on reducing EDSS score progression was not confirmed. On the other hand, disability showed a statistically significant change in favour of fingolimod treatment in the FREEDOMS II study [36]. Finally, the recently completed INFORMS trial showed no significant benefit of fingolimod on neurological disability in primary progressive MS patients treated for at least 3 years [37].

2.2.3. *Laquinimod*

Laquinimod (N-ethyl-N-phenyl-5-chloro-1,2-dihydroxy-1-methyl-2-oxo-quinoline-3-carboxamide) is structurally related to linomide, which was tested for efficacy in MS more than one decade ago, and discontinued after serious adverse events occurred in a Phase III trial [38, 39]. After an extensive screening of a large number of chemically modified quinoline-3-carboxamides, laquinimod was selected to have less toxicity and better efficacy than linomide in various experimental autoimmune inflammatory-mediated animal models, including experimental autoimmune neuritis in Lewis rats [40].

The precise mechanism by which laquinimod induces these beneficial effects is yet to be fully elucidated. Preclinical studies in EAE mice have shown that laquinimod might protect myelin and axons by decreasing pro-inflammatory cytokines such as IL-17 by T cells [41]. In addition, suppression of the nuclear factor-kappaB (NF-κB) pathway that concordantly led to the activation of apoptosis of immunocompetent cells was also induced by laquinimod, proving the anti-inflammatory potency of the drug [42]. Regarding the effects in the CNS, laquinimod treatment prevented the loss of brain-derived neurotrophic factor (BDNF) induced by the disease process. In EAE mice, laquinimod induced an elevation of BDNF expression in various brain regions to reach similar BDNF concentration as that of naïve controls [43]. In the human, a Phase II study undergoing laquinimod treatment showed a significant and specific elevation of serum BDNF levels compared to the placebo group after 3 months of treatment [44]. Whether laquinimod directly affects BDNF expression within the neurons, or induces bystander mechanisms that arrest the inflammatory progression and facilitates neuroprotection, needs to be further clarified.

Two Phase III clinical trials of laquinimod in RRMS (the ALLEGRO and BRAVO trial sponsored by TEVA) have been completed. In the first one, treatment with laquinimod as compared with placebo was associated with a modest reduction in ARR, decreased the risk of disability progression and reduced the number of gadolinium-enhancing lesions detected by MRI. However, the failure to meet primary end point in the BRAVO study led the manufacturer to delay requesting FDA approval. On May 2013, laquinimod was approved in Russia as a treatment for RRMS.

Nevertheless, in 2013 Teva Pharmaceutical and Active Biotech started the third Phase III trial of laquinimod in patients with RRMS. The study is designed to evaluate the safety and efficacy of laquinimod with a primary end point of time to confirmed disability progression, as measured by the EDSS (CONCERTO trial, ClinicalTrials.gov Identifier: NCT01707992). CONCERTO results are expected to be available towards mid-2017.

2.2.4. Anti-LINGO antibody

Nogo receptor-interacting protein (LINGO-1) is a transmembrane signal-transducing molecule, selectively expressed by oligodendrocytes and neurons and that associates with the Nogo-66 receptor (NgR1) complex [45]. NgR1 binds myelin-associated inhibitors of axonal regeneration such as Nogo-A, myelin-associated glycoprotein and oligodendrocyte myelin glycoprotein [46]. In response to CNS injury and demyelination, oligodendrocyte precursor cells and stem cells from the white matter become activated, migrate to the demyelinated area, proliferate and differentiate into oligodendrocytes that will remyelinate damaged axons. In chronic MS lesions, despite the presence of oligodendrocyte precursors in demyelinated plaques and the close proximity between pre-myelinating oligodendrocytes and demyelinated axons, axonal remyelination failed. This suggests that the differentiation process may be locally blocked by inhibitory factors [47].

In animal models, LINGO-1 expression is up-regulated in rat spinal cord injury, experimental EAE, 6-hydroxydopamine neurotoxic lesions and glaucoma models [48, 49]. Several works have reported the blockade of Nogo signalling as a therapeutic approach for neurological disorders such as spinal cord injury, traumatic brain injury, stroke, schizophrenia, amyotrophic lateral sclerosis and MS [50]. Animal models provide evidence that LINGO-1 is a potent inhibitor of axonal remyelination and regeneration in vivo. For example, transgenic mice overexpressing full-length LINGO-1 under the neuronal promoter of synapsin showed a significant reduction in the number of myelinated axons in the spinal cord and brain at P8 [51]. Other authors showed that neurite outgrowth inhibitor Nogo-A is involved in autoimmune-mediated demyelination in vivo [52].

BIIB033 is a monoclonal antibody that inhibits LINGO-1 and promotes axonal integrity/ remyelination in MOG-EAE mice [49]. In preclinical experiments, LINGO-1 antagonist antibodies did not alter EAE onset but did significantly mitigate disease severity across all stages of disease progression. This functional recovery in EAE correlates with improved axonal integrity as determined by magnetic resonance diffusion tensor imaging, and with newly formed myelin sheaths as determined by electron microscopy [53].

Biogen Idec Inc. started two different human studies with BIIB033 in 2010 (ClinicalTrials.gov Identifier: NCT01244139 and NCT01052506, respectively). Both studies finished in 2012 and BIIB033 showed favourable safety profile, desirable pharmacokinetic in healthy adults and MS patients and predicted brain penetration [53]. Based on these promising results, in 2013, Biogen started a Phase II dose-response study to assess the efficacy, safety, tolerability and pharmacokinetics of BIIB033 in 400 RRMS patients when used concurrently with Interferon β-1a (Avonex®) (SYNERGY, ClinicalTrials.gov Identifier: NCT01864148). SYNERGY results are expected to be available along 2016.

2.2.5. *(−)-Epigallotechin-3-gallate*

Green tea consumption has been associated to differences in the incidence of some diseases such as different kinds of cancer or cardiovascular pathologies [54]. Its composition includes, among other bioactive molecules, vitamins, pro-vitamins and antioxidants. Some of the more abundant components are tea polyphenols, also known as catechins, especially the (-)-epigallotechin-3-gallate (EGCG) [55]. EGCG has been profusely studied as an anticancer compound, as long as it can cause apoptosis and arrest cell cycle of tumoural cells [56]. As long as EGCG presents antioxidative properties, it can act as a chelator of neurotoxic metals and inhibit pro-inflammatory processes [57].

Efficacy studies in the EAE models for MS have shown that, alone or in combination with approved treatments for MS, oral EGCG ameliorated disease course and decreases EAE severity, preventing and reversing disability. This positive effect has been mainly attributed to the inhibition of NF-κB-mediated inflammation, cell proliferation, TNF-α secretion and Th1/ Th2 response. EGCG enhanced axonal preservation and inhibited neuronal apoptosis in treated animals [58]. The neuroprotective profile of EGCG has been attributed to its activity as a free radical scavenger [58]. Although this effect may be related with the inhibition of NF-κB pathway and glial reactivity, this indirect neuroprotection is also of main interest for the treatment of MS and other neurodegenerative diseases.

Several epidemiologic studies and clinical trials have been performed to test the preventive and therapeutic effects of EGCG in neurodegenerative diseases such as Alzheimer's, Parkinson's or Huntington's diseases [59]. In general, these studies show no EGCG-related prevention of neuronal and glial cell death in patients [59]. In 2013, a multicentric Phase II national study to investigate the anti-inflammatory and neuroprotective effects of EGCG in 120 RRMS patients was started (SuniMS Study, ClinicalTrials.gov identifier: NCT00525668, sponsored by Charite University, Berlin, Germany). At the moment, no results are available for this study.

Finally, to analyse the metabolic effects of EGCG and to assess the importance of lipid oxidation in fuel muscle's energy metabolism and its relationship with muscle weakness and fatigue in RRMS patients, the same institution completed a clinical research trial in 2013 (ClinicalTrials.gov identifier: NCT01417312). Results showed that EGCG given to MS patients over 12 weeks improves muscle metabolism during moderate exercise to a greater extent in men than in women, possibly because of sex-specific effects on autonomic and endocrine control. These results indicate that EGCG could be a promising treatment for MS, with a good- and well-known safety profile and an interesting combinability with other treatments. However, as the EGCG pass through the blood-brain barrier in humans is still controversial, its bioavailability remains to be characterized [60].

3. Effects of diazoxide in multiple sclerosis

3.1. K_{ATP} channels and neuroinflammation

Adenosine triphosphate (ATP)-dependent potassium (K_{ATP}) channels play important roles in many cellular functions by coupling cell metabolism to electrical activity. First detected in cardiac myocytes, they are also expressed in a wide number of cell types such as pancreatic β-cells, skeletal and smooth myocytes, neurons and microglia. In these cells, K_{ATP} channels regulate potassium fluxes across the cell membrane when glucose is available in sufficient conditions, which couple the electrical activity of the cell to energy metabolism [61, 62]. An increase in the cellular ATP concentration leads to channel closure and membrane depolarization. On the contrary, metabolic inhibition opens K_{ATP} channels and suppresses electrical activity.

Functional K_{ATP} channels in the cell membrane are assembled as a heterooctameric complex [63] from two structurally distinct subunits: the regulatory sulphonylurea receptor (SUR) and the pore-forming inwardly rectifying potassium channel (Kir) subunit 6.1 or 6.2. While ATP inhibits the K_{ATP} channel by directly binding to the cytoplasmic Kir6 domains, activators, such as potassium channel openers (KCOs), and inhibitors, such as sulphonylurea drugs [64], bind SUR to modulate the channel. Similar K_{ATP} channels have also been described in the mitochondria, located on the inner membrane of these organelles where they play a crucial role in the maintenance of mitochondrial homeostasis and function [65].

In recent years, K_{ATP} channels have attracted increasing interest as targets for drug development. Their pivotal role in a plethora of physiological processes has been underscored by recent discoveries linking potassium channel mutations to various diseases. The second generation of KCOs with an improved in vitro or in vivo selectivity has broadened the chemical diversity of K_{ATP} channel ligands. On the other hand, considering the unique role that K_{ATP} channels play in the maintenance of cellular homeostasis, KCOs add their potential in promoting protection against metabolic stress to the already existing pharmacotherapy. Studies in animal models showed KCO effects in several pathological situations such as hypertension, cardiac ischaemia or asthma, which indicates a broad therapeutic potential for KCOs. For example, in the smooth muscle of blood vessels and pancreatic β-cells, diazoxide (7-chloro-3-methyl-4H-1,2,4-benzothiadiazine 1,1-dioxide) binds with similar affinities to SUR1 and SUR2B subunits of K_{ATP} channels, increases membrane permeability to potassium ions and induces hyperpolarization [64]. In these cells, diazoxide-induced hyperpolarization inhibits the opening of voltage-gated calcium channels, and results in vasorelaxation and inhibition of insulin secretion [66]. As a consequence, diazoxide has been used since the 1970s for treating malignant hypertension and hypoglycaemia in the United States, Canada, and most European countries [67].

Our laboratory has described the expression of K_{ATP} channels in microglia [68–70], through which they control the release of a diversity of inflammatory mediators, such as NO, IL-6 or TNF-α [71, 72]. We also evidenced that reactive microglia increase the expression of the K_{ATP}-channel components Kir6.1, Kir6.2, SUR1 and SUR2B [69, 73]. With this increased microglial expression, KCOs may modulate neuroinflammation. In this line, we and other authors have documented that pharmacological activation of K_{ATP} channels with diazoxide can exert CNS neuroprotective and anti-inflammatory effects against excitotoxicity, ischaemia, trauma and neurotoxicants [71, 72, 74, 75]. For example, any rat brain microinjection of glutamate analogues triggers a persistent process that leads to progressive atrophy with a widespread neuronal loss and a concomitant neuroinflammation [76]. This neurodegenerative process is reduced by diazoxide oral treatment, which ameliorated microglia-mediated inflammation and reduced neuronal loss [73].

Controlling the extent of microglial activation may offer prospective clinical therapeutic benefits for inflammation-related neurodegenerative disorders [73]. In this context, increased expression of K_{ATP} channels by activated microglia and the specific anti-inflammatory actions of diazoxide reveal the use of this drug as a therapeutic agent to treat MS inflammatory processes.

3.2. K_{ATP} channel openers and experimental autoimmune encephalomyelitis

We analysed the putative neuroprotective effects of diazoxide on an EAE murine model of MS by its oral administration in the classical EAE MOG35-55 mouse model for preclinical studies of MS [72]. The doses tested (0.8 and 0.05 mg/kg) were below those that induce blood glucose increase (>1 mg/kg) and both of them ameliorated clinical signs of EAE, being 0.8 mg/kg more effective [72]. Then, this dose was tested in two different experimental designs: (a) a preventive paradigm, in which diazoxide was administrated daily starting on the same day animals were immunized and (b) a palliative paradigm, in which mice were treated with diazoxide daily starting when they reached a clinical score of ≥1. In both cases, the treatment showed similar effectiveness and mice treated with diazoxide obtained a lower clinical score during the chronic phase of EAE. However, in the preventive paradigm, diazoxide could not delay EAE onset or reduce the number of animals developing EAE. This indicates that diazoxide effects could be mediated mainly by neuroprotection rather than by immunosuppression. The histopathological analysis of injured spinal cords confirmed that diazoxide elicited a significant reduction in myelin and axonal loss accompanied by a decrease in glial activation and neuronal damage, but it did not affect the number of infiltrating lymphocytes positive for CD3 and CD20.

We then analysed the neuroprotective properties of diazoxide in vitro and ex vivo [77]. In this study, diazoxide effectively protected NSC-34 motoneurons against oxidative, excitotoxic and inflammatory insults. It also enhanced the expression and nuclear translocation of Nrf2 in these cells as well as in the spinal cord of EAE animals orally administered with diazoxide. This demonstrated that one of the mechanisms of actions implied in the neuroprotective role of diazoxide is mediated by the activation of Nrf2 expression and nuclear translocation. Finally, diazoxide decreased neuronal death in organotypic hippocampal slice cultures after excitotoxicity and preserved myelin sheath in organotypic cerebellar cultures exposed to pro-inflammatory demyelinating damage. Thus, diazoxide is a neuroprotective agent against oxidative stress-induced damage and cellular dysfunction.

We finally studied the putative actions of diazoxide on autoimmune key processes during EAE such as antigen presentation and lymphocyte activation and proliferation [78]. For this, we analysed K_{ATP} channel expression in CD4-positive T cells and the proliferative of lymphocyte response in the EAE model. When we used whole splenocytes to test whether diazoxide could modulate lymphocyte proliferation, results showed a significant inhibition of the lymphocyte proliferative rate both in vitro and in vivo. Also, the expression of dendritic cell activation markers such as CD83, CD80, CD86 or major histocompatibility complex class II was reduced in cultures treated with diazoxide. However, we observed no inhibition of cell proliferation when isolated CD4-positive T lymphocytes were used instead of whole splenocytes. Diazoxide also failed to inhibit the expression of lymphocyte activation markers. These results suggest that although diazoxide does not directly suppress lymphocyte activation and proliferation, it could modulate lymphocyte activity by regulating antigen presentation. These discrete effects indicate again that diazoxide treatment attenuates EAE pathology with no immunosuppressive effects.

Taken together, at the doses studied, our results demonstrate novel actions of diazoxide as an anti-inflammatory drug that present beneficial effects on EAE through neuroprotection. At the functional level, diazoxide is a neuroprotective agent against oxidative stress-induced damage and cellular dysfunction (**Figure 2**). It attenuates EAE pathology not by causing lymphocyte suppression but by modulating immune communication, decreasing glial harmful activation and promoting myelin and neuronal protection. Thus, treatment with this widely used and well-tolerated drug may be a useful therapeutic intervention in ameliorating MS disease.

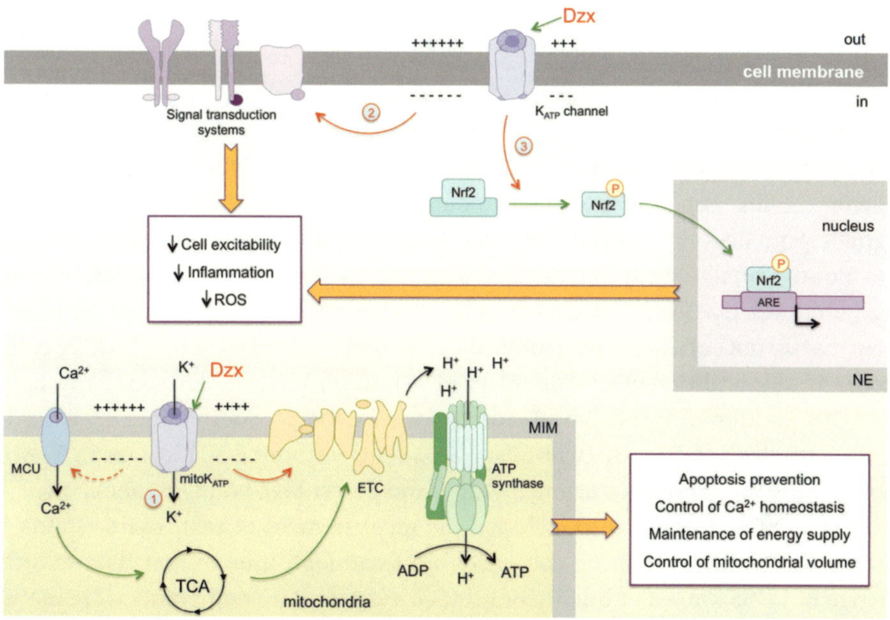

Figure 2. Diazoxide modifies microglial reactivity in brain. Drawing of the effects of diazoxide in the microglial reaction during MS. (1) Diazoxide (Dzx) binds to mitochondrial K_{ATP} channels, induces depolarization of the mitochondrial internal membrane (MIM) and potentiates the H^+ gradient generated by the electron transport chain (ETC). This enhances both ATP synthesis and calcium concentration by activation of ATP synthase and the mitochondrial calcium uniporter (MCU), respectively. Calcium in the mitochondria also increases the tricarboxylic acid cycle (TCA) flux by activation of deshydrogenases and enhances ATP production [73]. Dzx also activates K_{ATP} channels from the plasma membrane, which modifies the cell response to activation signals, (2) activates Nrf2 and (3) through a mechanism that remains to be described. ARE, antioxidant response element; NE, nuclear envelope.

3.3. Effects of diazoxide in MS patients

Based on the positive preclinical studies and considering that diazoxide has been on the market for decades with an excellent safety profile, two Spanish biotechnological companies, Neurotec Pharma and Advancell, performed a clinical development programme to assess diazoxide efficacy and safety in MS patients. NEUROADVAN trial (ClinicalTrials.gov identifier: NCT01428726) was initiated in 2011 and ended in 2014. NEUROADVAN was a Phase IIa, multinational, double-blind, placebo-controlled clinical trial to evaluate the efficacy and safety of diazoxide. The drug was orally administered at two different doses and compared in 103 patients with RRMS versus placebo (1:1:1). The total duration of the treatment was 6 months. Additionally, patients were allowed to continue during an optional extension period, in the same arm of the study, in a blinded way, until study finalization.

Men and women aged 18–55 years with RRMS (McDonald criteria 2010 [79]) and an EDSS score of 0–5.0 were eligible for the study. The inclusion criteria required at least one relapse in the previous 2 years or the presence of at least one Gad1 lesion in the previous year. During 24 weeks, patients received one daily oral tablet with 0.3 or 4 mg diazoxide. MRI scans were performed at baseline and every 4 weeks until the end of the study. Patients enrolled in the follow-up study were subjected to an additional scan at week 48.

The primary efficacy end point was that the number of new Gad1 lesions appeared on T1-weighted sequences from weeks 4 to 24. This end point has been validated in many previous 6-month MS trials and was based on the diazoxide effects on microglia activation and blood-brain barrier closing. Secondary MRI end points included cumulative number of lesions on T2-weighted sequences for all MRIs, cumulative number of lesions on T2-weighted sequences in the 6 months of the study (compared with the baseline MRI); cumulative number of combined unique active lesions (CUALs), addition of new or enlarged lesions on T2-weighted sequences that do not enhance with gadolinium and new Gad1 lesions for all MRIs; cumulative number of CUALs, addition of new or enlarged lesions on T2-weighted sequences that do not enhance with gadolinium and new Gad1 lesions in the 6 months after starting therapy (compared with the baseline MRI); number of patients without Gad1 lesions in T1-weighted sequences in the 6 months after starting therapy; and percentage brain volume change (PBVC). Secondary clinical end points also included the measurement of relapse-free status, relapse rate, number of relapses requiring corticosteroid treatment, time to first relapse during the trial, change in EDSS scale and quality of life. Secondary safety end points were monitorized during the 6 months of therapy up until 15 days after the last dose of diazoxide and included incidence, nature and severity of adverse events (AEs). Control of glucose levels, glycated haemoglobin and blood pressure were also monitorized.

The results of the clinical trial showed no differences in the diazoxide groups in the primary end point or in the other MRI variables associated with the presence of new lesions [80]. However, an interesting decrease in the PBVC in the patients who received diazoxide compared with placebo was found. The number of new T2/Proton Density lesions converting to black holes was not different between arms. Finally, in accordance with the small sample size of the trial, no differences were detected in clinical variables of relapse-free status, relapse rate, number of relapses requiring corticosteroid treatment, change in EDSS or quality of life.

There were six serious adverse events during the study but only a case with autoimmune hypothyroidism was considered to be related to the therapy that was not discontinued. Regarding the described clinical effects of diazoxide on glycaemia, the detected glucose blood levels were always within the limits of normality. This confirms that the diazoxide doses used in this trial were lower than those that induce hyperglycaemic and hypotensive effects.

As commented above, at the doses tested, diazoxide does not seem to have a significant effect that impedes the appearance of new Gad1 lesions. However, although patients were randomly distributed within the groups, at the beginning of the study those patients receiving diazoxide presented a higher number of Gad1 lesions than patients included in the placebo group. This initial higher disease activity in the group treated with diazoxide was maintained throughout the trial. These findings confirm the need to perform an extensive and accurate selection of patients, in terms of the activity of the disease, which must be carried out prior to the clinical trial.

http://dx.doi.org/10.5772/63730

Regarding the effects of diazoxide on brain atrophy, PBVC progressed more slowly in treated patients in a dose-dependent manner. This is consistent with a recent study that validates the measurement of brain atrophy as an outcome for Phase II trials in RRMS [81]. However, taking into account that treated patients had a more active disease, and that diazoxide presents vasodilator actions and peripheral resistance, the reduced atrophy found in patients treated with diazoxide may also be secondary to fluid shifts and not a true protection against brain injury. Nevertheless, the effects in slowing the progression of brain atrophy would require further validation.

To sum up, NEUROADVAN study indicates that diazoxide is a safe drug, well tolerated in patients with MS, but it was not possible to find evidence of efficacy in preventing the formation of new inflammatory lesions.

4. Conclusion

Neurodegenerative changes in MS such as demyelination and axonal loss take place early in the disease and independently from acute immuno-mediated inflammation. The reason why these focal demyelinating inflammatory lesions appear within the CNS still needs to be clarified, but diverse clinical presentations indicate the existence of different patterns of inflammation and neurodegeneration. Nevertheless, the molecular mechanisms underlying axonal damage in acute inflammation and chronic demyelination are potentially amenable to therapy. In this context, the pursuit of neuroprotective therapies in MS should provide new valid alternatives to significantly impact on disease progression. In this pursuit, the standard view of neuroprotection, which has long been mostly focused on neurons, is no longer valid. Instead, this view has been replaced by an integrative approach that recognizes the importance of dynamic interactions between immune cells, microglia, astrocytes and neurons.

A proper evaluation of neurodegenerative aspects in MS remains difficult. Also, for all mentioned drugs the neuroprotective effect has not been fully established. These issues could be better understood by applying well-established and new clinical and imaging parameters that require further preclinical and clinical investigations. Moreover, molecular characterization of the different MS clinical presentations must allow a pharmacogenomics classification of patients and development of personalized therapies. In this line, promising future approaches will combine high-throughput techniques such as proteomics and genomics to investigate further MS neurodegenerative processes, in particular neuroinflammation.

5. Disclosures

JFEP and MP have applied for a PCT application 'Diazoxide for use in the treatment of a central nervous system (CNS) autoimmune demyelinating disease' (application number PCT/EP2011/050049).

Acknowledgements

This research was supported by grant IPT-2012-0614-010000 from the Ministerio de Economía y Competitividad, and by grant 2014SGR1115 from the Generalitat de Catalunya, Spain.

Author details

Juan Espinosa-Parrilla, Marco Pugliese, Nicole Mahy and Manuel J Rodríguez*

*Address all correspondence to: marodriguez@ub.edu

Department of Biomedical Sciences, Institute of Neuroscience, IDIBAPS, University of Barcelona, and Center for Biomedical Research Network in Neurodegenerative Diseases (CIBERNED), Barcelona, Spain

References

[1] Katz Sand IB, Lublin FD. Diagnosis and differential diagnosis of multiple sclerosis. Continuum (Minneap Minn). 2013 Aug; 19(4 Multiple Sclerosis):922–43.

[2] Trapp BD, Nave K-A. Multiple sclerosis: an immune or neurodegenerative disorder? Annu Rev Neurosci. 2008 Jan; 31:247–69.

[3] Hohlfeld R, Dornmair K, Meinl E, Wekerle H. The search for the target antigens of multiple sclerosis, part 1: autoreactive CD4+ T lymphocytes as pathogenic effectors and therapeutic targets. Lancet Neurol. 2016 Feb; 15(2):198–209

[4] Krumbholz M, Derfuss T, Hohlfeld R, Meinl E. B cells and antibodies in multiple sclerosis pathogenesis and therapy. Nat Rev Neurol. 2012 Nov 5; 8(11):613–23.

[5] Losy J. Is MS an inflammatory or primary degenerative disease? J Neural Transm. 2013 Oct; 120(10):1459–62.

[6] Goverman J, Perchellet A, Huseby ES. The role of CD8(+) T cells in multiple sclerosis and its animal models. Curr Drug Targets Inflamm Allergy. 2005 Apr; 4(2):239–45.

[7] Lopez-Diego RS, Weiner HL. Novel therapeutic strategies for multiple sclerosis – a multifaceted adversary. Nat Rev Drug Discov. 2008 Nov; 7(11):909–25.

[8] Senanayake VK, Jin W, Mochizuki A, Chitou B, Goodenowe DB. Metabolic dysfunctions in multiple sclerosis: implications as to causation, early detection, and treatment, a case control study. BMC Neurol. 2015 Jan; 15:154.

[9] Luchtman D, Gollan R, Ellwardt E, Birkenstock J, Robohm K, Siffrin V, et al. In vivo and in vitro effects of multiple sclerosis immunomodulatory therapeutics on glutamatergic excitotoxicity. J Neurochem. 2016 Mar; 136(5):971–980

[10] Salter MW, Beggs S. Sublime microglia: expanding roles for the guardians of the CNS. Cell. 2014 Jul 3; 158(1):15–24.

[11] Block ML, Zecca L, Hong J-S. Microglia-mediated neurotoxicity: uncovering the molecular mechanisms. Nat Rev Neurosci. 2007 Jan; 8(1):57–69.

[12] Hellwig S, Heinrich A, Biber K. The brain's best friend: microglial neurotoxicity revisited. Front Cell Neurosci. 2013 Jan; 7:71.

[13] Lassmann H. Multiple sclerosis: is there neurodegeneration independent from inflammation? J Neurol Sci. 2007 Aug 15; 259(1–2):3–6.

[14] Ransohoff RM, Perry VH. Microglial physiology: unique stimuli, specialized responses. Annu Rev Immunol. 2009 Jan; 27:119–45.

[15] Kwilasz AJ, Grace PM, Serbedzija P, Maier SF, Watkins LR. The therapeutic potential of interleukin-10 in neuroimmune diseases. Neuropharmacology. 2015 Sep; 96(Pt A): 55–69.

[16] Tanaka T, Yoshida S. Mechanisms of remyelination: recent insight from experimental models. Biomol Concepts. 2014 Aug; 5(4):289–98.

[17] Vogel DY, Vereyken EJ, Glim JE, Heijnen PD, Moeton M, van der Valk P, et al. Macrophages in inflammatory multiple sclerosis lesions have an intermediate activation status. J Neuroinflamm. 2013 Jan; 10(1):35.

[18] Pugliese M, Espinosa-Parrilla JF, Bustos J, Campàs C, de Frias M, Sorrosal G. Novel therapeutic approaches to multiple sclerosis: neuroprotective drugs for relapsing-remitting multiple sclerosis. Adv Neuroimmune Biol. IOS Press; 2013; 4(3):187–204.

[19] Schweckendiek W. Treatment of psoriasis vulgaris. Med Monatsschr. 1959 Feb; 13(2): 103–4.

[20] Gold R, Linker RA, Stangel M. Fumaric acid and its esters: an emerging treatment for multiple sclerosis with antioxidative mechanism of action. Clin Immunol. 2012 Jan; 142(1):44–8.

[21] Ghoreschi K, Brück J, Kellerer C, Deng C, Peng H, Rothfuss O, et al. Fumarates improve psoriasis and multiple sclerosis by inducing type II dendritic cells. J Exp Med. 2011 Oct 24; 208(11):2291–303.

[22] Scannevin RH, Chollate S, Jung M, Shackett M, Patel H, Bista P, et al. Fumarates promote cytoprotection of central nervous system cells against oxidative stress via the nuclear factor (erythroid-derived 2)-like 2 pathway. J Pharmacol Exp Ther. 2012 Apr; 341(1):274–84.

[23] Licht-Mayer S, Wimmer I, Traffehn S, Metz I, Brück W, Bauer J, et al. Cell type-specific Nrf2 expression in multiple sclerosis lesions. Acta Neuropathol. 2015 Aug; 130(2):263–77.

[24] Gold R, Kappos L, Arnold DL, Bar-Or A, Giovannoni G, Selmaj K, et al. Placebo-controlled phase 3 study of oral BG-12 for relapsing multiple sclerosis. N Engl J Med. 2012 Sep 20; 367(12):1098–107.

[25] Groves A, Kihara Y, Chun J. Fingolimod: direct CNS effects of sphingosine 1-phosphate (S1P) receptor modulation and implications in multiple sclerosis therapy. J Neurol Sci. 2013 May 15; 328(1–2):9–18.

[26] Brinkmann V, Davis MD, Heise CE, Albert R, Cottens S, Hof R, et al. The immune modulator FTY720 targets sphingosine 1-phosphate receptors. J Biol Chem. 2002 Jun 14; 277(24):21453–7.

[27] Fujino M, Funeshima N, Kitazawa Y, Kimura H, Amemiya H, Suzuki S, et al. Amelioration of experimental autoimmune encephalomyelitis in Lewis rats by FTY720 treatment. J Pharmacol Exp Ther. 2003 Apr; 305(1):70–7.

[28] Kataoka H, Sugahara K, Shimano K, Teshima K, Koyama M, Fukunari A, et al. FTY720, sphingosine 1-phosphate receptor modulator, ameliorates experimental autoimmune encephalomyelitis by inhibition of T cell infiltration. Cell Mol Immunol. 2005 Dec; 2(6): 439–48.

[29] Rossi S, Lo Giudice T, De Chiara V, Musella A, Studer V, Motta C, et al. Oral fingolimod rescues the functional deficits of synapses in experimental autoimmune encephalomyelitis. Br J Pharmacol. 2012 Feb; 165(4):861–9.

[30] Cipriani R, Chara JC, Rodríguez-Antigüedad A, Matute C. FTY720 attenuates excitotoxicity and neuroinflammation. J Neuroinflammation. 2015 May 8; 12(1):86.

[31] Sato K, Ishikawa K, Ui M, Okajima F. Sphingosine 1-phosphate induces expression of early growth response-1 and fibroblast growth factor-2 through mechanism involving extracellular signal-regulated kinase in astroglial cells. Brain Res Mol Brain Res. 1999 Dec 10; 74(1–2):182–9.

[32] Choi JW, Gardell SE, Herr DR, Rivera R, Lee C-W, Noguchi K, et al. FTY720 (fingolimod) efficacy in an animal model of multiple sclerosis requires astrocyte sphingosine 1-phosphate receptor 1 (S1P1) modulation. Proc Natl Acad Sci U S A. 2011 Jan 11; 108(2): 751–6.

[33] Noda H, Takeuchi H, Mizuno T, Suzumura A. Fingolimod phosphate promotes the neuroprotective effects of microglia. J Neuroimmunol. 2013 Mar 15; 256(1–2):13–8.

[34] Cohen JA, Barkhof F, Comi G, Hartung H-P, Khatri BO, Montalban X, et al. Oral fingolimod or intramuscular interferon for relapsing multiple sclerosis. N Engl J Med. 2010 Feb 4; 362(5):402–15.

[35] Kappos L, Radue E-W, O'Connor P, Polman C, Hohlfeld R, Calabresi P, et al. A placebo-controlled trial of oral fingolimod in relapsing multiple sclerosis. N Engl J Med. 2010 Feb 4; 362(5):387–401.

[36] Calabresi PA, Radue E-W, Goodin D, Jeffery D, Rammohan KW, Reder AT, et al. Safety and efficacy of fingolimod in patients with relapsing-remitting multiple sclerosis (FREEDOMS II): a double-blind, randomised, placebo-controlled, phase 3 trial. Lancet Neurol. 2014 Jun; 13(6):545–56.

[37] Novartis. Novartis provides update on fingolimod Phase III trial in primary progressive MS (PPMS) [Accessed 2015-09-20]. Available from: https://www.novartis.com/news/media-releases/novartis-provides-update-fingolimod-phase-iii-trial-primary-progressive-ms-ppms.

[38] Wolinsky JS, Narayana PA, Noseworthy JH, Lublin FD, Whitaker JN, Linde A, et al. Linomide in relapsing and secondary progressive MS: part II: MRI results. MRI Analysis Center of the University of Texas-Houston, Health Science Center, and the North American Linomide Investigators. Neurology. 2000 May 9; 54(9): 1734–41.

[39] Noseworthy JH, Wolinsky JS, Lublin FD, Whitaker JN, Linde A, Gjorstrup P, et al. Linomide in relapsing and secondary progressive MS: part I: trial design and clinical results. North American Linomide Investigators. Neurology. 2000 May 9; 54(9):1726–33.

[40] Yang J-S, Xu L-Y, Xiao B-G, Hedlund G, Link H. Laquinimod (ABR-215062) suppresses the development of experimental autoimmune encephalomyelitis, modulates the Th1/Th2 balance and induces the Th3 cytokine TGF-beta in Lewis rats. J Neuroimmunol. 2004 Nov; 156(1–2):3–9.

[41] Wegner C, Stadelmann C, Pförtner R, Raymond E, Feigelson S, Alon R, et al. Laquinimod interferes with migratory capacity of T cells and reduces IL-17 levels, inflammatory demyelination and acute axonal damage in mice with experimental autoimmune encephalomyelitis. J Neuroimmunol. 2010 Oct 8; 227(1–2):133–43.

[42] Gurevich M, Gritzman T, Orbach R, Tuller T, Feldman A, Achiron A. Laquinimod suppress antigen presentation in relapsing-remitting multiple sclerosis: in-vitro high-throughput gene expression study. J Neuroimmunol. 2010 Apr 15; 221(1–2):87–94.

[43] Aharoni R, Saada R, Eilam R, Hayardeny L, Sela M, Arnon R. Oral treatment with laquinimod augments regulatory T-cells and brain-derived neurotrophic factor expression and reduces injury in the CNS of mice with experimental autoimmune encephalomyelitis. J Neuroimmunol. 2012 Oct 15; 251(1–2):14–24.

[44] Thöne J, Ellrichmann G, Seubert S, Peruga I, Lee D-H, Conrad R, et al. Modulation of autoimmune demyelination by laquinimod via induction of brain-derived neurotrophic factor. Am J Pathol. 2012 Jan; 180(1):267–74.

[45] Mi S, Miller RH, Lee X, Scott ML, Shulag-Morskaya S, Shao Z, et al. LINGO-1 negatively regulates myelination by oligodendrocytes. Nat Neurosci. 2005 Jun; 8(6):745–51.

[46] Liu BP, Fournier A, GrandPré T, Strittmatter SM. Myelin-associated glycoprotein as a functional ligand for the Nogo-66 receptor. Science. 2002 Aug 16; 297(5584):1190–3.

[47] Kuhlmann T, Miron V, Cui Q, Cuo Q, Wegner C, Antel J, et al. Differentiation block of oligodendroglial progenitor cells as a cause for remyelination failure in chronic multiple sclerosis. Brain. 2008 Jul; 131(Pt 7):1749–58.

[48] Inoue H, Lin L, Lee X, Shao Z, Mendes S, Snodgrass-Belt P, et al. Inhibition of the leucine-rich repeat protein LINGO-1 enhances survival, structure, and function of dopaminergic neurons in Parkinson's disease models. Proc Natl Acad Sci U S A. 2007 Sep 4; 104(36):14430–5.

[49] Mi S, Hu B, Hahm K, Luo Y, Kam Hui ES, Yuan Q, et al. LINGO-1 antagonist promotes spinal cord remyelination and axonal integrity in MOG-induced experimental autoimmune encephalomyelitis. Nat Med. 2007 Oct; 13(10):1228–33.

[50] Petratos S, Ozturk E, Azari MF, Kenny R, Lee JY, Magee KA, et al. Limiting multiple sclerosis related axonopathy by blocking Nogo receptor and CRMP-2 phosphorylation. Brain. 2012 Jun; 135(Pt 6):1794–818.

[51] Lee X, Yang Z, Shao Z, Rosenberg SS, Levesque M, Pepinsky RB, et al. NGF regulates the expression of axonal LINGO-1 to inhibit oligodendrocyte differentiation and myelination. J Neurosci. 2007 Jan 3; 27(1):220–5.

[52] Karnezis T, Mandemakers W, McQualter JL, Zheng B, Ho PP, Jordan KA, et al. The neurite outgrowth inhibitor Nogo A is involved in autoimmune-mediated demyelination. Nat Neurosci. 2004 Jul; 7(7):736–44.

[53] Mi S, Pepinsky RB, Cadavid D. Blocking LINGO-1 as a therapy to promote CNS repair: from concept to the clinic. CNS Drugs. 2013 Jul; 27(7):493–503.

[54] Mak JCW. Potential role of green tea catechins in various disease therapies: progress and promise. Clin Exp Pharmacol Physiol. 2012 Mar; 39(3):265–73.

[55] Balentine DA, Wiseman SA, Bouwens LC. The chemistry of tea flavonoids. Crit Rev Food Sci Nutr. 1997 Dec; 37(8):693–704.

[56] Lu Y-P, Lou Y-R, Liao J, Xie J-G, Peng Q-Y, Yang CS, et al. Administration of green tea or caffeine enhances the disappearance of UVB-induced patches of mutant p53 positive epidermal cells in SKH-1 mice. Carcinogenesis. 2005 Aug; 26(8):1465–72.

[57] Lin YL, Lin JK. (-)-Epigallocatechin-3-gallate blocks the induction of nitric oxide synthase by down-regulating lipopolysaccharide-induced activity of transcription factor nuclear factor-kappaB. Mol Pharmacol. 1997 Sep; 52(3):465–72.

[58] Aktas O, Prozorovski T, Smorodchenko A, Savaskan NE, Lauster R, Kloetzel P-M, et al. Green tea epigallocatechin-3-gallate mediates T cellular NF-kappa B inhibition and

exerts neuroprotection in autoimmune encephalomyelitis. J Immunol. 2004 Nov 1; 173(9):5794–800.

[59] Mähler A, Mandel S, Lorenz M, Ruegg U, Wanker EE, Boschmann M, et al. Epigallocatechin-3-gallate: a useful, effective and safe clinical approach for targeted prevention and individualised treatment of neurological diseases? EPMA J. 2013 Jan; 4(1):5.

[60] Zini A, Del Rio D, Stewart AJ, Mandrioli J, Merelli E, Sola P, et al. Do flavan-3-ols from green tea reach the human brain? Nutr Neurosci. Jan; 9(1–2):57–61.

[61] Kline CF, Kurata HT, Hund TJ, Cunha SR, Koval OM, Wright PJ, et al. Dual role of KATP channel C-terminal motif in membrane targeting and metabolic regulation. Proc Natl Acad Sci U S A. 2009 Sep 29; 106(39):16669–74.

[62] Nichols CG, Lederer WJ. Adenosine triphosphate-sensitive potassium channels in the cardiovascular system. Am J Physiol. 1991 Dec; 261(6 Pt 2):H1675–86.

[63] Proks P, Ashcroft FM. Modeling K(ATP) channel gating and its regulation. Prog Biophys Mol Biol. 2009 Jan; 99(1):7–19.

[64] Ashcroft FM, Gribble FM. New windows on the mechanism of action of K(ATP) channel openers. Trends Pharmacol Sci. 2000 Nov; 21(11):439–45.

[65] Kowaltowski AJ, Seetharaman S, Paucek P, Garlid KD. Bioenergetic consequences of opening the ATP-sensitive K(+) channel of heart mitochondria. Am J Physiol Heart Circ Physiol. 2001 Feb; 280(2):H649–57.

[66] Petit P, Loubatières-Mariani MM. Potassium channels of the insulin-secreting B cell. Fundam Clin Pharmacol. 1992 Jan; 6(3):123–34.

[67] Koch-Weser J. Diazoxide. N Engl J Med. 1976 Jun 3; 294(23):1271–3.

[68] Ramonet D, Rodríguez MJ, Pugliese M, Mahy N. Putative glucosensing property in rat and human activated microglia. Neurobiol Dis. 2004 Oct; 17(1):1–9.

[69] Ortega FJ, Gimeno-Bayon J, Espinosa-Parrilla JF, Carrasco JL, Batlle M, Pugliese M, et al. ATP-dependent potassium channel blockade strengthens microglial neuroprotection after hypoxia-ischemia in rats. Exp Neurol. 2012 May; 235(1):282–96.

[70] Ortega FJ, Jolkkonen J, Rodríguez MJ. Microglia is an active player in how glibenclamide improves stroke outcome. J Cereb Blood Flow Metab. 2013 Jul; 33(7):1138–9.

[71] Zhou F, Yao H-H, Wu J-Y, Ding J-H, Sun T, Hu G. Opening of microglial K(ATP) channels inhibits rotenone-induced neuroinflammation. J Cell Mol Med. 2008 Jan; 12(5A):1559–70.

[72] Virgili N, Espinosa-Parrilla JF, Mancera P, Pastén-Zamorano A, Gimeno-Bayon J, Rodríguez MJ, et al. Oral administration of the KATP channel opener diazoxide ameliorates disease progression in a murine model of multiple sclerosis. J Neuroinflammation. BioMed Central Ltd; 2011 Jan; 8(1):149.

[73] Rodríguez MJ, Martínez-Moreno M, Ortega FJ, Mahy N. Targeting microglial K(ATP) channels to treat neurodegenerative diseases: a mitochondrial issue. Oxid Med Cell Longev. 2013 Jan; 2013:194546.

[74] Robin E, Simerabet M, Hassoun SM, Adamczyk S, Tavernier B, Vallet B, et al. Postconditioning in focal cerebral ischemia: role of the mitochondrial ATP-dependent potassium channel. Brain Res. 2011 Feb 23; 1375:137–46.

[75] Roseborough G, Gao D, Chen L, Trush MA, Zhou S, Williams GM, et al. The mitochondrial K-ATP channel opener, diazoxide, prevents ischemia-reperfusion injury in the rabbit spinal cord. Am J Pathol. 2006 May; 168(5):1443–51.

[76] Espinosa-Parrilla JF, Martínez-Moreno M, Gasull X, Mahy N, Rodríguez MJ. The L-type voltage-gated calcium channel modulates microglial pro-inflammatory activity. Mol Cell Neurosci. 2015 Jan; 64:104–15.

[77] Virgili N, Mancera P, Wappenhans B, Sorrosal G, Biber K, Pugliese M, et al. K(ATP) channel opener diazoxide prevents neurodegeneration: a new mechanism of action via antioxidative pathway activation. PLoS One. 2013 Jan; 8(9):e75189.

[78] Virgili N, Mancera P, Chanvillard C, Wegner A, Wappenhans B, Rodríguez MJ, et al. Diazoxide attenuates autoimmune encephalomyelitis and modulates lymphocyte proliferation and dendritic cell functionality. J Neuroimmune Pharmacol. 2014 Sep; 9(4):558–68.

[79] Polman CH, Reingold SC, Banwell B, Clanet M, Cohen JA, Filippi M, et al. Diagnostic criteria for multiple sclerosis: 2010 revisions to the McDonald criteria. Ann Neurol. 2011 Feb; 69(2):292–302.

[80] Villoslada P, Rovira A, Montalban X, Arroyo R, Paul F, Meca-Lallana V, et al. Effects of diazoxide in multiple sclerosis: a randomized, double-blind phase 2 clinical trial. Neurol Neuroimmunol neuroinflammation. 2015 Oct; 2(5):e147.

[81] van den Elskamp IJ, Boden B, Dattola V, Knol DL, Filippi M, Kappos L, et al. Cerebral atrophy as outcome measure in short-term phase 2 clinical trials in multiple sclerosis. Neuroradiology. 2010 Oct; 52(10):875–81.